Beyond the Sage on the Stage

S.L. SEETHALER

Beyond the Sage on the Stage

COMMUNICATING SCIENCE AND CONTEMPORARY ISSUES EFFECTIVELY

UNIVERSITY OF TORONTO PRESS
Toronto Buffalo London

© University of Toronto Press 2024
Toronto Buffalo London
utorontopress.com
Printed and bound by CPI Group (UK) Ltd, Croydon, CR0 4YY

ISBN 978-1-4875-4748-6 (cloth)   ISBN 978-1-4875-4752-3 (EPUB)
ISBN 978-1-4875-4749-3 (paper)   ISBN 978-1-4875-4750-9 (PDF)

Library and Archives Canada Cataloguing in Publication

Title: Beyond the sage on the stage : communicating science and contemporary
    issues effectively / S.L. Seethaler.
Names: Seethaler, Sherry, 1970– author.
Description: Includes bibliographical references and index.
Identifiers: Canadiana (print) 20230529631 | Canadiana (ebook) 20230529674 |
    ISBN 9781487547486 (cloth) | ISBN 9781487547493 (paper) |
    ISBN 9781487547509 (PDF) | ISBN 9781487547523 (EPUB)
Subjects: LCSH: Communication in science. | LCSH: Communication.
Classification: LCC Q223 .S44 2024 | DDC 501/.4 – dc23

Cover design: Mary Beth MacLean
Cover image: iStock.com/Kateryna Kovarzh

We welcome comments and suggestions regarding any aspect of our
publications – please feel free to contact us at news@utorontopress.com
or visit us at utorontopress.com.

Every effort has been made to contact copyright holders; in the event of an error
or omission, please notify the publisher.

We wish to acknowledge the land on which the University of Toronto Press
operates. This land is the traditional territory of the Wendat, the Anishnaabeg,
the Haudenosaunee, the Métis, and the Mississaugas of the Credit First Nation.

University of Toronto Press acknowledges the financial support of the Government
of Canada and the Ontario Arts Council, an agency of the Government of Ontario,
for its publishing activities.

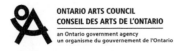

ONTARIO ARTS COUNCIL
CONSEIL DES ARTS DE L'ONTARIO
an Ontario government agency
un organisme du gouvernement de l'Ontario

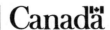

Funded by the   Financé par le
Government   gouvernement
of Canada   du Canada   Canadä

Dedicated to cherished Ruby, for being my guide on the side every step of the way.

Contents

Figures and Tables

Figures

Tables

Preface

My regal Vizsla mix seems to think that toys breed in trees. Using the same canine logic and extraordinary spatial memory that her ancestors (the aristocratic companion-hunters of the Carpathians) applied to return to nesting sites and breeding grounds of fowl and terrestrial game, she will repeatedly take me back to a tree in which we once found a tennis ball or the bushes where she rooted out her prized foam dodge ball. She is undaunted in her bright-eyed, tongue-lolling optimism even when, time and again, she comes up empty mouthed.

We humans can be similarly stubbornly persistent in the face of evidence that our strategy is not working. Take, for example, the deficit model of communication – the widespread assumption that we can get people to make choices more consistent with evidence by merely telling them what we think they should know. Research communication training programs and written guides are usually implicitly driven by this assumption. They focus on de-jargonizing explanations, sprinkling in colorful metaphors, and tying everything together into a nice narrative. This approach is logical, even necessary, but thinking that it is sufficient is as naïve as my canine companion's approach to hunting human-made suburban prey.

Like the hunting strategy engrained in a sporting dog's long genetic history, it is easy to see how the deficit model of communication comes about. The lecture being a favored mode of communication, all of us trained in science, technology, engineering, mathematics, medicine, and most other fields are products of it. The problem is that it does not work so well for changing minds, because most decisions are based on more than facts. Furthermore, even when the goal is constrained to conveying facts, the deficit model often fails. When we treat brains as empty vessels to be filled, valiant efforts at communication amount to barking up the wrong tree.

Just as scientists delve into the peer-reviewed literature before heading into the lab, communication strategies should be rooted in research. Neither in science nor in communication should we check our intuition at the door, but in both cases, intuitions must be checked against evidence. The scholarship that provides insight into how to communicate sprawls across multiple fields. It is (ironically, given the subject matter, but like other academic writing) filled with domain-specific terminology and dominated by implications for theory, rather than recommendations for practice. Yet, like the vast fields and forests where my dog's sleek ancestors earned their living, it is full of meat that a good nose can sniff out. Over the course of my career, I have been spurred on by the bright-eyed (but not, I hope, tongue-lolling) optimism that scholarship offers meaningful lessons for practitioners. This book compiles those lessons for educators, students, journalists, researchers, medical professionals, policymakers, changemakers, and anyone who wants to have more productive conversations about the science, health, environmental, and other complex issues of our times.

Acknowledgments

The research, writing, and revisions of *Beyond the Sage on the Stage* took seven years, a gestation period that does not include the journey leading to its conceptualization. As time travel movies remind us, our ability to recollect the multitude of forces, events, and people that influenced our trajectories is incomplete. These acknowledgements too are inevitably incomplete.

I limit my focus here to contributors to this most recent work, skipping the long list of individuals who were formative influences in my early years. That list I attempted in the acknowledgements to my first book, *Lies, Damned Lies, and Science*, which is complementary to *Beyond the Sage on the Stage*. The former is a book of tools to support consumers of information; the latter is a book of tools to support conveyers of information.

My friend and colleague, Cathy Gere, was the first person to read nascent chapters of *Beyond the Sage on the Stage*. Her insightful feedback helped shape it, and her encouraging words kept me going through the ups and downs of what (as all writers know) can be a lonely journey. Hildie Kraus added words of encouragement and helped ensure that the chapter on misconceptions was accessible to readers with or without a science background. The anonymous reviewers, who provided clear, constructive feedback on the manuscript, helped me hone the final product substantively.

The most arduous part of writing this book was the early research phase, when I was surveying books about communication, many of which left me frustrated. One day, an edited volume of reviews that failed to deliver the promised actionable recommendations made me leave the house in a huff. To my horror, I returned to a scene of destruction – books toppled from the shelves and bits of chewed pages strewn about the living room.

Panic gripped me. Leaving a stack of library books in reach of my usually angelic dog was going to nip (violently) in the bud my growing (through all those trips to the library) friendship with the charming librarian. Fortunately for me, my dog had selected and eaten only the immediate source of my anger, a book I owned. She spent the next two days straining to poop out those dry pages. Her indigestion inspired me to step back and reimagine the book I wanted to write.

All my books are rooted in my lifelong passion for science and for learning about how people learn, and in my career-long desire to bridge scholarship and practice, but I also had a pragmatic motivation for *Beyond the Sage on the Stage*. During the years that I was researching and writing this book, I was teaching in the Research Communications Program (RCP) that I helped found at the University of California, San Diego. RCP gave me the opportunity to see first-hand what researchers struggle with, and to design, test, and iteratively refine the strategies presented in the book.

Working with researchers and watching them learn to better communicate their discoveries and discovery process has been a joy and a privilege, as it has given me the opportunity to grow as a teacher and practitioner alongside the other talented members of our core RCP team, Mario Aguilera, Debbie Meyer, and Kim Rubinstein. RCP, funded by a grant from the Gordon and Betty Moore Foundation, has benefited from the support of many staff, campus leaders, especially the deans of the Schools of Physical and Biological Sciences, and our champions Kit Pogliano, Steve Briggs, Bill McGinnis, and Jeff Remmel. Jeff, I wish you could have seen it all come to fruition. Your vision, leadership, and sense of humor are sorely missed.

The University of Toronto Press brought my cellulose child into the world. Thank you to Stephen Jones, the acquisitions editor, for believing in the project; Meg Patterson for shepherding the manuscript through the review process; Jennifer DiDomenico for moving it through the U of T board's approval process; Stephanie Mazza and the marketing team; the editing team, Jodi Litvin, Janice Evans, and Leanne Rancourt; and everyone toiling behind the scenes. When I was an undergraduate, the University of Toronto launched my professional journey with a scholarship and a world-class education, so this has felt like a homecoming.

I want to acknowledge the many scholars whose work is not mentioned in this book. Most communication guidebooks cite no or few references. In bucking that trend, I have endeavored to honor the scholarly corpus, but this book was never intended to be a literature review. To provide evidence-based, actionable recommendations in an enjoyable format, it must cover much ground and draw from many fields judiciously. The resulting hard choices about what not to include do not reflect my esteem for your contributions to your field.

I also want to acknowledge all the hard-working communicators, the ones whose names you know and the ones you have never heard of but who educate, inspire, and advocate for their communities every day. I chose not to hold up specific individuals as models because we all need to find our own voice, learning from others without trying to emulate them, just as a golfer can learn from but should not try to emulate another golfer's swing.

Communication is always a work in progress, but my golf swing is much more a work in progress. When at the driving range with my friend Laura Weis, the charming librarian who is a lifelong golfer, she may say, with her back turned to me, "That was a good hit." She knows because her golf ears can hear it. I know, because the instant I connect a delightful zing passes through my entire body. In communication, as in golf, making that connection not only sounds right, it feels right. It keeps us coming back for more.

Introduction

"Think different." Apple's famous slogan could be proclaimed not only by an innovation guru or life coach, but also by this author. Succeeding as an innovator requires us to get past tired ways of looking at problems to unveil a path to a novel solution. Growing as a person requires us to abandon defeatist ways of thinking and adopt a self-affirming inner dialogue. Thus, both personal and professional change begin with overhauling long-held patterns of thought and adopting fresh perspectives that seem obvious in retrospect. It is like a game of "Where's Waldo?" Waldo can be painfully elusive, but once you spot him, you wonder how on earth you could have missed that hat and striped shirt. This book will help you think differently about communication, and the new way of thinking will be beautifully intuitive.

Drawing on an extensive research base that cuts across traditional disciplinary silos, *Beyond the Sage on the Stage* delivers practical, evidence-based communication strategies. It does not, as many communication guides do, waste pages of ink on lengthy discussions of the importance of effective communication; after all, that is preaching to the choir. It is not driven by a purely journalistic perspective, because that is too limited a view of communication. It is organized around principles, instead of being partitioned (as is common for communication guides) by communication format, because principles apply even when formats change. It is not simply a call to think differently; it is a guide to thinking differently, and it can meet you wherever you are on your personal or professional communication journey.

In treating the development of communication competencies as a professional journey, this book rejects the flawed assumption that some people are just bad communicators who are beyond help. Many of us are bad at chess and backgammon, but most of us would agree that we could become decent chess or backgammon players by studying the game and practicing. In educational psychology, this is known as a growth mindset of ability, in which ability is viewed as dynamic and incremental. Students who hold a growth mindset about school (math ability, for instance) work harder and are more successful than those who have a fixed ability mindset, in which ability is seen as a static entity.[1]

This is a guide to communicating about the sciences, social sciences, technology, health, the environment, and current issues related to these topics. Communication is conceptualized broadly to encompass lectures, science cafés, journalism, conversations between patients and medical professionals, blogs, vlogs, podcasts and emerging media, public health and environmental awareness campaigns, informal education at museums and aquariums, formal education such as teaching and mentoring students, fundraising, policy work, community engagement and action, responding to questions posed by the children in your family or circle of friends, and challenging conversations about substantive issues with the adults in your networks.

Now more than ever, dynamic, unstructured, multidimensional problems, such as health disparities and environmental degradation, are the focus of discussions in the public and private sectors locally, nationally, and globally. These are examples of "wicked problems" – a term that has many conceptualizations but refers to problems that are characterized by their inherent complexity and the need for solution approaches that draw on diverse expertise.[2] Wicked problems have social relevance but need not be characterized by social discord. The (socially unifying but wickedly challenging) race to beat cancer involves researchers from nearly every discipline in academia, industry, and government, as well as clinicians, patients, families, public health experts, the media, policymakers, funders, and those who will educate the next generation of researchers and leaders. Wicked problems make it clear that communication about science-related issues is not, and cannot be, the purview of a select few.

Becoming an effective communicator in any setting requires a combination of knowledge, skills, and ways of thinking. As we have seen with the pressing issues of our time, such as during the COVID-19 pandemic, communication can go terribly wrong. It can leave people with misconceptions about concepts or evidence and the process through which evidence was obtained. It can disempower people by confusing them and making them more reliant on reasoning shortcuts unsuited to the problem at hand. It can trigger any of several kinds of backfires. When science communication goes awry, it interferes with the right of everyone to "share in scientific advancement and its benefits," as stated in the Universal Declaration of Human Rights.[3]

Communication about science-related issues must therefore be inclusive – no one should be or feel excluded by their politics, religion, race, ethnicity, gender, sexuality, disability, national origin, socioeconomic status, or any other identities or circumstances. Inclusive communication is defined as being intentional (about reaching audiences), reciprocal (by valuing diverse expertise), and reflexive (with self-awareness and willingness to adapt).[4] Inclusive communication often means getting "beyond the sage on the stage." By drawing on scholarship across disciplines in the sciences, social sciences, and humanities, this book builds a foundation of knowledge, skills, and ways of thinking for making communication more effective and inclusive. The chapter-by-chapter summary provides an overview of the foundation to be built.

CHAPTER 1 – MAPPING THE LANDSCAPE OF AUDIENCES, CONTEXTS, AND GOALS

Communication may involve many kinds of audiences, and it may take place in a range of contexts or through various forms of media, with a plethora of possible goals. To make the craggy communication landscape easier to navigate, this chapter maps out the three-dimensional terrain of audiences, contexts, and goals. It explores the subdimensions within these three dimensions and provides tips on how to choose or take advantage of the context to reach the audience and meet your communication goals. The chapter also introduces a pedagogical framework, based on a hierarchal organization of communication goals, that provides a novel and productive way for conceptualizing the knowledge, skills, and habits of mind needed to be an effective communicator. The framework also provides a logical structure that underpins this book.

CHAPTER 2 – MASTERFUL USE OF WORDS AND IMAGES, THE FUNDAMENTAL TOOLS OF THE COMMUNICATION ARTISAN

Creative acts originate with a vision that is invariably shaped by external factors, but it all starts with mastering the basic tools of the trade. For the communication artisan, the fundamental tools are words and images, to be used alone or in combination in a wide range of mediums and settings. Communication training programs often repeat slogans, such as "de-jargonize," "distill" and "keep it simple." Such advice is mostly sound, but it is so incomplete that a communicator is left with more questions than answers. It ignores that jargon is often hiding in plain sight as terms that sound colloquial but are not, that simplification is not the same as clarification, and that visuals are not just pretty pictures – they can empower people to make sense of complex information when words are inadequate. This chapter goes beyond the simplistic advice with an eye-opening exploration of hidden jargon and concise lessons from research on multimedia learning.

CHAPTER 3 – METAPHORS AND ANALOGIES: UNCOVERING HOW THEY FRAME THOUGHT

The ubiquitous calls to reduce jargon and distill the message are oversimplified but nonetheless consistent with the research discussed in the previous chapter. Another strategy recommended by traditional communication training programs – using colorful metaphors – deserves scrutiny, because a poorly chosen comparison has the potential to create misconceptions or strengthen existing ones. Metaphors and analogies use words to create images by linking two ideas, and their explanatory power depends on the audience making the intended inferences. The use of metaphors and analogies comes with implicit, but potentially inaccurate, assumptions about the audience. Moreover, popular metaphors like the ones used to describe DNA and genes can become anachronistic in the wake of advances in the science. They can also arouse emotions that are antithetical to the goals of the communicator. This chapter takes a critical look at metaphors and analogies to help you avoid inadvertent self-sabotage and to be on the lookout for surreptitious hype.

CHAPTER 4 – SO WE LIVE IN A SNOW GLOBE? MISCONCEPTION MISHAPS AND DESIGNING STORIES FOR LEARNING

All of us come to any learning situation with prior conceptual knowledge that influences how we assimilate new information. To reduce the gap between what is taught and what is learned, communicators (and communication trainers) need to co-opt the lessons from an extensive body of education research on people's knowledge and misconceptions about a wide range of topics. This chapter summarizes current views on the nature of these ideas and how they arise. They can be quite wild. One example is that young children who, struggling to reconcile their experience of flat Earth with schooling telling them it is a sphere, imagine our planet as a souvenir snow globe with us situated inside. This chapter discusses current thinking on how people build knowledge and what strategies help them restructure their knowledge to integrate new information, without souvenir-snow-globe-like thinking mishaps. It also demonstrates how a well-crafted narrative structure can seize audiences' interest and support learning.

CHAPTER 5 – THE HIDDEN CLIMB REVEALED: GIVING VOICE TO PEOPLE AND PROCESS

Views of science and scientists held by students, teachers, and others are gleaned from formal education, the media, and popular culture. These depictions have not been static over time, but widespread perceptions of scientists and the nature of scientific research still often bear little relationship to reality. These myths are detrimental to publics and scientists alike, and many voices are needed to get us beyond them. Insights from across disciplines lay the groundwork for better portraying the human side of science and conveying the routinely hidden process through which scientific knowledge comes to be. Foreshadowing the thread that runs through the second half of this book, this chapter also explores perspectives on the role of dialogue with various stakeholders in communicating science. It ends with tips on how to productively bridge the cultures of research and policymaking.

CHAPTER 6 – NEGOTIATING UNCERTAINTY AND THE INTRICACIES OF TRADEOFFS

Researchers, journalists, and other communicators may have the goal of providing information to help people make sound decisions for themselves and for society. In theory, after elucidating the costs and benefits of a product, procedure, or other choice, individuals can weigh the costs and benefits and follow the most rational path. In reality, however, the process of identifying and comparing tradeoffs and assessing risk is inevitably subjective. Uncertainty presents a very real challenge for communicators. How does one talk about evidence in a way that does justice to the uncertainty without making people frustrated such that they throw their hands in the air and exclaim, "So-called experts don't know anything anyway!" It is a fine line to tread and raises knotty ethical questions. This chapter provides a detailed framework for identifying and discussing tradeoffs and uncertainty.

CHAPTER 7 – HOW (NOT) TO TRIGGER AUDIENCES' DECISION-MAKING SURVIVAL TACTICS

To navigate both the physical world and the world of ideas, we have little choice but to be decision-making machines, oblivious to the vast majority of decisions we make in a day. This is blissful ignorance, because we would be paralyzed into inaction if we truly sweated all the small stuff. Decision autopilot relies on reasoning shortcuts – heuristics. Heuristics are efficient, and can be perfectly effective, but they are also fallible when we rely on them blindly to make decisions about complex issues or to make sense of data. Much well-meaning communication is flawed in ways that stymie reasoners and make them more likely to fall back on heuristics. This chapter shows how recognizing these potential communication pitfalls can help you make the transition from a presentation that reasoners fail to assimilate to communication tailored to support decision-making about complex topics. This chapter also offers detailed guidance on communicating numerical and statistical information.

CHAPTER 8 – OBVIOUS BUT WRONG: THE PERILS OF THE BACKFIRE EFFECT AND TIPS TO PREVENT IT

An attempt at providing information can lead people to believe misinformation more strongly than before. It can even make people more likely to take the action (or the inaction) the communication was trying to prevent. In other words, communication can backfire, resulting in a situation in which communication is not merely unproductive – it is counterproductive. The assumptions underlying communication often ignore the possibility of the backfire effect, but the effect is common, robust, and comes in many flavors. This chapter builds on the research introduced in the previous chapter by exploring how information processing is influenced by individuals' group affiliations and identities. It also identifies contexts in which backfires occur for reasons that have nothing to do with ideology. It concludes with a detailed description of practical, evidence-based communication approaches that help minimize or eliminate each type of backfire.

CHAPTER 9 – CRUCIAL CONVERSATIONS, TRUST, AND THE DARK MATTER OF COMMUNICATION

So much is left unsaid, or at least unspoken. Our eyes, facial expressions, postures and movements, breathing patterns, and other nonverbal cues say quite a lot, without us saying anything at all. This dark matter of communication not only (often to our dismay) reveals us to others, it can reveal us to ourselves. The dark matter of communication arises at the confluence of complex psychological and physiological factors that control our emotional states, which in turn determine our ability to be active, empathetic listeners. Thus, better understanding the confluence of psychological and physiological factors, and how they interact to give rise to the dark matter of communication, is essential to becoming a more effective communicator. This chapter offers techniques that can help you develop the habits of mind and body needed for handling stage fright, maintaining composure in a difficult conversation, and being perceived as credible and trustworthy.

CHAPTER 10 – COLLECTING THE TOOLS INTO THE TOOLBOX

The final chapter synthesizes the book's lessons and reinforces them with examples and exercises. You can deepen your personal and professional growth by working through them individually or with colleagues. Teachers and communication trainers can use the exercises and examples in courses and workshops. Checklists as well as a taxonomic organization of the knowledge, skills, and habits of mind built across the chapters provide opportunities for reflection and the scaffolds to help you apply what you have learned.

Getting communication wrong puts our individual and collective futures at risk. This book presents a new vision for communication and the tools to bring it to life.

- *Informed by an extensive evidence base.* It draws from a cross-disciplinary body of research that is not typically used to inform communication teaching and practice.
- *Conceptualized as a professional journey.* It adapts a powerful educational framework to teach how to build communication knowledge, skills, and habits of mind along a meaningful learning trajectory.
- *Applies to communication about complex issues in challenging times.* It offers guiding principles and practical strategies to not only be an excellent presenter, but also to get "beyond the sage on the stage" and reach common ground through dialogue.

The first half of this book (Chapters 1–5) lays the groundwork to make communication efforts about any topic more conducive to learning. The second half (Chapter 6–10) digs into how people reason about complex and controversial issues and identifies strategies for discussing tradeoffs and uncertainty, negotiating heuristics, avoiding backfires, and perceiving unspoken nuances. Research demonstrates that it is surprisingly easy to get communication wrong. Fortunately, the same research also tells us how to get it right. Now is the time to start building the toolkit for success.

1

Mapping the Landscape of Audiences, Contexts, and Goals

If you zoom in on the intricacies of a fractal landscape, successive levels of the fractal world unfurl before your eyes. For a chemist, this world may be the fractal patterns in crystals. For a biologist, it may be the branches of a tree or an animal circulatory system. For an astrophysicist, it may be superclusters of clusters of galaxies of stars. The father of fractal geometry, Benoit Mandelbrot, coined the term "fractal" to describe shapes that are irregular and fragmented with the same degree of irregularity and fragmentation across scales.[1] Fractals are magnificent, mindblowing, amazeballs – no superlative seems out of place to describe their power to inspire awe. They are also accessible to everyone, out in nature or through images, animations, and soundscapes that put the microscopic or astronomical fractal pattern on a human scale.

Fractals are an apropos way to start this first chapter for several reasons. Awe enhances creative thinking.[2] So we begin with awe-inspiring fractals to awaken our minds for the creative act of communication. Fractals are a reminder that information is never received by empty brains. Not everyone has heard the word "fractal," but most everyone has encountered fractal patterns – snowflakes, veins in a leaf, Romanesco cauliflower, bolts of lightning in the sky, river systems glimpsed from a plane, as well as musical fractal soundscapes. Fractals also exemplify how one topic has many levels of depth, from the "gee whiz" to cutting-edge scientific and mathematical research. These beautiful and mysterious objects epitomize the rewards that come from probing beneath the surface. Zooming in on a fractal landscape can serve as a metaphor for how this book delves into communication to get beyond superficial perspectives.

Like fractals, communication is set in three-dimensional landscape – the audience (who), the context or medium (when and where), and the goals (why). All three of these dimensions interact and should shape the "what" of communication, which is why this book does not follow the common approach of building the chapter structure around communication context. A particular context or medium may be used to reach various audiences or achieve various goals, and communication within that context must be adapted accordingly. Furthermore, communication contexts change unpredictably, whether due to the arrival of a new social media platform or a pandemic that plunks us all into Zoom boxes. Therefore, this book provides strategies that can be flexibly applied, guided by the three dimensions of the communication landscape. We begin our journey by mapping out the audience, context, and goal dimensions and exploring the dimensions within these dimensions.

CHAPTER LEARNING OBJECTIVES: MAPPING THE LANDSCAPE

Knowledge: What are the affordances and constraints of potential communication contexts?
Skills: Begin to optimize communication for the audience and to design for diversity.
Habits of Mind: Compare goals of all involved in the communication and assess outcomes.

DIMENSION 1: THE WHO OF COMMUNICATION

> Every one of us is an outsider to all but a few aspects of modern life.[3]

Reconceive Expertise from Dichotomies to Degrees

The quotation that begins this section is a reminder that all of us, including those with graduate training in a science discipline, have narrow expertise. An interdisciplinary collaboration on a curriculum project is one experience that has driven this home to me. The project involved developing a set of short lesson videos to help undergraduate students come to a deeper understanding of rates of change, such as population growth in biology, reaction kinetics in chemistry, and velocity and acceleration in physics. The focus was on the first-year undergraduate curriculum, and the project team consisted of eight PhD scientists and mathematicians at a major research university, but it was a struggle for team members to grasp the nuances of each other's disciplines, which use different language, notations, and conventions. The experience, described in a paper, helped us recognize how instructors' communication shortcomings can directly contribute to students' difficulties learning the material.[4] Despite humbling experiences like these, experts in a discipline may still hold biases about what "the public" knows.[5] To avoid underestimating what nonspecialists can bring to the conversation or overestimating what colleagues know, take a nuanced view of audiences that allows for different kinds and gradations, or degrees, of expertise.

Do Your Homework to Get to Know Your Audience

The list of categories of potential audiences for science and health communication is long and diverse (see Table 1.1). (Note: For lack of a better term, I will tend to use "audience" or "learners" to describe those "receiving" communication, but with the understanding that roles shift dynamically in multidirectional communication.) Some of these categories can be parsed into subcategories. Funders of science may be government agencies, philanthropic donors, or venture capitalists. Likewise, policy decisions are typically made by collections of people, some with formal responsibility and others with informal influence; therefore, "policymaker" is a catchall category that includes those who are elected to office and those, such as civil servants, who are not. Individuals may fall into multiple categories (such as parent/patient/community organizer/blogger), and their communication needs and expectations differ according to what hat they are wearing at the time. A bit of sleuthing can help you better prepare to reach your audience. Ask the teacher what the class is studying. Research what legislation the policymaker has sponsored. Explore the previous investments of the philanthropic donor or the mission of the corporate sponsor. For a live

Table 1.1. Potential Audiences for Science and Health Communication

Education	Health Care	Media	Policy/Advocacy	Others
– K–12, undergraduate, and graduate students – Teachers – Administrators – Curriculum designers – Parents	– Patients and families – Doctors, nurses, pharmacists, and other health care providers – Hospital administrators – Insurers	– Consumers of specialist and nonspecialist publications – Mainstream media (print, radio, television) – Emerging media and social media	– Legislators and other policymakers – Judges and lawyers – Regulatory agencies – Activists and community organizers – Local, national, and global nonprofits	– Scientists in various fields – Potential funders – Collaborators in industry or the arts – Consumers, voters, and all others

audience, consider using an app that permits you to ask a few questions at the beginning of a talk. Before an interview with a journalist, take a look at their previous work.

Remember Your Audience's Audience to Avoid "Broken Telephone"

Journalists are audiences with their own audiences to reach. When speaking with someone from the media, know the target audience of their publication or broadcast to avoid getting caught off guard. I can say from personal experience that it is easier to roll with a DJ's bawdy question when you know that is part of the schtick the audience is expecting! Policymakers and program officers are other audiences with audiences. Elected policymakers are beholden to all their constituents, not only the constituents who share their viewpoints. Familiarity with a policymaker's constituent base can help you frame arguments and evidence in a way that the policymaker will be able to envision making a case to the constituencies back home. Similarly, program officers do not usually hold the purse strings; they may need to defend the projects they want to fund to a board of directors. Be strategic by giving the program officer arguments suitable to take back to the board. A grant proposal should draw on language (e.g., headings) from the request for proposals and review criteria. Doing so will help reviewers summarize for program officers and program officers summarize for those who hold the purse strings. To avoid the situation where the message gets distorted like in the children's game of broken telephone as it is passed from your audience to their audience, keep your message clear and concise and structure it how it will be used.

Accept that Your Communication Intuitions May Mislead You

We have all had frustrating conversations. Perhaps you felt bowled over by someone who was loud and gesticulating, interrupted before you could finish speaking, and asked you rapid-fire questions. Alternatively, perhaps you had a conversation where no matter how hard you tried, the person to whom you were speaking seemed reticent to respond to your enthusiastic interest, making the conversation feel like you were pulling teeth. Regardless of which of these two situations you found yourself in, you likely thought the other person was rude. It may never have occurred to you that there exist differences in conversational style.

These are examples of "high-involvement conversational style" and "high-considerateness conversational style."[6] Compared to a high-considerateness style, high-involvement style is animated, fast-paced with very little or no pause between speakers, and often involves more personal topics and storytelling.[7] Despite the name, "high-considerateness" is not inherently more polite than "high-involvement." When speakers share the high-involvement style, they view it as a sign of enthusiasm and engagement, and they regard those who do not share their style as withholding. Also, these styles are relative – Sam may have a high-considerateness style compared to Leo, but a high-involvement style compared to Riley.

Another aspect of conversational style is directness versus indirectness. Indirect speakers hint at what they want but do not state it directly. Like involvement, directness varies across cultures and among individuals within a culture, and it often leads to conflicts in married couples.[8] One partner gets angry that hints are being ignored, and the other partner gets angry at being expected to read minds. Because people rarely discuss communication processes – metacommunication – conversational style is often invisible.[9]

We take our own styles as self-evident and are quick to draw unflattering conclusions about the personalities and intentions of those with different

Figure 1.1. The Developmental Model of Intercultural Sensitivity

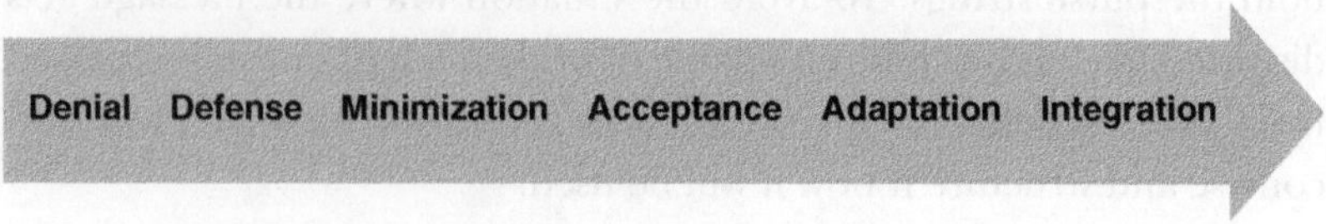

Denial   Defense   Minimization   Acceptance   Adaptation   Integration

conversational styles. Without knowing it, we may react in the moment by intensifying our own styles, for instance, trying to be even more excited and animated when confronted by a "withholder," who, in response, experiences a rising desperation to crawl under the nearest rock. The expanding schism generated when two parties increasingly fall back on their own opposite styles is known as **complementary schismogenesis**.[10] Knowing that bit of jargon may not help you become a better communicator, but it will be a balm for those who share my cocktail party angst.

Question Your Assumptions to Build Intercultural Sensitivity

The everyday example of conversational styles illustrates a recurring theme in this book – the importance of developing the habit of mind of questioning your assumptions and endeavoring to view things from another's vantage point. Milton James Bennett's developmental model of intercultural sensitivity, a continuum of six stages from ethnocentric to ethnorelative views of culture, is a useful tool for reflecting on your understanding of the individuals and groups with whom you communicate (Figure 1.1).[11] The model takes a broad view of culture (not equating it with nationality) and is relevant to moving between any cultures or subcultures, such as demographic groups or demographically diverse communities united by shared interests.

In the first stage, **denial**, one has only a vague category of "otherness" and is lacking the tools to deal with cultural diversity. In the second stage, **defense**, the "other" category is more fully perceived but still in stereotypical ways, with one's culture seen as superior to another. In the third stage, **minimization**, cultural differences are obscured to keep the focus on cultural similarities. The fourth stage, **acceptance**, is marked by a curiosity about culture and cultural differences, but knowledge about them is limited. By the fifth stage, **adaptation**, one is able to see the world as if participating in a different culture and to respond with empathy. In the final stage, **integration**, one is comfortable moving in and out of different cultural worldviews without sacrificing authenticity.

Given that most of us move among many cultures and subcultures, reaching the final stage is a high bar, but cultivating acceptance and adaptation is a worthy aspiration in a world of division. Adaptation makes it easier to follow Bennett's **Platinum Rule**: Instead of treating others as we would like to be treated (the Golden Rule), we should treat others how they would like to be treated (the Platinum Rule).[12] Although this may not always be possible, it is a reminder to seek others' perspectives instead of assuming we know. On the journey to build intercultural sensitivity, communication scholarship can buttress your personal research on the audience, provide insight into what would otherwise be hidden, and reveal how your current approaches to communication can be counterproductive. The box lists what the different areas of scholarship discussed throughout the book reveal about the audience.

AUDIENCES DO NOT COME AS EMPTY VESSELS TO BE FILLED

Audiences bring their own ways of making sense of the world, including the following:

- Perceptual filters for processing verbal and visual information (Chapter 2)
- Cultural knowledge to interpret metaphors and analogies (Chapter 3)
- Knowledge and misconceptions about specific concepts and topics (Chapter 4)
- Understandings and misunderstandings of the process of research (Chapter 5)
- Ways of evaluating tradeoffs and thinking about uncertainty (Chapter 6)
- Heuristics for handling complex and ambiguous information (Chapter 7)
- Ideologies and worldviews that may clash with specific framings (Chapter 8)
- Nonverbal cues that interplay with emotions and empathy (Chapter 9)

DIMENSION 2: THE WHEN AND WHERE OF COMMUNICATION

Identify the Affordances and Constraints of Each Communication Context

The communication context sets communication parameters in the form of directionality, modes, time, story (indirectly), and style. Properties of a tool or context that enable ways of interacting with it are called "affordances."[13] What is an affordance naturally depends on the individual interacting with the tool or context. For example, a basic image-editing tool may have a few affordances that allow users to crop, resize, or recolor an image; professional image-editing software may have an overwhelming number of affordances. Both tools are useful but suited to users with different purposes. A novice may not perceive the affordances of the complex software, and thus they are not an affordance for that user. The affordances of the medium or context should be optimized for the audience and goals.

DIRECTIONALITY

The term "audience" comes with less baggage than "public," but it too implies something about the nature of the communication interaction that may or may not be accurate. Audience suggests directionality to the flow of information. A lecturer stands in front of an audience. The followers of a vlog are an audience. The readers of a magazine article are an audience. In each case, the information flow is typically unidirectional, from a communicator to a passive listener or reader. Audience questions or comments may introduce some bidirectionality, but the communication still aims to confer knowledge from an expert onto those lacking that knowledge.

In contrast, in a citizen forum or brainstorm with colleagues, information flow is multidirectional and any participant may contribute expertise. This is also true for asynchronous communication forums. For example, regulatory agencies may solicit feedback through their websites on proposed regulation changes. When seeking input, be aware of barriers to participation. For example, face-to-face citizen forums privilege those with time, transportation, and child care, and technology-mediated communication privileges those with access.[14] Seeking out the underrepresented voices may require partnerships with local communities, such as through local business leaders, religious leaders, health professionals, schools, and libraries. These types of partnerships can also help inform a culturally sensitive communication plan.

MODES

Communication contexts often afford the engagement of multiple sensory modes. Most permit the presentation of visual information along with text or audio. When optimized, visuals are powerful communication tools. Nowadays, video allows you to see, in three-dimensional dynamic glory, processes that students would once have had to imagine in their heads based on textbook passages. Do not overlook the power of a universal speech-accompanying visual – gesture. Speakers are often unaware of what gestures they are using, or that they are gesturing at all.[15] Gesture is so integral to speech that people still gesture when the listeners cannot see them, and congenitally blind people also use gesture. Conscious development of gestures can help the speaker as well as the audience, because gesture is not merely a reflection of our cognitive processes; it drives them.[16]

When possible, take advantage of the sense of touch. From my days in graduate school, I remember a talk in our departmental colloquium to which the speaker brought an example of the model organism he worked on, tobacco hornworm (*Manduca sexta*). As the plastic cup containing the enormous horned green caterpillar was passed around the audience, the creature was regarded with fascination. It was undaunted by the many curious pokes, as well as the horrified recoiling of the student beside me. I enjoyed and learned from our biology colloquium series, but all these years later that is the only lecture of which I have a conscious memory. This is consistent with research that shows information processed through multiple modes is more likely to be retained in long-term memory.[17]

Practical matters may preclude researchers from bringing an actual sample to a public talk, but the prevalence of 3-D printers is making it increasingly feasible to create replicas for people to hold, rotate, and scrutinize. Many university and public libraries have maker spaces with 3-D printers. With these tools, an obscure-sounding molecule can instantly become tangible and memorable, or a cell can be opened and its organelles understood as shapes and textures. It is worth noting that multimodal communication can support audience members with learning differences or disabilities – neuro-diverse learners, to use a more inclusive term.

TIME

Like the affordances already mentioned, time (duration/length and repetition) varies by context and influences what goals can be achieved. Repetition of interactions is an essential consideration for building relationships and fostering trust. Another time consideration is whether the audience or the communicator controls the pacing. For example, would your audience be better served by a self-paced lesson than by a live presentation (or by a combination of both formats)? Also, based on the material and the audience's attention span, consider whether multiple shorter pieces or presentations would be more effective than one long piece or presentation.

Tempo is an important aspect of timing. Introducing judicious pauses for emphasis and clarity will improve your public-speaking experience. Also, in an interview that will be edited, your interviewer will appreciate pauses in your speech that provide natural break points. Without them, the interviewer may be forced to make the cuts where you happen to take a breath, instead of making the editing decisions based on the message content. Moreover, if anxiousness about public speaking tends to leave you feeling lightheaded, it may be because you are either hyperventilating or forgetting to breathe as you attempt to cram too much information into too short a time. (For why hyperventilation and holding your breath both result in lightheadedness, see Chapter 9.)

STORY

Within any scientific advance are multiple stories. The length of a presentation or written piece will determine how much of a story you can tell, but the context also sets the story parameters indirectly. Consider the stories told about the detection of gravitational waves by the Laser Interferometer Gravitational-Wave Observatory (LIGO). In September 2015, the two LIGO instruments registered a transient signal that, after careful data analysis, was determined to be gravitational waves emanating from the merger of two massive black holes. It was a discovery that the physics community had been working toward for 100 years, ever since Einstein published his theory of general relativity, which predicted black holes and gravitational waves. The LIGO discovery yielded nearly 1,000 front-page newspaper articles and lit up Facebook, Twitter, YouTube, and other social media.[18]

LIGO stories emphasized the historic nature of the discovery and made reference to Einstein, but the stories had unique takes depending on the readership of the publication. Space enthusiasts, likely to be seeking a more in-depth understanding, were greeted by the headline "Epic Gravitational Wave Detection: How Scientists Did It."[19] Readers of *The Guardian*, seeking to grasp fundamentals, were treated to "Explain It to Me Like I'm a Kid: Scientists Try to Make Sense of Gravitational Waves," in which scientists made comparisons to toy dogs, spinning games, and boats.[20] The *Washington Post* gave their politically minded audience a story that, while positive, vied for readers' attention in the opening paragraph with mention of the "controversial" experiment and its billion-dollar price tag.[21] The first paragraph of the *Huffington Post* blog, "What Are Gravitational Waves and Why Should You Care?" emphasizes humanity's power to achieve when we focus on "constructive rather than destructive purposes."[22] It is worth noting that behind this richness of stories was the carefully coordinated effort of the scientific researchers and their institutions. They provided a lay-language summary of the peer-reviewed scientific paper – a press release – translated into 18 languages, a press conference, an education guide, animations, and more.[23]

STYLE AND TONE

Is the blog, vlog, podcast, or other setting to which you plan to contribute formal or informal? Does it call for a concise presentation of your methods and findings or a humorous account of your trials and tribulations in the laboratory? Audiences vary by context, and the same audience will have different expectations in different contexts. Allow the context to be your guide. In some cases, your technical choices about how content is presented and organized must be informed by formal rules described in style guides for a publication. The degree of objectivity, speculativeness, emotionality, intimacy, and humor – the tone – is partly determined by the context, but also by the topic. Of course, there is always room for your unique, creative voice. Although it is easier to let your personality shine through in less formal communication contexts, give yourself permission to be your authentic self in both informal and formal communication settings. Also, even in formal communication settings, you may have more flexibility than you think; for example, you may have been taught that academic scientific writing must use the passive voice, but style guides increasingly encourage the use of the active voice (and the strategic use of both active and passive).[24]

TITLE STYLES EXEMPLIFY THE EXPECTATIONS OF AUDIENCES, CONTEXTS, AND GOALS

Consider the titles of two articles: "Goldilocks Black Holes" and "A New Sample of Candidate Intermediate-Mass Black Holes Selected by X-Ray Variability."[25] They were published the same year (2012) and are on the same topic. It will come as no surprise that the first is from a popular science magazine, *Scientific American*, and the second is from a specialist publication, *Astrophysical Journal*.

An analysis that compared a quarter century of astrophysics titles in *Scientific American* to the titles of research papers published in the most prestigious journals in astrophysics during the same period documented striking differences:[26]

- The popular science titles were more than three times shorter.
- References to journalistic discourse, such as idioms ("The Cosmic Reality Check"), and cultural references, including literature ("The Little Spacecraft That Could" and "A Hundred Billion Years of Solitude") and popular culture ("Here Come the Suns" and "The Biggest Bang Theory"), were common in the *Scientific American* titles but nonexistent in specialized journals.
- Also common in *Scientific American* but nearly absent in specialist journals are rhetorical strategies, such as personification ("Star Gobbler"), metaphor ("Stellar Bells"), and double entendres ("Catching the Wave").

Article titles in specialist journals must be clear and informative (and achieve search engine optimization) to reach a narrow target audience. In contrast, popular science titles invite audiences to use their background knowledge to guess at the meaning and to attract the widest possible audience, including nonscientists and scientists in other fields. The titles in one context are not "smarter" than those in the other; instead, they capture different audiences and achieve different goals.

Recognize the (Potentially Deadly) Dangers of a Poorly Optimized Tool or Context

Individual tools have inherent affordances and constraints that make them unsuited for particular tasks. A tragic example is the use of PowerPoint summaries in place of technical reports in the assessment of damage to the space shuttle *Columbia*. In January 2003, a piece of foam insulation fell from *Columbia*'s fuel tank just after liftoff and hit the wing. Two weeks later, during *Columbia*'s re-entry, the shuttle burned up, because the damage caused by the foam insulation had been more serious than thought, despite the extensive risk analysis undertaken by NASA during the two-week period. As Edward Tufte documents, the constraints and affordances of PowerPoint (or at least the poor optimization of the medium) seem to have been pivotal in the underestimation of the damage caused by the falling debris.[27] Default constraints on the amount of text per slide encouraged the use of acronyms and fragmented explanations. Additionally, the affordance of hierarchical bulleted lists led to slides where reassuring large bullets dominated lower-level bullets that contained critical information about the possibility of much greater risk. Tufte's analysis of the *Columbia* tragedy suggests that the kind of bad presentations we have all seen can have far worse consequences that just boring audiences.

Support Accessibility for Audiences with Diverse Needs

The principles of universal design, developed at North Carolina State University, are a set of seven overarching principles with accompanying finer-grained guidelines to make products and environments widely useable and accessible for as diverse a population as possible.[28] The idea is not to retrofit designs for accessibility, but to take a proactive approach. The universal design guidelines that are potentially relevant to communication in different contexts include the following:

- Eliminate unnecessary complexity.
- Be consistent with the expectations and intuitions of audiences.
- Maximize the legibility of essential information.
- Arrange information according to its importance.
- Support compatibility with devices used by people with sensory limitations.

An example of the latter is pauses in soundtracks that provide time for audio descriptions for the blind. Another is keeping essential visual content above the lower third of the video screen to make room for closed captions for the hearing impaired.[29]

Instructors or others who are designing curricula or engaging in other ongoing communication efforts should also become familiar with a second (distinct, despite the similar name) set of accessibility guidelines, universal design for learning guidelines.[30] These guidelines focus on the need to offer options for neuro-diverse learners. Options include ways to engage with the materials through different senses and different kinds of representations. The guidelines also emphasize providing learners with options for expression, self-regulation, and executive function.

Take Advantage of (but Do Not Feel at the Mercy of) the Evolving Media Landscape

New media creates new opportunities and challenges. I often hear from graduate students and postdocs who feel pressured to promote their work through their own social media blogs, vlogs, or podcasts. These are fantastic ways to reach people, but they take time to do well and require balancing competing personal and professional obligations that may already feel overwhelming. Do prioritize self-care. They can have other downsides as well; social media controversies have sometimes hindered individuals' career advancement.[31] When using social media for professional purposes, the goal should be providing quality material and a unique personal voice, not pumping out material from a sense of obligation. Choose the platform most suitable to your work. Contributing individual pieces or interviews to established platforms, such as those through your professional society or by hosts you admire, can be a happy middle ground that shares your work widely without the constant pressure to create content for your own feeds. Also, if your work gives you a unique perspective on a timely issue, you may expand your reach by contributing a perspective piece, such as a newspaper op-ed or an opinion piece for a new media outlet you respect.

Whether or not you are active on social media, do make available nontechnical entry points to your work. If you are a researcher, be sure to create lay-language abstracts for your peer-reviewed publications. These can be shared by interested bloggers and can allow reporters from traditional and new media to find you. Likewise, for your website, a brief public-friendly video about your research is helpful for the media, other publics, and prospective students, who will feel more comfortable approaching you when they gain a basic understanding of your work and can see that you want to make it accessible. Think of these materials as inviting audiences into a conversation, rather than trying to summarize all you do. They are effective if they whet the appetite of those who see them. Science communication frequently fails to be inclusive.[32] Consider how strategically expanding the contexts through which you communicate can help you reach underserved audiences.

DIMENSION 3: THE WHY OF COMMUNICATION

Identify Your Communication Goals

Consider a list of possible communication goals:

- Increase appreciation for and excitement about science.
- Teach a concept.
- Realistically portray the research process.
- Be a role model.
- Attract or retain students.
- Appeal to potential collaborators in other disciplines.

- Secure funds for a research project or increase investment in the field.
- Be accountable to those whose taxes fund federal and state agencies.
- Gain public input to shape the priorities of the work.
- Inform consumer or medical decisions.
- Inform citizen participation in democratic processes.
- Raise an alarm or initiate emergency action.
- Advocate for or inform particular policies.
- Debunk misinformation or challenge implicit assumptions.
- Build relationships and trust.
- Collaborate to find solutions to a community problem.

These goals have several features worth noting. First, they can overlap. An article debunking claims made by the manufacturer of a product may inform consumer decisions and generate consumer discontent that leads to new legislation. Second, some of these goals may be achievable in the short term, such as holding an event about fossils to excite young people about geology, while others, such as building relationships and trust, require repeated, sustained interactions over the long term. Third, some goals, such as informing consumer decisions and promoting healthy lifestyle choices, are based on the hope that changing people's knowledge can influence their actions. Fourth, the goals may be centered on advising, advocating, or a mix of advising and advocating. Finally, the goals may be personal, such as securing funds to advance your own work, or they may have societal implications, such as ensuring that diverse voices inform research priorities. When planning communication, consider what is the desired outcome for you and the audience.

Communicate to Bridge Divides

Subsequent chapters provide in-depth guidance on bridging divides when discussing potentially contentious issues, but more attention also needs to be placed on bridging divides between research disciplines. Such divides even exist between fields that would seem closely related, like science education and science communication. Research silos are detrimental, because advances in one field have the potential to advance other fields, often in unforeseen ways. For example, our astrophysics graduates are in demand at biotechnology companies because the big data skills needed to answer fundamental questions about the universe turn out to be applicable to drug development. Combining knowledge, techniques, and tools from different disciplines can lead to remarkable research advances. At such junctures, the scientific breakthrough is inextricably linked to a communication breakthrough, because it is already challenging to keep up with the ever-burgeoning literature in one's own field. Researchers largely keep up with other fields the same way as do nontechnical audiences, through the media and other secondary sources.

Media coverage increases citations of research papers, an effect not simply attributable to the media earmarking papers that would have received attention anyway. During a strike at the *New York Times* in which an "edition of record" continued to be produced but not distributed (to control for the "earmarking hypothesis"), it was demonstrated that popular press coverage (i.e., coverage in the editions that were actually published) does in fact amplify transmission of scientific findings to the research community.[33] The amplification was seen in total citations and was even more pronounced for citations in the most prestigious scientific journals. Other work shows that use of specialized terminology and acronyms in research papers, especially in the title and abstract, reduces the number of citations, because jargon is an impediment to interdisciplinary collaboration.[34]

Consider the Audience's Communication Goals and Assess Communication Accordingly

Take care not to assume that your goals and the audience's goals overlap. For events with live audiences, promotions should be transparent about the communication goals. If attendees are offered a public forum to voice their concerns about an issue, they will feel cheated if the format is instead a scientist-led presentation with little opportunity for questions or discussion. On the other hand, participants in dialogues express frustration when they attend an event seeking specific information and experts fail to provide it.[35] In terms of interacting with the media, researchers may judge a finding to be newsworthy, but journalists have different goals and accordingly different criteria for newsworthiness, which typically include timeliness (the finding was published recently, possibly even today), superlativeness (biggest, fastest, etc.), unexpectedness, impact, human story, and geographical/cultural proximity.[36]

A large body of research on learning supports the importance of audience "relevance" as a motivational factor, where relevance includes any of three overlapping dimensions: individual (curiosity and interests and the knowledge and skills to cope with daily life), societal (knowledge and skills to contribute to humanity and society's sustainable development), and professional (relevance for current or future careers).[37] Thus, relevance can be individual or collective, and it can be focused on the immediate or the longer term. Consider how to enhance relevance. For example, a talk to youth about the neural mechanisms that enable monarch butterflies to set their flight path should be more than a watered-down version of the technical talk. It can include personal stories that give insight into career paths or offer ways for the students to get involved in creating local certified monarch waystations that provide milkweed habitat for migrating monarchs.

Obtain feedback from the audience to the extent feasible within the constraints of the mode of communication. In formal educational settings, midterms, finals, and other summative assessments are the norm, but adding more frequent lower-stakes formative assessments allow an educator to take stock of learning and adjust instruction as needed. In other contexts, short surveys or feedback forms can be useful. In live settings, attend to the body language of the audience, as well as the questions asked, to gain a sense of engagement and comprehension. Make a note of anything that should be changed for next time and aim for cycles of improvement in your communication efforts.

Be Transparent about the Difference between Advising and Advocating

Communication may be approached with the goal of providing "neutral" information–advising–or with the goal of shaping outcomes–advocating.

As illustrated by the three cases below, the line between these two communication goals is not always apparent to the audience.

1. Health care
   Advising: Helping patients understand the available treatment options.
   Advocating: Guiding patients toward a particular treatment option.
2. Academia
   Advising: Giving a seminar to teach students a newly developed lab technique.
   Advocating: Pitching your research with the aim of recruiting students to your lab.
3. Government
   Advising: Providing policymakers with a summary of the state of knowledge in your field.
   Advocating: Providing policymakers with evidence to encourage them to adopt a particular policy.

Even when researchers see themselves as advisors rather than advocates, their own values can be acting in subtle ways to influence their communication efforts. Ethical communication involves reflecting on your goals, implicit assumptions, and values and being transparent with the audience.[38] The call for transparency, however, should not be taken as an argument against any kind of advocacy. Those communicating about pressing public health issues and natural disasters, for example, may find it ethically questionable to remain silent about what they believe is necessary action.[39]

Thanks to the Truth Tobacco Industry Documents, we now know that tobacco companies have long sponsored extensive psychological and sociological research to better market their products.[40] This is a reminder of the power of using research findings to inform communication. As discussed in Chapter 8, however, the research-informed savvy used by the tobacco companies is often absent from public health campaigns. Most science and health degree programs place minimal emphasis on communication skills, and do not so much as address the existence of communication scholarship. In writing *Beyond the Sage on the Stage*, it is my goal to help well-meaning health and science experts understand this research and its implications for their advising and advocacy efforts. The Truth Documents are also a cautionary reminder that communication scholarship can inform ethical goals as well as non-ethical ones.

Your field, professional society, and organizations that publish your work almost certainly have established lists of ethical principles (e.g., journalism ethics, research communication ethics) with which you are familiar. The discussion of ethics in this book should complement any ethics training you have already had. Because ethics are a complex aspect of communication, especially communicating to inform personal and societal decisions, discussions of them are threaded through this book as they pertain to the specific topics covered in each chapter. Compared to lists of principles that make it seem as if ethics is black and white, the interwoven approach to communication ethics is designed to encourage ongoing reflection and provide the opportunity to consider more nuanced ethical questions.

Conceptualize Goals Hierarchically and Use Backward Design to Plan

When I think about science and health communication that has changed my life, three moments stand out:

• In the first, alone in my tiny college bedroom reading about proteins in a textbook, I had a sudden epiphany that sent shivers down my spine. I realized that I am only alive because the protein molecular motors in my cells are marching along like the workers in the classic science fiction movie *Metropolis*, and enzyme proteins are functioning independently yet in sync, like the workers of different trades on a major construction site. I credit that moment with sparking my lifelong fascination with biochemistry.
• In the second, I was in office hours with a chemistry professor who went on to win many awards for her teaching, and she read my mind! Of course, she did not actually read my mind, but she accurately predicted what error I would make (while drawing a resonance structure of the nitrate ion) before I made it. I credit that moment with my lifelong curiosity about how people learn science.

- The third occurred in the office of an orthopedic surgeon who had the good sense to counsel me by simultaneously explaining the relevant biomechanics of my injury and speaking to my fear of taking time away from exercise. He was not more compassionate than doctors whose advice I did not follow, but as someone who spent time around athletes, he knew how to relate to someone who was compulsive about exercise. Besides helping me heal, that moment was a personal demonstration of the importance of connecting through core identity when communicating potentially threatening or unwelcome information.

In the first anecdote, I was trying to learn scientific facts, and a well-written textbook supported that goal. In the second, I was struggling to gain conceptual understanding and needed a two-way interaction with someone who knew her audience and knew how to build on what I already knew. In the third, I was a stubborn patient who was not going to let pain hold me back from my lifestyle, and changing my mind required more than an exchange of knowledge. It involved a carefully tailored explanation as well as a short dialogue to find a collaborative solution in the form of a safe exercise plan. To my mind these three anecdotes fall along a continuum of increasing complexity of goals for the audience.

A useful way to think about audience goals (both the communicators' goals for the audience and the audience's goals for the communication) is through the lens of a hierarchical ordering of cognitive skills known as **Bloom's Taxonomy**. Bloom's Taxonomy was originated by Benjamin Bloom in 1956 and revised in 2001.[41] It is widely used in formal educational settings as a common language for communicating about learning goals and to ensure that students are given opportunities to go beyond memorization to building critical thinking skills essential for lifelong learning. Here I have adapted Bloom's Taxonomy into Bloom's Taxonomy of Communication Goals. In this book, the communication strategies are presented in an order consistent with Bloom's hierarchy of goals for audiences.

Complementary to Bloom's Taxonomy is the strategy of **backward design**. Also widely adopted by effective educators, backward design of curriculum has three stages: (1) Establish your learning goals; (2) determine how you will know the goals have been achieved; and (3) plan the

Figure 1.2. Bloom's Taxonomy of Communication Goals

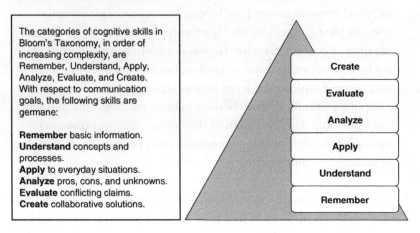

The categories of cognitive skills in Bloom's Taxonomy, in order of increasing complexity, are Remember, Understand, Apply, Analyze, Evaluate, and Create. With respect to communication goals, the following skills are germane:

Remember basic information.
Understand concepts and processes.
Apply to everyday situations.
Analyze pros, cons, and unknowns.
Evaluate conflicting claims.
Create collaborative solutions.

Create

Evaluate

Analyze

Apply

Understand

Remember

instruction and learning experiences.[42] It is backward design because planning typically starts with what material needs to be covered or what the instructor will do or say. In contrast, backward design entails defining your desired outcomes before you start planning how to get there. An example from my own experience can help clarify the distinction. Embarrassingly, I was an adult before I understood the importance of studying history, because my history classes did not show me that history explains the present. I imagine that my teachers thought they were teaching a history of the present, but that is not how the material was communicated or assessed. Their focus was on curriculum materials and activities to transmit information (forward design) instead of what they wanted us students to do with that information (backward design). Backward design is thus a shift of intentionality. Bloom's Taxonomy provides a way to conceptualize the goals that start the process of backward design (Figure 1.2).

A communicator's work becomes more complicated as the expectations for audiences step higher up Bloom's Taxonomy. It is one thing to communicate with the goal of having an audience remember a few fun facts. It is more difficult to help audiences truly understand concepts and more difficult still to help people make decisions that involve complex tradeoffs or to work with others to create collaborative solutions. The purpose of the taxonomy of goals is not for readers to try to figure out the minimum skills needed based on the goals (because it is easy to underestimate). Instead, it is a logical structure for the progression of topics in the book, and it is a map for a communicator's professional journey – a holistic journey, not just the basics covered in other communication guides and trainings. To achieve successively more challenging outcomes, communicators' professional journeys must help them build the needed knowledge, skills, and habits of mind. This book is thus designed with that professional journey in mind – although the chapters are also deliberately self-contained so that they are amenable to being revisited and can be consumed in a different order. (For example, those who find themselves in anxiety-provoking communication situations may find it helpful to read Chapter 9 next.)

NAVIGATING THE THREE-DIMENSIONAL AUDIENCES, CONTEXTS, AND GOALS LANDSCAPE

Optimize the Mutable Dimensions for the Immutable Dimensions

Sometimes choosing the communication context is an option. In other cases, for example when you are invited to give a lecture or contribute an editorial to a particular publication, the context is already set. Figure 1.3 presents the interrelationships among audiences, contexts, and goals, which shows how your communication decisions must vary depending on whether the context is predetermined or not. The goals for the communication should drive the content and format of the communication. Both the communicator and the audience should contribute to setting the goals, but the context of the interaction, if immutable, will constrain what goals may realistically be achieved. Choose the best contexts for your audience and goals, but if the context is already fixed, modify your goals to ensure they are achievable within the limitations of the context. Here are four questions to consider (the numbers align with the numbers used in Figure 1.3):

1. To reach this audience, what context should I choose?
2. In this context, what audiences can I reach?
3. With these goals, what context should I choose?
4. In this context, what goals can I achieve?

Figure 1.3. Interrelationships between Audiences, Contexts, and Goals

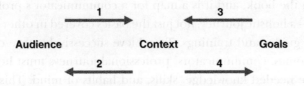

Table 1.2. Reflecting on the Three-Dimensional Communication Landscape

Audience	Context	Goals
– Who are my audiences? – Who are their audiences? – What knowledge and values do my audiences bring? – What assumptions am I making about them and how can I learn more about them?	– Where and how will the communication take place? – What are the affordances for inclusive communication? – What constraints may inhibit effectiveness or inclusivity? – How can the context be optimized?	– What are my goals? – What are my audience's goals? – How can I better align our goals or enhance transparency about the difference? – What does success look like and how can I assess it?

Table 1.2 provides some questions to consider when reflecting on the three-dimensional communication landscape.

This chapter has focused on getting our bearings in the audiences, contexts, and goals of the three-dimensional landscape. Now it is time to craft something beautiful with that knowledge. To get started, the next chapter explores the basics of tailoring communication according to where you end up in the landscape. Humans are verbal and visual creatures, so learning to optimize communication starts with learning to tailor and combine words and images. Chapter 2 will provide a solid grounding in these aspects of tailoring. Like a beautiful fractal pattern, no matter how intricate the surface, there is always depth beneath. The remaining chapters of the book will continue to spiral us deeper into strategies for making communication effective for different audiences, contexts, and goals, particularly as the substance of communication becomes more complex and as the stakes for communication increase.

Masterful Use of Words and Images, the Fundamental Tools of the Communication Artisan

Every architect, artisan, and artist has an individual creative vision that is guided by many factors, such as the purpose of the project, the desires of their clients, local regulations, the topography of the terrain, and the shape and texture of the source material. In other words, even the most creative acts are shaped by audiences and contexts. The shaping may occur organically. The unique underwater sculptures of artist Jason deCaires Taylor arise as a mutual collaboration between the artist's handiwork and the sea, as marine plants and animals take up residence on and transform each sculpture into something new, something alive. This beautiful ongoing interaction is akin to how a conversation evolves and shapes us. Because artists must master the tools of their trade before their amazing visions can come to life, this chapter lays the groundwork for communicators to optimize the use of their fundamental artisanal tools – words and images.

CHAPTER LEARNING OBJECTIVES: WORDS AND VISUALS

Knowledge: What cognitive and perceptual principles are relevant to multimedia learning?

Skills: Optimize your verbal and visual language to reach the audience and meet the goals.

Habits of Mind: Distinguish clarification from simplification to maximize comprehensibility.

LANGUAGE: PREVENT WORDS FROM GETTING IN THE WAY

Cats and dogs do not speak the same language. My dog apparently had no experience with cats during her puppy years and felines still flummox her. When one of the confident neighborhood cats sashays up to her, this bold act completely overrides her hunting dog prey drive. She wags her tail, sniffs, lets the cat rub on her legs, and then, at the risk of anthropomorphizing, she looks embarrassed. She looks exactly the way people look when they meet someone who does not speak their language. After the initial friendly gesturing, one gazes awkwardly at one's feet as if pages from a foreign language phrasebook might be levitating around one's toes.

Scientists speak their own language. If you have a science background, it is probably not readily apparent to you just how much specialized vocabulary you have learned over your years of training. The number of vocabulary terms introduced in high school physics, chemistry, biology, and earth science textbooks ranges from around 1,000 to 3,000.[1] The recommended upper limit for foreign-language textbooks is 1,500. Science is indeed a foreign language. It is not surprising that when the conversation turns to science, those not conversant in science-ese are left staring awkwardly at their toes. As business gobbledygook generators on the internet humorously demonstrate, this problem is not unique to the sciences. The language recommendations below can help you break down language barriers.

Language Recommendation 1: Balance Efficiency, Precision, and Comprehensibility

A major focus of science communication training is de-jargonizing, and communication coaches' favorite recommendation is "Don't use jargon!" Although this is sound advice, it is oversimplified and may be served with a side order of condescension. Calls for specialists to de-jargonize sometimes imply that they are deliberately using unfamiliar terms instead of plain language to sound smart. Communication coaches need to concede that science-ese was not born of hubris. It is a matter of both efficiency and precision. Just as saying "the thick, woody part of the tree that grows up from the ground" is much less efficient than saying "the trunk," specialists need names for their methods, tools, and discoveries. Furthermore, although basophils, eosinophils, lymphocytes, monocytes, and neutrophils can all be lumped under the umbrella of "leukocyte," or white blood cell, they have distinct roles. Lumping them together reduces precision.[2]

People do find it satisfying to learn new words, but avoid the temptation to "geek out." So how much is too much? Human long-term memory is seemingly limitless, but short-term or working memory is extremely limited in its ability to grapple with new information. On average, people can hold onto seven independent pieces of information in working memory at one time, but keeping things in working memory is an active process involving rehearsal.[3] As you present conceptual information between definitions, you will be disrupting rehearsal and leading to split attention, so be judicious in your use of unfamiliar vocabulary.

Language Recommendation 2: Identify Hidden Jargon and Distinguish Its Technical and Everyday Meaning

Communication coaches' favorite recommendation implies that jargon is easily identified. Specialized science words, like "eosinophil," will immediately jump out to members of the audience, and with minimal reflection, to the speaker. Unfortunately, not all terminology is easily recognizable as such. Those who have taken a foreign language course will be familiar with "false friends" – words that look or sound the same in both languages but mean different things. False friends can trip you up, leading to hilarity or disaster. In France it would be obnoxious to request to borrow a book from a *librairie*, which is a bookstore. If you hear French teenagers complaining about their *boutons*, they are not wishing for zippers. *Boutons* means buttons in French, but it also means pimples. Expect furrowed brows if you ask a French shopkeeper about preservatives in your strawberry jam, because *préservatif* means condom. If you head for the land of tapas because your French language faux pas leave you a little embarrassed, your new Spanish friends may be left smirking when you tell them you are *embarazada* (pregnant). If you put the romance languages behind and head for Germany, you may be surprised your hosts look offended when you say you have a gift for them. In German, *gift* means poison.

Science is also full of false friends or terms that have been referred to as "paradoxical jargon."[4] It is jargon, but it is familiar and thus hidden. Hidden jargon is more insidious than regular jargon because communicators are more likely to unwittingly let hidden jargon slip through. Slips of hidden jargon are compounded by audiences' familiarity with a word, which prevents them from noticing it is a technical term.[5] In short, the hidden jargon communication gap is harder to detect, which can lead to the communicator and audience going off in different directions, unbeknownst to one another. Over 50 common examples of hidden science jargon with everyday and scientific meanings are shown in Table 2.1. This list is not comprehensive, nor does it include all the alternative meanings of each term, but it will help you develop a keen eye and ear for hidden jargon.

It is easy to see how any of the terms listed in the table above could slip through undefined into communication intended to be nontechnical. In some cases, the terms could inadvertently inspire fear (e.g., chemical, radiation), make researchers seem dishonest (e.g., bias, manipulation, plot, scheme), encourage unwarranted actions (e.g., significance), or lead audiences to be unfairly dismissive of research (e.g., theory). Hidden jargon should thus be treated the same way as more easily recognizable jargon. Hidden jargon can also be ambiguous to other researchers. Always be sure to provide sufficient context. When speaking about a control, for example, do not merely refer to it as a "control." State the control condition.

Language Recommendation 3: Beware of Hidden Jargon that May Raise Hackles

Specialists should thoroughly scan their own field-specific vocabulary to ferret out hidden jargon. Furthermore in certain cases, such as in the field of sociobiology, where terms like "rape," "cuckoldry," "adultery," and "harem" have been used to describe animal behaviors, researchers also need to determine whether everyday meanings of paradoxical jargon may interfere with scientific objectivity.[6] If these examples

Table 2.1. Hidden Jargon

Term	Everyday Meaning	Scientific Meaning
Aerosol	Spray can	Particles in the atmosphere
Anomaly	Oddity, peculiarity	Deviation from a trend
Artifact	Archeological artifact, such as Stone Age tools	An observation is an artifact if it is due to problems with the experimental setup
Bias	Prejudice	Form of experimental error
Carbohydrate	Starchy foods such as pasta	Cell-surface molecules involved in recognition and adhesion
Cascade	Water rushing downhill over rocks	Chain of actions in which the previous causes the next
Cell	*See discussion in text below.*	
Checkpoint	A location, such as a border crossing	A time, such as in the cell cycle
Chemical	Toxic substances in our environment	Any element or molecule
Confound	Perplex	Lurking variable, factor that affected the outcome
Control	Limit freedom	Comparison group in a study
Culture	Way of life	Grow cells outside the body
Date	Meeting with a romantic interest	Determining the geological age of an object
Differentiate	Distinguish the difference	A mathematical operation to find slope
Dirty/Promiscuous	Sexual/many sexual partners	A drug that activates nontarget receptors
Error	Mistake	Range of values in which a measured quantity may fall
Expression	Phrase, a look on one's face	Result of gene activity
Fitness	Athleticism	Reproductive success
Fix	Repair	Preserve (e.g., tissue)
Gene	*See discussion in text below.*	
Integrate	Bring together and merge	A mathematical operation to find the area under a curve
Law	Societal rule	A fundamental principle of nature
Manipulation	To control or misuse	Processing scientific data
Marker	Something with which to write	A chemical that labels cells or cell components
Media	Channels of communication	Substance to grow cells or microbes

(*Continued*)

Table 2.1. (*Continued*)

Term	Everyday Meaning	Scientific Meaning
Model	Replica, ideal	Computer simulation, mathematical expression
Mutant	Abnormal, freak of nature	Genetic variant that may or may not be physically distinct from "normal"
Negative/positive feedback	Bad/good feedback	Self-diminishing/self-reinforcing cycle
Negative/positive trend	Bad/good trend	Downward/upward trend
Noise	Loud sound	Spread or variation in data
Normal	Usual	Perpendicular or bell-shaped distribution
Nucleus	*See discussion in text below.* (Also, note pronunciation is *nu-cle-us* not *nu-cue-lus*)	
Organic	Method for growing food, or food grown by that method	Molecule containing carbon
Perturb	Annoy	Alter a system from baseline
Phase	A time period in life that one may grow out of	Distinct layer in a liquid; a period in the cell cycle
Plastic	Most widely used synthetic material	Readily moldable, for example, the developing nervous system
Plot	Scheme, storyline of a narrative	A graph or the act of organizing data on axes
Positive/negative feedback or trend	*See negative/positive feedback and trend above*	
Protein	A nutrient that builds muscle	Large molecule composed of amino acids with structural and metabolic (i.e., enzymatic, messenger) roles in living organisms
Radiation	Cancer-causing rays	Emitted particles or energy transferred in the form of waves
Radical	Someone with extreme political views	Reactive compound with a free electron; a square root sign
Salt	Table salt or road salt, sodium chloride is most familiar	Any neutral compound made of positively and negatively charged ions
Scheme	Devious plot	Diagram; systematic plan
Sensitivity	Emotionality	Limit of detection of a measurement
Significant	Important	Meets statistical threshold

(*Continued*)

Table 2.1. (*Continued*)

Term	Everyday Meaning	Scientific Meaning
Tag	Price, information or warning label on clothes or consumer goods	Chemical that binds to cells or cell components to help identify them (e.g., fluorescent tag)
Transcript	Written record	RNA copy of a gene
Theory	Speculation or hypothesis	Scientific explanation supported with evidence
Uncertainty	Doubt	Statistical range
Value	Monetary worth or ethical principle	Data point
Viable	Feasible	Able to survive

sound dated, consider the widespread use of "geriatric pregnancy" to describe a woman over 35 who is expecting, despite the fact that geriatric is typically used to refer (sometimes in a derogatory way) to ill or feeble elderly populations. The use of the offensive term has led to anger and resistance in the popular press and has only served to stymie conversation about age as a risk factor in pregnancy.[7] Besides the public backlash, health care professionals may want to ask themselves if use of the term places so much focus on age that its use risks eclipsing each individual's unique combination of risk factors.

More generally, these examples serve as a reminder that language can have a negative impact on an audience when the communicator's intended meaning and the audience's received meaning differ. This situation can arise with no ill intent on the part of a communicator, and it does not mean that the audience is being "too sensitive." When we become familiar with our discipline's hidden jargon, we may develop tunnel vision as to the other nuanced meanings of the terms. Therefore, if an audience reacts negatively, it is best to take a step back, address the concerns with empathy, and reconsider the use of that term in future communication.

Language Recommendation 4: Eliminate It or Use a Synonym, but If You Say It, Own It!

In any communication situation, consider your three options for handling terminology: (1) define it; (2) find a synonym for it; or (3) remove it entirely. Removing technical words entirely can support the purging of details only relevant for researchers, so think of it as an opportunity to streamline. If a term cannot be removed, consider substituting with a more familiar word or phrase. When selecting the best synonym, balance functionality and zest. Zesty words are the bomb – except when they are distractingly jarring or poor synonyms. Journalists and communication trainers should avoid erring in the direction of choosing style over substance. In contrast, scientists and other specialists may want to push themselves a little more (while prioritizing accuracy) to select vivid language.

At times, you may have a calculated reason to introduce terminology. Perhaps your audience members are fans of crime shows, medical dramas, or science fiction where the terms have been thrown around. Maybe these are terms they need to understand literature about their medical condition or relevant published decisions of regulatory agencies. Perchance you want to write a blog post describing the specialized equipment in a lab to provide insight into why research in the field is expensive. It is also possible that a term is pivotal for describing the research in any depth. The option you select to handle terminology should therefore be a strategic decision based on the audience, context, and goals. If you do use terminology, avoid the all-too-common tendency to rush through and mumble as though you are embarrassed about using it.

In the absence of audible cues that segment speech, listeners must rely on word recognition – lexical cues.[8] Lexical cues usually play the primary role in helping listeners parse speech, but they are hard to discern in the case of unrecognizable words.[9] If you use terminology, slow down and clearly articulate each syllable. For example, speakers distinguish "grey tie" from "great eye" using allophonic variation – the difference in the way letters or groups of letters are pronounced in words.[10] In American English, the "t" in "top" is pronounced with an accompanying forceful expulsion of air, while the "t" in "stop" is not. These consonant pronunciations are referred to as aspirated versus unaspirated, respectively. In the example of "grey tie" and "great eye," the "t" in "tie" is aspirated and the "t" in "great" is not. Deliberately enunciate unfamiliar words and briefly pause before and after each to parse it into a distinct unit.

Language Recommendation 5: Provide the Definition *before* the Term

If you must use terminology, hidden or otherwise, be sure to define it. Note that people tend to define words by first giving the term and then saying what it means, but this is the opposite of how we learn language as toddlers. We point to a big round object and are told that it is a "ball." Fido sidles up to lick our ever-sticky hands and we are supplied with "doggie." Before we are given the word, we are presented with the thing that the word describes. Thus, we only learn the word when we need it. This way of learning language is not only effective for toddlers. It works for grown-ups too.

People develop a better conceptual understanding when they are exposed to a concept (e.g., what a nucleic acid is) before they are given the technical vocabulary (i.e., the term "nucleic acid") to describe it.[11] It is helpful to separate initial exposure to new concepts and new terms because it reduces information processing requirements imposed on learners at any one time. Before introducing new terminology, aim to familiarize the audience with the concept by describing it, showing an image of it, or otherwise setting up the need for it.

Language Recommendation 6: Avoid Assuming that Others (Including Colleagues) Know What You Mean or Will Speak Up When They Do Not

Science lingo has disciplinary dialects. To illustrate, think about the following: What is the meaning of the word "nucleus" in everyday language and in anatomy, astronomy, biology, chemistry, geology, meteorology, and physics?
Answers are in Table 2.2.

The statement made near the beginning of the chapter, "Scientists speak their own language," is not entirely accurate. Scientists speak their own *languages*. Each discipline has its own language, and sometimes the same words have different meanings in different disciplines.

Table 2.2. Meaning of "Nucleus" in Different Disciplines

Discipline	Meaning
Everyday	A central hub in a network (e.g., with respect to social interactions or economic activity)
Anatomy	Clusters of nerve cell bodies in the central nervous system
Astronomy	Core in the head of a comet or central dense portion of a galaxy
Biology	A spherical structure in the cell that contains the genetic material
Chemistry and physics	The positively charged center of an atom or the seed of crystal formation
Geology	Large area of rock from which the continents are thought to have grown
Meteorology	A particle on which water vapor condenses to form droplets or ice

For example, a researcher who works on plasma could be a biologist studying the liquid portion of the blood or a physicist studying the fourth state of matter. "Cell" is an even richer example. To a biologist, cells are the fundamental parts of the body, or they are the bacteria in a Petri plate. Biochemists may work with living cells, while their physical chemistry neighbors may study battery cells. Over in atmospheric sciences, a group may be tracking storm cells. Colleagues in electrical or computer engineering may work on the kind of cells that humans cannot look up from when walking down the sidewalk.

Even when a term refers to the same thing in different fields, scientists may be interpreting it in distinct ways depending on their disciplinary perspectives. An example is "gene," which is a heritable trait to a geneticist, a segment of DNA to a molecular biologist, instructions for protein to a biochemist, a developmental switch to an embryologist, and a selfish entity to some evolutionary biologists.[12] The possibility for confusion, even within a scientific setting, is thus real. Exacerbating the situation, people are loathe to speak up when they think they are the only one who does not understand, just like in the children's story, "The Emperor's New Clothes." Undergraduates, graduate students, and anyone struggling with imposter syndrome may be too afraid of revealing their ignorance to ask for clarification when someone's presentation is incomprehensible. Everyone just pretends to get it, creating a vicious cycle where speakers think they need to up the jargon ante to be one of the gang.

Language Recommendation 7: Take a Lesson from the Arts to Reach Mixed Audiences

In *Hamlet*, after an intense night out on the battlements of Denmark's royal castle, the character Horatio sees the sun rising and describes the dawn in poetic language as a person cloaked in russet walking across the dewy hills in the east. It is just the kind of fancy language we expect from Shakespeare, right? Not exactly. Shakespearean director, Barry Edelstein, contrasts Horatio's personification of dawn to the direct statement about dawn's arrival spoken by Duke Vincentio in *Measure for Measure*.[13] In this comparison, the contrasting height of language reflects both the emotional state of the characters and their educational levels. Individual characters also juxtapose high and low language in the same speech. An example is when Hamlet opens a scene on the battlements with, "The air bites shrewdly. It is very cold."[14] By mixing language of different heights, Shakespeare appealed not only to elite Elizabethans but also to commoners. The juxtaposition strategy is common in literature and popular culture, and many other forms of art can be interpreted on concrete and abstract levels. You can use the strategy when communicating research to mixed audiences that include fellow specialists and those unfamiliar with the language and conventions of the field. For example, for each slide or transition point, provide a clear statement that gives a conceptual overview before you introduce any technical details (see Figure 2.1).

Language Recommendation 8: Be Aware of What Terms in Your Discipline Are (and Are Not) in the American Sign Language (ASL) Dictionary

For those who use ASL, discipline-specific terminology presents unique challenges. When signs for technical terms do not exist, as is often the case, signers must resort to finger spelling, which dramatically slows communication. Creating an inclusive environment for deaf participants is thus another reason for eliminating unnecessary terminology in your talks, and for slowing down and articulating each syllable when you do use new terms. You may also consider giving a list of unfamiliar terms with definitions to interpreters ahead of a talk (check with your host for details).

Figure 2.1. Reflection Chart for Finding the Right Words

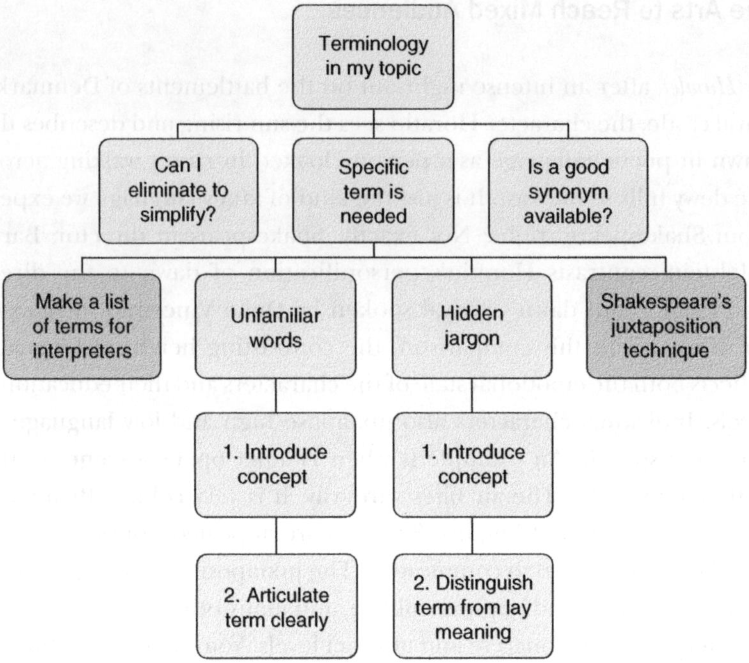

ASL-fluent scientists are developing more and more science-specific signs. These signs often visually represent the concept they depict; for instance, the sign for DNA delineates its double helical structure. Because a term may have different meanings in different fields, signs can also differ across fields. For example, the word "molecule" has one sign in physics, one in chemistry, and three in biology.[15] Another challenge is that ASL interpreters often do not have the disciplinary expertise to know the signs and use them appropriately. If you have students who rely on ASL to communicate, consistency of interpreters and time for sign development (allowing students and interpreters to work together to invent or converge on the signs they will use) is highly beneficial.

VISUALS: PAINT A CLEAR PICTURE

Scientific research explores aspects of our world that are too small or too large to be visible to the naked eye, and processes that are on too short or too long a timescale to be directly observed. It also generates multidimensional datasets that cannot readily be visualized in raw form. Researchers regularly create visuals as part of the discovery process and to communicate findings. Visuals are important in helping students learn, including successfully addressing their misconceptions.[16] Compelling visuals can also influence policy. Among the earliest examples are physician John Snow's maps of cholera incidences during London's 1854 epidemic, and nurse Florence Nightingale's "rose diagrams" showing causes of death and death rates of soldiers during the Crimean War.[17] Snow's and Nightingale's visuals helped advance measures that reduced the spread of infectious disease.

The design of visuals is both an art and a science. Visuals can take many forms, from static graphics, such as illustrations, charts, and data displays, to dynamic graphics, such as animations, multimedia presentations, and interactive displays. The audience, context, and goals may not dictate the exact form a visual should take, but they should inform the options. As with the selection of language, cognitive demands placed on the audience must be carefully considered in the design of visuals. The visuals recommendations below provide guidance on how to apply research on perception and attention to inform a design aesthetic.

Visuals Recommendation 1: Recognize the Challenges of Your Discipline's Visual Vocabulary

To save space, figures in research articles are often intended to show multiple things, and researchers have a bad habit of repurposing their jam-packed journal figures for all audiences and contexts. Experts in a field have not only learned a vast verbal vocabulary, they have learned a "vocabulary" or repertoire of visual representations. Using their background knowledge, they are able to process domain-specific visuals efficiently because they can group visual elements that a novice would have to make sense of in a piecemeal way. An example of domain-specific knowledge supporting visual processing is that chess experts who are briefly shown an image of a chessboard can readily recall the positions of the various pieces.[18] A novice chess player performs much worse on this recall task; however, it is not that experts have better memories or more processing capacity in general. The difference is task specific. Chess experts only outperform novices when the pieces on the chessboard are arranged in an actual game pattern. Experts leverage their knowledge of game patterns to simplify the memory task. If the pieces on the chessboard are randomly arranged, experts cannot recall the positions of the pieces any better than novices can. Likewise, scientists' content expertise allows them to identify and recall patterns and relationships in the visual representations of their fields, while nonspecialists may not see past the superficial design elements.[19]

In addition to proficiency at gleaning information from individual visual representations, scientists have learned how to move fluidly between the different types of visual representations used in their fields. For example, to gain insight into chemical reactions, chemists may make use of the periodic table, static drawings of molecules, physical molecular models, dynamic computer simulations of molecular interactions, graphs, and mathematical formulae. Chemists do not need to explain to one another that these are all tools to understand atoms, molecules, and interactions within and between molecules. For scientists, moving among the canonical representations of the discipline becomes so natural that they tend to forget how difficult it was to achieve fluency in representation-ese. Moving among representations is especially challenging when it entails making links between the observable human-scale world and the unobservable world (microscopic/submicroscopic or astronomical/planetary) and symbolic abstractions.[20] Nonspecialist audiences cannot be expected to do so without substantial support, which is best provided by designing visuals specifically for them, rather than repurposing the visuals from research papers.

Visuals Recommendation 2: Balance the Design Elements that Influence the Complexity and Depth of a Graphic

Designing a graphic, such as a data display or a mechanistic representation, involves important decisions regarding inherent complexity. The aim of a graphic may be to support analytical thinking about evidence, or it may be to present a concept, but either way it must clarify things for the audience. Clarification is not the same as simplification. Simplifying a message often helps clarify it, but when simplification leaves out elements that would contextualize or otherwise make sense of the information, simplification interferes with

Table 2.3. Facets of Visualizations

	Increasing Complexity and Depth
Concrete	Abstract
Familiar	Original
Redundant	Nonredundant
Unidimensional	Multidimensional
Light	Dense
Unadorned	Decorated
	Increasing Cognitive Demands

attempts to clarify. When tailoring for nonspecialist audiences, be aware of not only what confusing details are present, but also what details are confusing by their absence.

In his book, *The Functional Art: An Introduction to Information Graphics and Visualization*, Alberto Cairo introduces a visualization wheel with six dimensions or facets that together determine the depth and complexity of graphics.[21] For simplicity (and clarity), Cairo's dimensions can also be viewed along a continuum of increasing depth, with concurrent increase in the cognitive demands placed on the audience (Table 2.3).

CONCRETE VERSUS ABSTRACT

Graphics differ as to whether they present a copy of reality or portray underlying concepts without actually physically resembling the original. For example, a realistic drawing of an airplane wing is relatively concrete, and a vector diagram showing how forces create lift is relatively abstract. Audiences may need to invest significant cognitive resources to make sense of an abstraction.

FAMILIAR VERSUS ORIGINAL

Bar graphs and pie charts are widespread and familiar graphical forms today. In contrast, Florence Nightingale's rose diagrams were original in her time and remain unfamiliar today. Although original graphical forms place more cognitive load on the audience, they may be the best option to meaningfully display certain datasets.

REDUNDANT VERSUS NONREDUNDANT

An otherwise similar graphic can depict different things once each, or can depict one thing redundantly in different ways. For instance, a map may represent population by using both shading and numbers. The shading could allow viewers to see patterns across a region; the numbers could allow them to home in on a location of interest. Because each of the redundant representations can support understanding of the others, redundant graphics are less cognitively demanding than equally detailed graphics that depict multiple unique things.

UNIDIMENSIONAL VERSUS MULTIDIMENSIONAL

This refers to the number of layers of depth that are available to be explored and is especially relevant for interactive information graphics. A multidimensional display allows a viewer to dig into the data. A unidimensional graphic focuses the audience on a main take-home message.

LIGHT VERSUS DENSE

The density of a graphic refers to the amount of information displayed in a given amount of space. Figure panels in *Science* and *Nature* are often extremely information dense and require a time investment to comprehend. Density also varies with representation style. A photograph is more information dense than a corresponding sketch. The former is more suitable for showing how things look, but the latter may better reveal how things work, because unessential details can be stripped away. This can support comprehension, albeit with the potential caveat of making things overly abstract.

UNADORNED VERSUS DECORATED

Decorations are visual elements included purely for aesthetics. Strategic use of fonts, spacing, and color to clarify information (not merely for art's sake) are not decoration. Decoration is the most debated of Cairo's dimensions. Because decoration demands attention without conveying information, it would be reasonable to conclude that it interferes with functionality and should be avoided. Indeed, that is the position of visualization expert Edward Tufte, who refers to artistic embellishments of graphics as "chart junk" and considers them insulting to the audience.[22] He argues for the minimization of non-data ink. This position, however, ignores the relationship between emotion and cognition. Aesthetic features, such as color and appealing graphics, influence the audience's motivation.[23] When aesthetic features generate positive emotions, audiences are more likely to continue to work with the materials.[24] To balance the cognitive demands with these benefits of engagement, the aesthetic embellishments should relate to the graphic's essential content, drawing attention to, not away from, it.[25]

In designing a graphic, these six facets can be used strategically. For instance, a designer may want to develop an original way to display patterns in data because no familiar graphical display is adequate for the dataset. To offset the greater attention required to process an unfamiliar graphical form, a designer can simultaneously increase redundancy or decrease density. In addition to considering the cognitive demands on the audience, the context in which the graphic will be presented must also be considered. An information graphic that individuals will be able to peruse or interact with at their own pace can be more complex than a graphic intended to be briefly displayed on a screen during a presentation.

Visuals Recommendation 3: Apply the Principles of Gestalt Psychology

If we mix two wavelengths of light, we see an intermediary color, not the component colors. This is utterly intuitive, but contrast the sense of vision with the sense of hearing. If a high sound and a low sound are played simultaneously, we hear the sounds played, not an intermediary sound. The fact that vision is a synthetic sense gives rise to our propensity to see optical illusions. The whole is greater than the sum of parts. This is the central tenet of the theory of perception known as Gestalt psychology.[26] Its laws of grouping – similarity, proximity, closure, enclosure, connectedness, figure/ground, good continuation, and common fate – should inform design of visual representations.

SIMILARITY

Similar elements are perceived as belonging to the same form. For example, in viewing a grid filled with dots and Xs, our perceptual system will automatically group the dots together and the Xs together and see the pattern formed by the dots as distinct from the pattern formed by the Xs. Likewise, in a set of items distinguished by color, items that are the same color will be perceptually grouped together. Designers can exploit this effect by making sure to use symbols and color palettes that help audiences see the relevant patterns. Each color should be used to show only one thing, and all things of the same type should be the same color.

PROXIMITY

Elements that are closest together are seen as belonging together. For example, when dots are arranged in a grid pattern, they will be seen as a set of dotted horizontal lines if the space between the rows is larger than the space between the columns. They will be seen as a set of vertical dotted lines if the space between the rows is smaller than the space between the columns. This principle can be applied in graphic design by organizing visual information from left to right (the way we are accustomed to reading), aligning related information horizontally or vertically on an imaginary grid, and using white space strategically to group related elements.

CLOSURE

Our perceptual systems often supply missing information to fuse lines or elements into a figure and relegate the rest of the image to the background. Try zooming out on a figure you have designed to see if your use of color, space, patterns, lines, and symbols is inadvertently triggering closure where it is not intended.

ENCLOSURE

Objects within the same enclosed region are viewed as grouped together. Therefore, borders can be used to indicate that the contained objects are related or should be considered as a unit. Use the practice sparingly, however, because being confronted with a plethora of rectangular frames in a figure can monopolize viewers' attention and cause them to relegate the actual content to the background.

CONNECTEDNESS

Objects or regions that are connected are viewed as being part of a unit. Content should be organized thoughtfully, with juxtaposition and links that help the viewer follow the relevant relationships.

FIGURE/GROUND

This principle determines how we perceive the relative location of shapes. The object with the simplest, uninterrupted boundary is perceived as being closer. A tip to make something jump out to the viewer is to choose the region or elements that contain the focal details and to fade (or change to grayscale) the rest of the image.

GOOD CONTINUATION

One of the ways our perceptual systems distinguish two objects from one another when they intersect is to group lines and curves that follow a smooth and established direction, rather than an abrupt turn. If a sharp turn is in fact part of the same shape, color or shading can be used to help the viewer make the appropriate distinction.

COMMON FATE

Elements that move in the same direction are perceived as belonging to the same object or collective, such as a partially hidden predator or a flock of birds. Motion used in dynamic visualizations should be well thought out and coherent.

   Apply the principles of Gestalt psychology in your designs for both specialist and nonspecialist audiences. For important or challenging figures, it may be helpful to hire a graphic designer to bring an experienced eye to your work. It is also useful to compare before

Figure 2.2. Applying Strategies to Focus Visual Attention

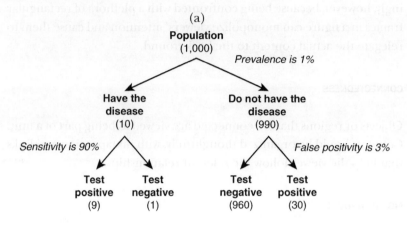

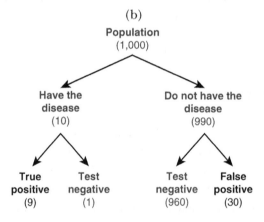

Note: The top diagram (used in Chapter 7 – see Figure 7.3) is intended to dispel the misconception that a positive test result means one has the disease. It is deliberately detailed (multidimensional) to allow the reader to work through it and learn how to create data trees like it. When used in a slide presentation, however, it can induce cognitive overload. You can avoid this by introducing the figure row by row and explaining as you go. Alternatively, you can modify the graphic to call attention to the specific elements that demonstrate your point (the number of true positives compared to false positives). The bottom diagram does that by fading everything but the focal information (exploiting the Gestalt principle of figure/ground) and removing and altering text (reducing dimensions to reduce complexity).

and after versions of scientific figures that have been improved by graphic designers. Examples that reveal common mistakes scientists make when designing figures, as well as fixes for those errors, can be found in books by award-winning science photographer Felice Frankel, including *Visual Strategies: A Practical Guide to Graphics for Scientists and Engineers.*[27] Also examine textbook figures in and outside your discipline to consider how they do (or fail to) use the Gestalt principles and balance complexity.

See Figure 2.2 for an example of how to apply strategies to focus visual attention.

Visuals Recommendation 4: Design for Limitations in Color Perception

The most common form of color blindness, red/green color blindness, affects about 8 per cent of men and 0.5 per cent of women.[28] If problematic color pairings cannot be avoided, combine lightness/darkness contrasts with color contrasts to help those with color blindness make the relevant distinctions between elements. Doing so is also helpful if your audience will print out your papers in grayscale. Try using one of the many web tools that predict how a graphic will look to people with various forms of color blindness.

Not all color palettes are equally effective at displaying data, even for those with normal color vision. Because two-thirds of retinal cone cells process longer wavelengths of light (red, orange, yellow), we perceive more detail along the warmer end of the spectrum than along the cooler. So, for instance, red stands out more than blue. Data displays that use a rainbow color gradient are common across fields, but a given data variation is underrepresented by a blue-green color gradient compared to a yellow-red one.[29] If you rely on color gradients to make decisions about the data, the perceptual distortion can lead to inappropriate conclusions. Select from one of the scientifically derived color maps – that is, maps that take into consideration the quirks of the human perceptual system, including the most common forms of color blindness. Color maps should be optimized for different types of datasets (such as cyclic versus sequential, or continuous versus categorical). A list of publicly available scientifically derived color maps and selection guidelines are provided in the paper "The Misuse of Colour in Science Communication" by Crameri and colleagues.[30]

WORDS AND VISUALS: COORDINATION FOR COMPREHENSION

When combining words and visuals, strategically focus the audience's attention to maximize comprehension. The theoretical underpinning for the effective design of multimedia is that memory, attention, and mental processing power are limited at any given time, and that learning is diminished when a task exceeds a learner's available cognitive resources – cognitive load theory.[31] This theory, along with extensive empirical research in multimedia learning, provides five rules of thumb to be applied when combining audio and visuals in videos, slide presentations, or other multimedia forms: synchronize, eliminate interference, signal, segment, and weed.

Combining Words and Visuals Recommendation 1: Synchronize

Audiences learn better when both words and images are provided because connecting information through multiple modalities makes for a richer mental model.[32] Specific meaningful gestures can also be used consciously to improve learning by supporting thinking that involves both mind and body – embodied cognition – in the speaker and the listener.[33] The following are examples of gestures that are potentially useful for communicating about science and natural phenomena. Unless you are miming your work to entertain an audience of young children, only use gestures that feel natural and relevant, and use them strategically, not repetitively.

- *Size and scope.* Stretch out your arms to remind us of the vastness of the range of options. Show us how tiny your prototype is by bringing together your fingers and thumbs.

- *Layout of a space.* Point out the positions of and connections between the parts of a system you are describing to help us imagine it in three dimensions.
- *Actions in your work.* Show a task such as assembling components or preparing samples, or signal the ebbs and flows of the research process.
- *Processes you study.* Use your hands or body to indicate how entities separate, integrate, transport, shapeshift, communicate, and so on.
- *Emphasis.* Lean forward toward your webcam or audience to let us know you are about to communicate key information. Use your fingers to count off the steps you are describing.

Words and gestures or images should be presented in sync – with temporal contiguity – to help audiences more readily store them together in long-term memory. This is because when words and images are presented sequentially instead of simultaneously, extra cognitive demands are placed on the audience to do the work of integrating the audio and visual material.[34] Spatial contiguity also improves learning, because processing images in more than one location at the same time divides visual attention. For this reason, media formats that use multiple windows are distracting.[35] Animations with changes happening simultaneously in different parts of the animation also divide attention.[36]

Combining Words and Visuals Recommendation 2: Eliminate Interference within and between Channels

Although humans are adept at simultaneously processing information through the visual and auditory channels, the visual channel becomes overloaded if both images and text need to be processed through it. Therefore, it is more effective to present graphics and narration than to present graphics and written text.[37] With closed captions, the implication is that when an important figure is shown, hearing impaired audience members need to be given time (a gap in your narration) to examine the figure without the captions competing for their visual attention.

Furthermore, we are not capable of simultaneously processing different verbal information through audio and visual channels, because working memory has just one verbal processing center.[38] Our comprehension suffers because while we are reading text on slides we inadvertently tune out the speaker, unconsciously flipping our attention back and forth between slides and speaker. Limit text on slides. Slides are not meant to be notes. If using any longer bodies of text (such as quotations), provide the audience time to read it. Take care to make certain the font size is readable, including when you adapt a presentation for the greatly reduced screen size of a virtual environment.

Combining Words and Visuals Recommendation 3: Signal to Point Out Key Features ...

... TO THE EYE

For audiences to create appropriate referential connections between visuals, the connections need to be drawn to their attention, using some combination of verbal guidance and visual cues, such as arrows and highlights.[39] Cues can themselves be troublesome, however, because their meaning is not always clear. For example, not only do students interpret arrows in unintended ways, textbooks and other curriculum materials vary the size, shape, and intended meaning of arrows with little rhyme or reason.[40] Variations, such as in color, size, or motion, attract the audience's attention to the varying feature, which means that unintended inconsistencies may inadvertently emphasize unimportant features.[41] Use arrows, colors, font sizes and styles, and other signals judiciously and coherently.

... TO THE EAR

Theater director Barry Edelstein teaches actors to add extra emphasis to words or phrases, such as the name of a place or person, when first introduced. He uses the apt term **billboarding** to help actors imagine acoustically illuminating a word.[42] For example, if I were introducing the term "billboarding" in a talk, I would use slight pauses before and after the term to bracket it, and I would slow down to articulate each syllable. Variations in volume and pitch are other vocal cues that can be used to billboard. This echoes the advice given under Language Recommendation 4 above, but billboarding can also be applied in various ways to signal in multimedia presentations. For instance, in addition to highlighting new terms or important words, you can use billboarding to highlight a key idea or step as it appears on screen. It can also emphasize contradiction in a line of reasoning. Edelstein uses the example of a circus performer spinning plates as a metaphor for how to emphasize temporally separated contrasting ideas. When spinning plates on sticks, the circus performer must give the first plate a strong spin so that it continues to spin as the performer gets to the other plates. When planning your presentation, think about what ideas are in opposition so that you can billboard the contrasts, potentially combining them with visual cues (such as gestures, color, or a transition slide) that further emphasize the progression of logic.

An indirect form of signaling is the quality of the signal. Although audience engagement with multimedia is not contingent on high production value, poor quality has a negative influence on audience perceptions of research and researchers.[43] A related finding is that the auditory medium affects attitudes toward the communicator.[44] When the listener uses headphones instead of an amplifier, the listener feels closer to the communicator and the communicator is judged to be warmer and more empathetic, which in turn increases message persuasiveness.

Combining Words and Visuals Recommendation 4: Segment Information into Logical Chunks

Some speakers seem to talk in rapid-fire mode, without ever stopping to breathe. At disciplinary conferences, sequences of short talks are referred to as fire-hose sessions in reference to how they make listeners feel – mowed down by a fire hose. To not exceed cognitive load, learners need time to process information, with increasing time needed for information that is especially complex or new to the learner.[45] To reduce the fire-hose feeling, presenters can segment their presentations by identifying the key points within the overall story and giving the audience a moment to digest the point. When possible, use of interactive modes of communication, in which learners can view material at their own pace, are also conducive to learning.

Combining Words and Visuals Recommendation 5:
Weed Out Extraneous Information

Learning is enhanced when the cognitive demands placed on a learner are germane, and extraneous processing – that which does not serve instructional objectives – is minimized.[46] All of us have seen presentations in which the slides sidetracked us from what the speaker was saying, with undecipherable graphics or too much text. Irrelevant sounds and music in multimedia presentations can also impede learning.[47] Logos and background graphics are other distractions to be avoided or constrained to the acknowledgments slide. Even when a presentation is for colleagues, the slides should be as clear as possible, not as jampacked with information as space permits.

The slide in the "Woe is the slideument!" illustration (Figure 2.3) is not an exaggeration of the kinds of confusing, overloaded slides I often see in presentations, including those by experienced, otherwise engaging speakers. Even when I am familiar with the research, I find myself struggling to know where to look, especially (as is often the case) when the speaker talks without specifically referring to the things on the slide. A slide-document

Figure 2.3. Woe Is the "Slideument! Need to Weed (and Synchronize, Eliminate Interference, Signal, and Segment)

(a)

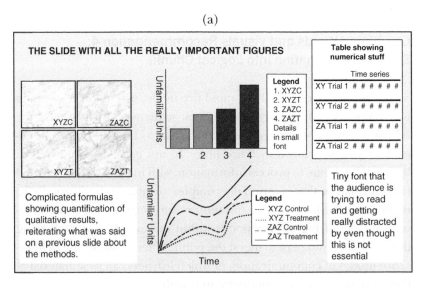

(b)

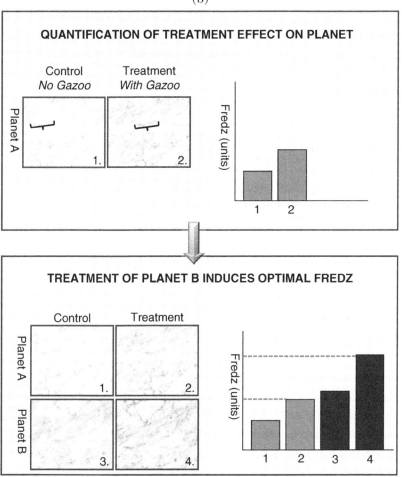

Note: The "slideument" (a, on the previous page) has graphics showing mock qualitative and quantitative data for three variables: location (planet), treatment condition, and time. The audience needs to be stepped through each. The first step (b, upper box) shows the control and treatment conditions for one planet. The outcome variable is an imaginary phenomenon called "Fredz," and the braces are animated in to help the viewer understand how the qualitative Fredz data were quantified to generate the graphed data. Once the viewer is oriented to the representations, the speaker can add the data for the second planet (b, lower box). Here dotted lines are animated in to call attention to the treatment condition for the two planets. Another slide could show the variation of the response to the treatment over time (i.e., a line graph or table). Use the presentation software's affordances and thoughtful choreography to guide the viewer through each set of results.

hybrid may work as a take-home document, or as a panel of figures in a journal article where space is limited, but it is far too confusing (even for others in your field) to be projected on a screen while you are speaking.

Multifigure panels, like the slideument shown in Figure 2.3, ask audiences to make sophisticated connections among representations and among variables.

- Representations
  - Qualitative data (e.g., images)
  - Quantitative data
    - Graphical data (e.g., bar, line)
    - Numerical or tabular data
- Variables
  - Independent
    - Objects of study (e.g., locations, populations, materials)
    - Condition (e.g., chemical, physical, or behavioral treatment)
    - Time
- Outcome

In the slideument figure in Figure 2.3 (which uses imaginary data and omits error bars, numbers, and tick marks for ease of viewing in book-sized grayscale slides), the independent variables are location (planet), condition (Gazoo treatment), and time, and the outcome is measured in Fredz. You may have many objects of study (e.g., wild type and multiple mutants) and conditions (e.g., multiple drug dosages), but the strategy is the same. Decide what are the key results you want to communicate. Choose the best representations available to do so. Introduce the variables in steps. Avoid acronyms, and make sure you have already defined any unfamiliar terms (e.g., Fredz, Gazoo treatment). Show the relationships between representations. Use the affordances of slide presentation software to signal important features and to synchronize what we see with what you say. Any set of data can be presented in various ways to shift the audience's attention and influence their interpretations. Therefore, your choices as a presenter are not only about cognitive load but also about clarity, honesty, and transparency. Table 2.4 outlines some common presentation pitfalls and practices you can adopt

Table 2.4. Prevalent Presentation Pitfalls and Preferred Practices

Prevalent Pitfalls	Practices to Adopt
Slides are text heavy and use small font.	*Pare text ruthlessly. Replace with images when possible.* Audiences cannot simultaneously process different words through visual and auditory systems.
Labels use unfamiliar names and acronyms.	*If you must use it, define it first.* Jargon monopolizes people's cognitive processing power.
Laser pointer is waving wildly.	*Use pointer sparingly and with purpose.* Good slide layout is the first choice to direct audience attention.
Slides are busy, like a multifigure journal panel.	*Streamline or segment into separate slides.* Visuals and narration should always be presented in sync.
Order of items on slide is not apparent.	*Group related items using proximity, with intervening white space to separate rows or columns of items.* Critique figures and slides using the principles of Gestalt psychology.
Audiences are expected to move between multiple representations on a slide.	*Introduce representations stepwise (with animation or individual slides) and separately explain each.* Remember that disciplinary visual conventions are a form of unfamiliar terminology.
A complex figure is shown without any orientation to it.	*Take the time to explain and build the figure step by step.* If constructing a figure stepwise is not an option, consider masking parts of the figure with opaque rectangles that you remove as you explain that portion.
Color is used excessively or inconsistently.	*Assign each color to mean only one thing and do not vary the meaning.* Color variation should be a signal to draw attention, not for flair.
Flashy slide transitions are distracting/nauseating.	*Choose simple transitions between slides. Apply embellishments sparingly and strategically.* Viewers on the autism spectrum and others can be sensitive to sudden movements, flashes, and loud sounds.
Presenter starts talking about something else while previous slide is showing.	*Insert a placeholder slide (blank or with a nondistracting image, such as a picture of you doing your work).* The synchronization principle applies here. The audience cannot mentally move on from the slide if it is still on screen.

in their place. Mastering these recommendations for language, visuals, and combining language and visuals will not only steer you clear of all-too-common communication pitfalls, it is the foundation for much more. The next chapter builds on this foundation by exploring how language is used to create images in the audience's mind with metaphors and analogies. Metaphors and analogies can introduce artistic flair while simultaneously improving comprehensibility. They are also unruly beasts that can come back to bite you.

3

Metaphors and Analogies: Uncovering How They Frame Thought

> Like the army of White Walkers who march haltingly across the tundra in the HBO series "Game of Thrones," cancer cells trudge along in a menacing, but hobbled, state. The same genetic defects that help them proliferate also render them vulnerable to attack. Find the right molecule for the right weak point, and it's like charging the White Walkers with knives made of dragonglass: They're done for.[1]

War. What is it good for? Whether you consider yourself a hawk or a dove, chances are you are oblivious to many of the wars raging around us. Long-standing wars on cancer, drugs, terror, poverty, and crime are likely familiar, but what about the wars on illiteracy, plastic bags, traffic, sunshine, gluten, salad, soap operas, video games, and leg warmers?[2] We are bombarded by combat metaphors in public discourse. Nowhere is this onslaught more aggressive than in the biomilitarism of biomedicine.[3] Heroic researchers rally fellow troops and soldier on in the trenches to achieve the next breakthrough. They are engaged in an arms race to spearhead the campaign against superbugs and cancer, and to develop a more powerful armamentarium before our deadliest adversaries gain ground. Besieged physicians on the front lines are trained to use every weapon in their arsenal to attack the enemy, defending brave patients who fight valiantly, holding out for a magic silver bullet. The situation leaves little hope of a détente, let alone lasting peace. This invasion of war imagery, and the observation that it largely flies under our radar, emphasizes two important facts. First, metaphor litters our speech. By some estimates 20 per cent of our language consists of metaphor.[4] Second, we are often oblivious to it and its power to influence thinking.

CHAPTER LEARNING OBJECTIVES: METAPHORS AND ANALOGIES

Knowledge: How do metaphors and analogies shape thought and when do they go awry?

Skills: Craft comparisons that offer productive frames and make the intangible tangible.

Habits of Mind: Beware of anachronism and other potential metaphor and analogy pitfalls.

COMPARING COMPARISONS

This chapter synthesizes relevant research to offer guidance for comparisons in general, but it is useful to start by distinguishing metaphors and analogies. An **analogy** is an explicit comparison between two things that draws inferences from one to explain the other. For example, a hydraulic/electric analogy is commonly used in introductory physics classes to help students make sense of electricity concepts by capitalizing on their familiarity with water flowing through pipes:

> Similar to the way a water pump applies a pressure that pushes water through a pipe, a battery provides a voltage that drives electrons through a circuit. Like how the flow of water slows when the diameter of the pipe is constricted, a thin wire acts as a resistor that slows the flow of electric charge.

This analogy may be extended to other components of an electric circuit, such as capacitors, inductors, and transistors. Electrons in a wire, of course, behave differently from water molecules in a pipe. Cutting a wire breaks the flow of electrons in an electrical circuit, whereas water gushes from a severed pipe. Electrons experience drag everywhere, but water molecules only experience drag along the inner walls of the pipe. Also, this analogy only works for direct current; high-speed current reversals in an alternating current circuit cannot be achieved in a water pipe. An analogy invites us to compare specific features of one thing to specific features of another.

Metaphor is derived from the Greek words "meta," meaning "over," and "pherein," meaning "to carry."[5] Metaphor is a figure of speech in which a word or phrase is used to suggest similarity between two things. When we are speaking about metaphor in the context of learning and communication, we are not usually concerned with the specific turn of phrase; we are interested in the concept at the heart of it – the underlying **conceptual metaphor**. The opening section to this chapter contains many metaphorical figures of speech all based on the same conceptual metaphor, the same as in the sentence below:

> The novel antibiotic is a silver bullet in the control of hospital-acquired infections.

Saying "silver bullet" is more vivid than using the more literal "solution," and it encourages the audience to draw on the underlying conceptual metaphor of combat or war. Unlike an analogy, however, metaphors do not invite us to explicitly compare how antibiotics are like bullets. Metaphor is more surreptitious than analogy, because a metaphor can be a single word that is any part of speech, including nouns (weapon, arsenal), verbs (spearhead, fight), and adjectives (brave, besieged). Although metaphors are often shorter than analogies, they can be extended into a longer passage, as in the passage on war metaphors above, or seeded throughout a piece. A **simile** is closely related to a metaphor, but more transparent to the audience because it uses "like" or "as" to introduce the comparison. The quotation that begins this chapter has two similes ("Like the army ..." and "like charging the White Walkers").

The distinction between comparisons is easy to make on paper, but when an audience's knowledge elaboration is factored in, the boundaries can become blurred. Consider Arthur Eddington's famous comparison between the expanding universe and the inflation of a balloon:

> We must therefore picture the stars and galaxies as embedded in the surface of a rubber balloon which is being steadily inflated; so

that, apart from their individual motions and the effects of their ordinary gravitational attraction on one another, celestial objects are becoming further and further apart simply by the inflation.[6]

The purpose of this comparison is to provide a way of thinking about how the universe is expanding in all directions without any center of expansion. Since Eddington first devised it, his comparison has been helping cosmology students around the world grasp the mysteries of the universe.[7] So is this famous comparison an analogy or a metaphor? It is explicit, and we are invited to draw specific inferences from one thing (balloon) to another (celestial objects), which fits the criteria of analogy. What if a writer uses the same comparison, but without explicitly providing the details? For example, "the ballooning universe" or "the universe is inflating like a party balloon." On their own these two balloon references would appear to be, respectively, metaphor and simile. Yet they invite readers to conjure up Eddington's analogy, and if they are familiar with it, their thought processes extend the metaphor or simile through analogical reasoning.

HIDDEN POWER

Metaphors Underpin Our Conceptual Systems

Once thought of as mere rhetorical flourishes, it is now clear that metaphor is a natural part of our workaday speech. More striking than the ubiquity of metaphorical reasoning is the way in which it appears to underpin our thought processes. One example is the directional metaphors that we use to describe our emotions. We use these kinds of directional references so automatically that they do not seem like metaphor:

> I *fell* into a depression when I got the results. My spirits *sank* to a new *low*. Then, I called my sister, which really *boosted* my mood. Talking to her always puts me in *high* spirits. It is hard to believe I was so *down* yesterday and today I am practically *soaring*.

Why do sad-down and happy-up pairings feel natural? In *Metaphors We Live By*, Lakoff and Johnson argue that everyday metaphors emerge

instinctively from our life experiences.[8] In the case of directional metaphors to describe our moods, we may take the cues from our own posture, which is upright when we are feeling happy and slumped down
when we are feeling sad. In other words, cues from our environment
mediated through our senses give rise to metaphorical ways of thinking. The study of how sensory and kinesthetic feedback from our bodies influences our thinking has become a popular subfield of cognitive
science known as *embodied cognition*. Our brains control our bodies, but
our bodies also control our brains. Once these metaphorical ways of
thinking about the world become internalized, we intuitively extend
them to new experiences.

We Are Not Always Conscious of How Metaphors Sway Us

Comparisons form boundaries that highlight features and constrain
interpretations; they frame reality. Single word metaphors have been
shown to significantly alter how people think about issues. Not only
is the impact large, it is covert. Consider a study that compared how
people reason about crime when it is described either as a virus or as
a beast.[9] In an experiment, participants read a paragraph-long report
about crime in a fictional city in which, in the first sentence, crime was
referred to either as a virus or as a beast. When people read the article
in which crime was described as a beast, they were more likely to suggest solutions that involved hunting down, capturing, and locking up
criminals – a response consistent with what would be done to contain
a literal beast on the loose. In contrast, when people read the article
in which the word "virus" was used in place of the word "beast," they
were more likely to suggest solutions that involved identifying root
causes and protecting communities against crime by reducing poverty and improving education – an approach comparable to a health
campaign. The difference between the group of participants reading
the virus version of the article and the group reading the beast version was twice as large as the initial difference between Democrats'
and Republicans' views on how to solve crime. Furthermore, when
asked to explain the reasons for their views, study participants pointed
not to the virus or beast metaphor, but rather to the crime statistics
presented in the article, which were identical in both virus and beast
versions.

Because metaphors can exert their influence covertly, care must be taken to use them ethically. This may raise the question of whether it is ever ethical to deliberately use metaphors to evoke a response that is based on emotion or gut reaction instead of logic. Such tactics may seem like the purview of advertisers and others with self-interested goals, but consider, as a foreshadowing of ethical questions to be revisited in the second half of the book, what if this kind of persuasion is done with the goal of saving lives through communication about risks, such as evacuating people in the path of a wildfire? Metaphor can be a titanic gift to a science communicator just as fire was a Titan's gift to humankind. Yet, like the flames that got Prometheus chained to a rock, metaphors can be difficult to control and their consequences unpredictable. Metaphors can become so embedded in the lexicon of popular science and even scientific research that we use them reflexively without fully considering their implications.

ANALOGICAL REASONING IN SCIENCE

The Imagination Personifies

In one of our communication workshops, a researcher who works on molecular transport said there are "literally" highways in cells and that molecular motors walk along these highways. Highways? Motors? Walk? Surely these are metaphors, not literal descriptions? Indeed. The metaphorical highways are fine protein filaments that form a structural framework within the cell called the cytoskeleton. The molecular motors the researcher studies – kinesin and dynein – move along the cytoskeleton carrying nutrients and manufactured goods around the cell. Needless to say, "manufactured goods" is another metaphor. It reflects the widespread notion of cells as factories, and it is a nod to the challenge of talking about these complex ideas without resorting to metaphorical language.

The researcher's use of "literally" in this context in part reflects the current linguistic quirk of declaring it for emphasis when speaking figuratively; however, as slips of the tongue often are, it is revealing. Someone asked if molecular transporters really "walk." The researcher responded that the transporters have leg-like appendages, and their movement closely resembles walking, and emphasized this with hand motions to depict their bipedal shape and "ambulation." The research is cutting edge, and new imaging techniques show kinesin and dynein with unprecedented clarity, but the cellular highways and walking molecules metaphors are long-standing. For example, my graduate neuroscience textbook alluded to little feet walking along the cytoskeleton.[10] The molecular motor researcher and I overlapped in graduate school at the same university (and presumably used the same well-known textbook). In short, metaphorical language is not something the researcher adopted for a nonspecialist audience. It is how she thinks about her molecules because she was introduced to the molecules and the metaphors at the same time. As such, it feels literal.

Chapter 2 highlighted how disciplinary experts move fluidly among the various kinds of visual representations used in their fields and link the human-scale world and the microscopic/submicroscopic or astronomical/planetary worlds of their research. Describing molecules as busy homunculi is another form of fluency with representations, in this case an imagined world. In my own experience as a scientist and in working with other scientists, these shifts from one representation to another – from the literal to the metaphorical and from one metaphorical comparison to another – are so natural that we are not always conscious of them. In a presentation about the role of one molecule in a cell-signaling cascade, a researcher may discuss genes and proteins; show gene maps, schematic representations of protein structure, and cell wiring diagrams; and use the metaphors of relay racers, toppling dominos, and colliding billiard balls. As the researcher shifts comfortably among a plethora of images and comparisons, however, the audience must make leaps to keep up. Therefore, support comprehension by strategically selecting your examples and by pointing out what you want the audience to see – "world building," as you would if you were taking us to Middle-earth or Narnia.

Comparative Reasoning Is at the Very Core of the Scientific Enterprise

The history of science is replete with examples of scientists tapping into the power of analogical reasoning. For example, in 1801 Thomas Young used the analogy of water waves to explain what he observed in his now famous double-slit experiment, in which fine light beams inter-acted to produce repeating contours of light and dark.[11] To explain the patterns, he drew inspiration from the crests and troughs of water waves, and he developed a demonstration tank to show the analogous constructive and destructive interference patterns in water. In another example, Robert Hooke reported in *Micrographia* in 1665 that, while looking at a thin piece of cork through a microscope of his own invention, he saw a large number of little boxes.[12] He called these walled spaces "cells" because they reminded him of the small rooms, or cells, in monasteries.

The metaphorical roots of another familiar scientific term, the green-house effect, are readily apparent. Jean-Baptiste Fourier suggested the comparison between the atmosphere and the glass lid of a plant starter box in 1824.[13] Svante Arrhenius, who was the first to recognize that release of carbon dioxide from the burning of fossil fuels could lead to global warming, credits the work of his predecessors and then elaborates on the analogy, which he referred to as "hot-house theory," in this passage from his book *Worlds in the Making*:

> Their theory has been styled hot-house theory, because they thought that the atmosphere acted after the glass panes of hot-houses. Glass possesses the property of being transparent to heat rays of small wave lengths belonging to the visible spectrum; but it is not transparent to dark heat rays ... The heat rays of the sun now are to a large extent of the visible, bright kind. They penetrate through the glass of the hot-house and heat the earth under the glass. The radiation from the earth, on the other hand, is dark and cannot pass back through the glass, which thus stops any losses of heat ...[14]

Today the term "greenhouse effect" has largely been replaced by "global climate change" to encompass a broader range of climate-related phenomena, including severe weather events and sea-level rise. This shift also acknowledges that global warming plays out with great variability at the local level, as certain regions may even experience cooling if ocean currents shift as a result of changes in ocean surface temperature or the influx of freshwater from melting ice. The greenhouse effect is still taught in schools, however, and in the scien-

tific literature the metaphor lives on in the widely used term "greenhouse gases."

Comparisons Bring It to a Human Scale

The scientific metaphors discussed in this section relate the unfamiliar
to the familiar. One way they do this is by comparing things that are
on a nonhuman scale to those on a human scale. Microscopic cytoskel-
etons are scaled up to highways. Plant cells are inflated to rooms in
a monastery. The vastness of the earth's atmosphere is brought down
to the size of a greenhouse. This graspable world of time, size, speed,
weight, and temperature dimensions familiar to human perception has
been dubbed the **mesocosm**.[15] When scientists model reality, they often
turn to metaphors and analogies rooted in the mesocosm to make the
intangible tangible.[16]

The Comparisons in Use Can Constrain or Advance Scientific Thinking

The power of metaphors and analogies to advance science comes from
their ability to depict the familiar in new ways, but scientists' starry-eyed
enthusiasm for a comparison can hinder scientific progress. A case in
point is J.J. Thompson's plum pudding model of the atom – a continuous distribution of positive charge in which electrons are embedded
like plums in a pudding. In the wake of Ernest Rutherford's now-famous
experiment, in which alpha particles were fired at a thin sheet of gold
foil and (contrary to what Thompson's model would predict) most of
the particles passed right through the foil except for a few particles
deflected at large angles, Thompson clung to the plum pudding model.
He continued to lecture about it for years after Rutherford's findings
were published.[17] The results of Rutherford's alpha particle experiment
are consistent with the nuclear model of the atom – wherein the positive charge is concentrated in a tiny, massive nucleus (which strongly
deflects the alpha particles) that is surrounded by a large volume of low-
mass electrons (through which the alpha particles pass). Yet, instead of
a eureka moment, Rutherford himself may have struggled to abandon
Thompson's model, taking more than a year of rumination to publish
the results.

Metaphors and analogies in science are not merely created for the purpose of explaining to others; they play an important role in the development of scientific theories. Thomas Kuhn argued that scientific language is rooted in metaphors and analogies, and that in scientific theories these comparisons, along with nature and the language used to describe it, are tied together into an interconnected network.[18] New scientific discoveries perturb this network, driving conceptual changes, which alter the connections between scientific phenomena and the language used to describe them. Changes in metaphor and analogy are thus a crucial part of theory change in science, and new metaphors and analogies provide new ways of not only talking about the world but also understanding it.

LEARNING BY ANALOGY

One intriguing and pedagogically useful type of comparison is called a **bridging analogy**. It helps teach a scientific concept by bridging the gap between the concept and learners' prior intuitions. A study that pioneered bridging analogies in education was concerned with helping high school students understand a deceptively simple physics concept: whether a table exerts a force on a book that is placed on the table.[19] All of us have an intuitive physics that is rooted in a lifetime of experience in the world. Before learning Newtonian mechanics, and even after, the vast majority of us view static objects, like the table, as barriers that do not exert forces. Students correctly believe that a book exerts a downward force on a table, but when they are taught that the table exerts an equal and opposite force on the book, they disbelieve it.

Using an intuitive idea that is largely in agreement with currently accepted science – an **anchoring conception** – the study introduced a way to bridge from the idea to the troublesome scientific concept. In this case, the anchoring concept is a hand pushing down on a spring, a situation in which students intuitively understand that the spring exerts an upward force on the hand. Unfortunately, most students cannot make the intellectual leap from the spring to the table because they do not see these situations as analogous. With the introduction of an intermediary concept, however, students see the connection. In this case, the intermediary or bridging concept is a book on a thin, flexible board.

The flexible board's springiness connects it to the anchoring concept; likewise, its "boardness" connects it to the table. Students exposed to the bridging analogy during their unit on Newtonian mechanics were far more likely to have a scientifically accurate view of the forces involved in the book on the table situation than were students who had not seen the analogy. Variants of this lesson use a book on a foam pad as an additional bridging concept. A further benefit of this bridging analogy is that teachers can build on it to introduce the microscopic model of rigid objects that consist of atoms connected by spring-like bonds.

The difficulty of making intellectual leaps is also the focus of a different area of research on analogical reasoning, one that examines how people learn to solve problems by analogy with problems they have already encountered. Known as **analogical transfer**, an often-cited example is the physician's dilemma, in which a doctor must use radiation to obliterate an inoperable tumor.[20] The problem is that the dosage of radiation that must be administered in each treatment is so high that it would destroy any tissue it passes through on its way to the tumor. How can the doctor cure the patient? Most people find this problem challenging, but they solve it more readily when they have been exposed to an analogous problem – one that involves the same underlying strategy.

Analogous to the physician's dilemma is the following military problem: A general needs to get troops and equipment to a battleground, but the bridges on any of the roads that lead there are not strong enough to support the passage of everyone. How can the general proceed? The solution to the problem is that the company can be divided, sent along different roads, and reunited on the battleground. The basic strategy here is one of diverge and converge. By analogy, the solution to the doctor's dilemma becomes apparent: The doctor should use multiple beams of lower dose radiation, sent along different paths, that all converge onto the tumor.

Bridging analogies help people bridge between intuitive and scientific concepts. Analogical transfer is the transfer of ways of thinking from one problem or context to another. Research in both areas converges on the same lesson for communicators: People unfamiliar with a situation or concept need help to make connections that can seem obvious to people with relevant prior experience or expertise. Through successive approximations or drawing attention to the underlying analogous features, communicators offer bridges, steppingstones, or a trail of breadcrumbs for their audiences.

HOW MINDS MAP

Analogical and metaphorical reasoning is a process of mapping from one domain to another. In the mapping, the more familiar domain, the source domain, is drawn upon to provide insight into the less familiar domain, the target domain.[21] For example, when Young made inferences about light based on an analogy with water, light was the target domain and water was the source domain. In the case of the virus or beast metaphor for crime, a virus or a beast was the source domain and crime was the target domain.

Mapping refers to the process by which attributes from the source domain are used as metaphorical lenses through which to view the target domain. In the light and water analogy, as well as the crime and virus or beast metaphor, it is readily apparent that only certain attributes from the source domains should be mapped onto the target domains (see Figure 3.1). Young's reasoning was kindled by the way water waves interfere constructively and destructively. Wave interference was the attribute he conferred to light. The fact that water is wet or that its boiling point drops with elevation had no place in his analogical reasoning, and such irrelevant attributes could simply be ignored. For thinking about crime, the relevant attributes of viruses are that they cause illness, are contagious, and that inoculation campaigns can protect a population against them. Irrelevant attributes include the mechanism through which viruses infect cells and the fact that viruses are made of protein and DNA or RNA.

The trick, of course, is getting the mapping right. The individual doing the mapping must select the relevant attributes of the source domain and ignore the irrelevant attributes. In some cases, such as a carefully presented analogy in a science class, the mapping may be made explicit by the presenter. Often, the mapping is left to the audience, which means the usefulness of a comparison is determined by the beholder. Like a mariner unfurling the sails and hoping the winds will be favorable, launching a metaphor leaves much to chance. Reasoning about metaphors and analogies is not a rote, mechanical process: It is a

Figure 3.1. The Mapping Process in Comparative Reasoning

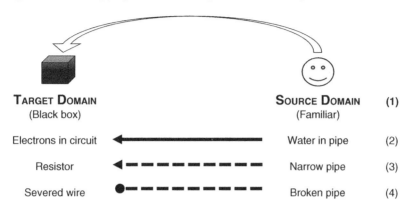

Note: The figure shows the mapping from a source domain to a target domain for the hydraulic/electric analogy commonly used in introductory physics courses. For learners, the target domain may be a black box (1). Mapping from the source domain opens the black box. Flowing water is tangible and provides a way of thinking about intangible flowing electrons (2). The audience must select, or be guided to select, the relevant attributes from the source domain to map onto the target domain (3). This process can break down if the audience does not know enough about the source domain (i.e., that water flows more slowly through a narrow section of pipe) or does not know enough about how to map from the source domain to the target domain (i.e., narrow pipe maps to resistor). Another type of breakdown occurs if the audience overextends the comparison (4). To avoid this, the audience needs to know what features of the source domain are detrimental to the mapping (i.e., the behavior of broken pipes).

creative act. Different ways of applying paint to a canvas do not simply give rise to different kinds of Impressionist paintings. A Jackson Pollock may come along, or things may get completely Dada or Cubist.

Emotion plays a role in the persuasive effects of metaphor. Neuroimaging studies have shown that, compared to their literal counterparts, metaphorical expressions cause more activity in the amygdala and hippocampus, regions of the brain associated with emotion.[22] Consistent with the notion that metaphorical thinking is an embodied experience, neuroimaging studies have shown that action metaphors engage sensory-motor regions of the brain. For example, the metaphorical "grasp an idea" and the literal action "grasp a hammer" both activate the motor cortex, but the literal nonaction "understand an idea" does not.[23] Novelty of a metaphor increases its persuasive effects.[24] Again, neuroimaging sheds light on why. As an expression becomes well established, it may no longer activate the same neural pathways.[25] In a study that compared literal, metaphorical, and idiomatic action sentences, activity was observed in the sensory-motor regions for the literal and metaphorical sentences, but not for the idiomatic ones.[26] This is likely because repeated experience with the co-occurring words in idioms like "spill the beans" leads to them being processed as a unit. Thus, when stirring emotion is the goal, it may be useful to craft a novel metaphor.

AVOIDING THE POTENTIAL HAZARDS

Whether a comparison is meant to do heavy lifting or is merely icing on the cake, be clear-headed in your choices. Because the communicator's intent does not constrain the comparison, to unleash metaphors and analogies into the world is to open Pandora's Box. The prior knowledge of each audience member will yield a kaleidoscope of interpretations. Comparisons may be taken more literally than intended or may be creatively extended in unanticipated ways. When using them, watch out for the following five potential pitfalls.

Beware of How Comparisons May Be Overextended

Rhetorical flourishes may compare things that bear no resemblance for the sake of adding color or humor. So cheers to the educators whose culinary comparisons regarding the mysteries of the cosmos, like supernova soufflés and pizza-pie galaxies, leave their students with appetites for both astronomy and lunch. If, instead of garnishing, a comparison is meant to do real explanatory work, it should be apt. For example, consider an analogy commonly used in middle and high school, the atom as a solar system. Students are told that in the Bohr model of the atom, electrons orbit around the nucleus like planets orbiting around a sun. At first glance, this comparison gives students a nice visual way to think about the atom. Niels Bohr's contemporary, Max Born, called the theory's symmetry between these vastly different scales of our universe "remarkable and alluring" and stated that it "exercises a great magic on mankind's mind."[27]

Yet the dissimilarity between the solar system and atomic orbitals is considerable:[28]

- Electrons are uniform in size and appearance. Each planet is distinct.
- Planetary orbits are largely in a plane. Atoms are spherical.

- Planets and stars interact through gravitational forces. Electrons and nuclei interact through electromagnetic forces.
- Electrons repel each other. Planets attract each other.
- Planets, unlike electrons, are composite bodies.
- Planets often have moons.
- Planetary orbits are relatively stable, but electron orbits can change rapidly.

One of the unintended consequences of the use of this analogy is that students extend the comparison in both directions. In addition to using the solar system to think about the atom, they take their new knowledge of the atom and apply it to the solar system. They suggest, for instance, that planets will repel each other or that inner planets will shield the outer planets from the gravitational pull of the sun. This is just what one would expect from thoughtful learners who are actively constructing their own knowledge.

Tip: Choose suitable comparisons, and when dealing with popular but less apt comparisons, use them as teachable moments. Calling attention to the similarities between the source and target domain is instructive, but spelling out the differences may be more enlightening still.

Avoid Anachronism

The atom as solar system is part of the beautiful history of progression of thought from Rutherford to Bohr to Schrodinger. It is also, like a Torino in the Tesla lot, an anachronism. Anachronisms are common in science education and communication. As scientists move on in their thinking, textbooks and popular science articles often cling to those antediluvian metaphors and analogies. In fact, scientists themselves may hang onto them for want of suitable up-to-date options. This is apparent in the transition from classical to molecular genetics.[29] In both popular science and research papers, it is still common to come across the shorthand "gene for X" or metaphors like code, program, map, or blueprint to describe genetic material. Contrary to popular belief, researchers who fall back on these expressions are not speaking literally.

In the years after Watson and Crick proposed the double-helical structure of DNA, a reductionist concept of genes prevailed: The gene was a material unit forming the instructions for a protein that carried out the function of the gene.[30] DNA was indeed perceived of as a kind of blueprint. The modern view of genetics is one of systems that cannot be reduced to the function of a singular macromolecule (except in the case of certain diseases, such as sickle-cell anemia, which are caused by single-point mutations). Proteins function as part of pathways and networks, often with feedback loops. Single genes can give rise to multiple different proteins, but not all genes even code for proteins. Furthermore, the environment plays a role in gene expression, a phenomenon explored in the growing field of epigenetics. In short, the deterministic view inherent in the DNA–blueprint metaphor bears little relation to reality, which has led to arguments that the reductionist concept of the gene has no place in twenty-first century biology.[31]

New metaphors for genetic material have been coined, such as genes as recipes or musical scores. The winner of a DNA metaphor contest held by Toronto's *The Globe and Mail* newspaper was "DNA: The web that spins the spider," contributed by a reader named Trevor Spencer Rines.[32] It is a profound comparison that could be a tantalizingly thought-provoking way to introduce a talk or story about genetics, but original metaphors have their own drawbacks. Originality may divert the attention of the audience from the main point. It may not be practical to explain a novel metaphor, especially if the complexity of the modern notion of a gene has no real relevance to a story that your editor is going to trim to 750 words. On the other hand, if the very topic of the communication is epigenetics or another aspect of gene regulation, the prevalence of the DNA blueprint metaphor is a problem that needs to be tackled directly, potentially with a contrast to a newer metaphor.

Tip: Carefully consider the implications of an anachronistic metaphor to determine whether it will derail your communication goals. If it might, substitute a more up-to-date comparison or stick with a literal explanation of how things work.

Be Mindful about Oversimplifying Complexity

More often than not, the point of using a comparison in research communication is to simplify complexity. For instance, what are telomeres?

> Telomeres are structures that hold the ends of chromosomes together in the way that the plastic caps on shoelaces keep the ends from fraying.

Telomere as plastic shoelace cap is a clear, compelling visual that can pique an audience's interest. Compared to a literal definition, it reduces cognitive load and sends the message that this science concept can be grasped by a lay audience. Telomere as plastic shoelace cap is simultaneously misleading. Upon learning that telomeres get shorter as we age, one might think by analogy with old shoelaces that bits of the telomeres break off as they bump around. Instead telomeres, which are not caps but repeated sequences of DNA, get shorter as the cell divides because the DNA replication machinery cannot copy all the way to the end of the chromosome.[33] An enzyme called telomerase can restore the length of the telomeres, but telomerase is only active in certain cells of the body. Thus, on the one hand, if the goal is to acknowledge the role of telomere length in cancer and other diseases, the simplistic comparison is an efficient way to lay the groundwork. On the other hand, if the goal of communicating about telomeres is to explain exactly how they work, telomere as shoelace cap is overly limiting.

While oversimplifying a concept is a potential hazard of any metaphor, for some classes of metaphor, most notably machine and information metaphors in the life sciences, the oversimplification may have far-reaching implications. Widely used in education and communication, mechanistic metaphors for biological systems include (to name just a few) DNA replication machinery, barcoding organisms, cells as factories, brains as computers, metabolisms kicked into gear, and the gene-editing tool CRISPR as "scissors." Interestingly, research on cells is dominated by two very different classes of metaphors – cells as machines and cells as social organisms – which can be compared to lenses of different magnifying power that focus attention on specific aspects of cells and give rise to different research programs.[34]

Oversimplified comparisons can be the result of anachronism, as with the gene as blueprint metaphor that represents a twentieth-century view of genetics. Mechanistic metaphors do have a long history, dating at least as far back as the Middle Ages.[35] Their prevalence, however, cannot be explained by anachronism, because these metaphors are constantly being reinvented and applied to new contexts. One example is the software and hardware metaphor applied in synthetic biology.[36] This metaphor was repeatedly used in the widespread media coverage of the creation of *Synthia* at the J. Craig Venter Institute in 2010.[37] *Synthia*, a bacterium, is the first organism with a fully synthetic genome. The software (genome) of *Synthia* is synthetic, but its hardware (the rest of the bacterial cell) was a naturally propagated bacterium with its genetic material removed to make room for the synthetic genome.

Machine and information metaphors provide a misleading view of the complexity of biological organisms and have been borrowed by advocates of intelligent design to support their arguments.[38] Together with metaphors that portray researchers working in synthetic biology as architects, engineers, and designers, mechanistic and information metaphors also portray living systems as being far more controllable than they are in reality.[39] Scientists criticize each other for overly simplistic metaphors, particularly when they think the metaphor is promulgating an unrealistic view of the science that is attracting investors. Craig Venter has been criticized for overly promotional use of metaphor, as has "the father of DNA barcoding," Paul Hebert, since the publication of his paper "Biological Identifications through DNA Barcodes."[40] Barcoding organisms does not refer to labeling them with stickers, but rather to standardizing taxonomy by using a particular DNA sequence to differentiate among species. The dream of inventing a real-life Star Trek tricorder – the handheld instrument used to scan alien environments to identify lifeforms – could understandably tickle investors' fancies, but twenty-first-century barcoding science has a lot of bugs that need to be worked out, hence the love-it-or-hate-it reaction to the metaphor.[41]

Tip: Decide to what extent a metaphor simplifies its target concept, and whether that level of simplification is appropriate for your audience, context, and goals. Look beyond the specific concept and consider the message the metaphor sends about the field more generally.

One way to make accessible the complexity that the simple metaphor obscures (if suitable alternatives are not available) is to use it as a starting point to build on. For example, if calling a receptor protein a "dock" would be too limiting because the work you are describing is about the dynamic, shapeshifting ability of the receptor, start with the notion of the dock and invite the audience to reimagine it with you. Perhaps you need us to visualize something like a dock but made of modeling clay, not wood, and you use body movements or pictures to show us how the protein shifts its shape. Audiences are happy to enter imagined worlds as long as you help them see what you see.

Consider the Familiarity of Comparisons

Comparisons use familiarity with the source domain to illuminate the target domain. The source domain "ripples on the surface of a pond" provides a concrete way of thinking about the target domain "light waves." Although not everyone has access to a pond or a lake, ripples in the dog's water bowl or the bathtub provide similar first-hand experience. Unfortunately, most source domains are less broadly familiar across demographics. To the youngest generation, a world of rotary phones, transistor radios, analog clocks, and fax machines is like a plasticized version of steampunk science fiction. Furthermore, any reference to literature, popular culture, sports, or other pastimes will appeal to some audience members and fly over the heads of others.

If you choose to wink, wink, nudge, nudge to a subset of your audience members by dipping into a source domain that is familiar to them, try to provide sufficient context to avoid alienating the rest of the audience. The quotation that begins this chapter is a good example. The article's author knows that plenty of the folks who make up the publication's readership do not watch *Game of Thrones.* For them, the author has elegantly inserted helpful cues. Not sure what White Walkers are? No problem. Whatever they are, they march haltingly and are hobbled but menacing. Clearly and uncondescendingly, the writer is saying, "And this, dear reader, is what you need to know about why I am comparing cancer cells to White Walkers." Those who watched *Game of Thrones* will be able to conjure up a more vivid image, but at least those less tuned in to popular culture are not left lost in The Land of Always Winter.

Tip: Reflect on the source domain of a comparison and the degree to which your audience will be familiar with it. For a source domain that may be unfamiliar to a subset of the audience, make explicit the essentials of the likeness between source and target.

Match Your Metaphors in Framing Problems and Solutions

The spatial metaphor, which characterizes depression as "down," is one of two common metaphorical ways of talking about depression. The second is a luminosity metaphor in which depression is "darkness." A study examined how these distinct metaphorical framings influenced people's preferences for a hypothetical drug to treat depression.[42] When the spatial metaphor was used, people preferred a drug called Liftix. When a luminosity metaphor was used, people preferred a drug called Illuminix. This illustrates an important strategy for using metaphor: When framing a problem with a metaphor, be sure to use the same metaphor to frame the solution.

A mismatched construal of problem and solution can undermine communication efforts, as demonstrated by a health messaging study about skin cancer prevention.[43] Study participants read a literal or metaphorical paragraph about the risks of sun exposure. The literal framing described the damaging effects of ultraviolet rays. The metaphorical framing was similar but compared the sun to an "enemy." Then study participants read a literal or metaphorical paragraph about prevention. The literal framing described the protective effects of sunscreen, sunglasses, hats, and clothing. The metaphorical framing talked about these same protective items in terms of "a suit of armor." When the risk and prevention framing were consistent (literal for risk and literal for prevention, or metaphorical for risk and metaphorical for prevention), participants were more concerned about sun exposure and had greater intentions of protecting themselves than participants in the inconsistent condition (literal for risk and metaphorical for prevention, or metaphorical for risk and literal for prevention). In other words, it was better to use no metaphor at all than to use metaphor in a way that framed a problem inconsistently with the framing of the solution.

Tip: When using a metaphorical framing for a particular problem, determine whether your proposed solution is congruent with the comparison. If not, choose a different metaphor, or reframe the solution to be consistent with the metaphor. Do not feel that you always need to use a comparison, especially if the literal explanation provides the most clarity or helps you match the framing of problems and solutions. (For a summary of tips, see Table 3.1.)

Returning to the question that began this chapter – "War. What is it good for?" "Absolutely nothing" is not the answer. For example, one study found that an article advocating war on climate change created more sense of urgency and willingness to increase conservation efforts than did an otherwise identical version promoting a race against climate change or a version that did not use metaphor, although the war advantage was small.[44] Another example is that President Nixon's 1971

Table 3.1. Troubleshooting Comparisons

Problem	Possible Fixes
Overextendable	Could it be turned into a teachable moment, for instance by having students identify the similarities and differences of the concept and comparison?
Anachronistic	How does the comparison fit into the history of thought in the field? Can you concisely sum up the gap between the comparison and the current thinking?
Oversimplified	Is the comparison something that can be built upon to make it more consistent with the target concept?
Unfamiliar	What likenesses are you drawing between the concept and comparison? Can an image or description provide sufficient background for the audience?
Mismatched	Is there a metaphorical problem frame that is consistent with the proposed solution? Can you generate alternative problem frames to unconstrain solutions and invite new perspectives?

declaration of war on cancer resulted in large increases in funding and zeal for cancer research, and some cancer patients find the war metaphor empowering.[45]

The war on cancer metaphor has a darker side, however, because patients may feel guilty when they are "losing the war." One study reported that patients had more depression and anxiety during treatment when they viewed cancer as a battle rather than a journey.[46] Another study demonstrated that a war framing reduced people's intention to engage in lifestyle changes that help to prevent cancer, such as quitting smoking.[47] Yet, consistent with the recommendation above on matching metaphors, this effect was reversed when preventive behaviors were also framed as fighting an enemy. The war on invasive species is another example of a potentially counterproductive militaristic metaphor, because it may promote a short-term and unholistic view of conservation biology.[48] Violently ripping out kudzu vines is consistent with a war metaphor, but taking care to learn about and cultivate only native species in your garden is not.

In short, instead of asking whether a metaphor or analogy is good or bad, we need to ask whether it serves its intended purpose. Sometimes you just want to have fun, laugh at your own corny jokes, and hope someone will laugh along with you. Hey, you do you! Laughter is infectious and it sure feels exhilarating to make people laugh. More often than not, however, the metaphors and analogies we use are meant to do real work in communication. The example of the nuanced effects of the war metaphor underscores a central theme of this book about tailoring communication. Because the effectiveness of a comparison depends on the prior knowledge and perspectives of the audience, you need an in-depth understanding of the knowledge and the misconceptions that audiences may bring. The next chapter provides that background through an exploration of the literature on what people know about a range of everyday science topics and how they construct conceptual understanding. It also provides strategies for designing stories that support learning.

4

So We Live in a Snow Globe? Misconception Mishaps and Designing Stories for Learning

In the second autumn of the COVID-19 pandemic, a gleam of light in the darkness was the arrival of *Voyage*, the first ABBA album in 40 years. The cover art featured solar eclipses instead of an iconic portrait of the band (the one on the *Voulez-Vous* album cover mesmerized me as a child!), but the music is "As Good as New." About Frida's and Agnetha's exquisite harmonies, I could go "On and On and On," but I had a nerdy "Disillusion" with one of my favorite songs on the album, "Bumblebee." I reasoned that the bumblebee in Frida's garden could not be a "he" (as Frida sang), because nearly all bees in a hive are worker bees, who are female, and male bees are only produced to "I Do, I Do, I Do, I Do, I Do" with the queen and then die. In searching for a reference to point out ABBA's mistake, however, I learned that sex ratios in bee species are variable and at times a hive's male bumblebees outnumber females.[1] The lyrics did not take artistic license; I had been carrying around a misconception since childhood.

It is not the first time my conceptual understanding was "Under Attack." The papers on scientific misconceptions I was assigned early in my doctoral work gave me "Just a Notion" that despite all my years of science classes, I had no reason to be smug about the Harvard and MIT graduates who said that it is warmer in the summer because the Earth is closer to the sun, that the Earth's shadow causes the phases of the moon, and that the mass acquired by a tree as it grows comes from the soil.[2] Delving into the vast and fascinating body of research on people's misconceptions in science leaves "No Doubt about It" that this work is an indispensable resource for improving communication, because naïvely failing to take people's ideas into account can leave their misconceptions intact or even generate a new "Crazy World" in their heads.

CHAPTER LEARNING OBJECTIVES: MISCONCEPTIONS AND STORY

Knowledge: How is conceptual understanding constructed and what misconceptions arise?

Skills: Develop preview, pitch, and plot stories with logical progression, without logic gaps.

Habits of Mind: Recognize, respect, and build on knowledge assets that others bring.

One (literal) example of a crazy world is alluded to in the title of this chapter. Young children believe that the Earth is "flat" – it extends along a plane (but not necessarily a plain) in the shape of a disc or rectangle and by traveling far enough one could reach the edge of it.[3] Exposed to the fact that the Earth is a sphere, children must reconcile the science with their intuitions. They synthesize and conclude that Earth is a flattened sphere, like a thick pancake, or that the Earth sphere consists of a bottom portion of terrain with the sky above forming the top half of the sphere, as if we are living in a souvenir snow globe. The active construction of logic stories like this is a normal part of the learning process. This chapter is about stories – stories of sensemaking. It is a *Voyage* into a fruitful body of research that upended commonly held perspectives on teaching and learning, while remaining largely unknown to communication trainers and others outside the field of education.

"THE NAME OF THE GAME" – FROM KNOWLEDGE ACQUISITION TO CONCEPTUAL CHANGE

The previous chapter explored how metaphor shapes thought, not only in daily life, but also in framing intractable problems at the frontiers of research. Although the Nobel Prize–winning work of Eric Kandel and colleagues provides insight into how, at the level of individual proteins, long-term memories are formed in the brain, much of this understanding comes from poking and probing sea slugs.[4] It remains a leap away from the acquisition of conceptual understanding in humans. Thus, the latter is largely the territory of educational psychology, and with limited insight into the neural substrates of learning, researchers, educators, and publics alike are highly reliant on metaphorical ways of thinking about learning.

While common enough to seem literal, "acquisition" is a metaphorical way of conceptualizing learning as the accumulation of units of knowledge, the way we acquire material goods, and implies that the learner is a blank slate or a container to be filled.[5] The acquisition metaphor of learning is thus consistent with the deficit model of communication. The field of education was decades ahead of the field of communication in raising the alarm about the blank slate/deficit view of learners because research on the "acquisition" of concepts makes it abundantly clear that learning is not simply the incremental accretion of knowledge. Misconceptions can and do arise at any stage of the game.

Misconceptions Can Arise Directly from Experience

The idea that the Earth is flat reflects children's common sense that unsupported objects would slide off a sphere, and it is consistent with their experience in the world. People of all ages have experiential misconceptions. Another common experiential earth science misconception is that soil, rocks, and landforms are unchanging, and that no new mountains are forming today.[6] The misconception that the Earth is closer to the sun in summertime may be rooted in day-to-day experience with intensity variations in heat (and light) with proximity to stoves and lamps. Familiarity with the use of force to move objects makes it difficult for people to accept the notion of a passive force, such as the fact that when a book is on a table, the table exerts a force on the book.[7]

The spotlight on experiential misconceptions is not meant to suggest that people's experiences in the world are a hindrance to science learning. They can also be conducive to science learning. One example is the intuitive idea that more effort or force brings about greater results and more resistance leads to less results, which applies equally well to physics and psychology and facilitates the learning of Ohm's law of electrical circuits, which relates voltage, current, and resistance.[8] The term "prior conception" is used to refer to any idea, accurate or not, an individual might bring to a learning situation, whereas "misconception" or "alternative conception" refers to those ideas that are not scientifically normative. Familiarity with people's prior conceptions is a key ingredient in effective communication.

Misconceptions Can Grow from Specific Gaps in Understanding

Compilations of misconceptions often include facts of which students, teachers, and publics have been found to be unaware, such as that genes and chromosomes are related and that nearly all cell types contain genes.[9] Another example is that both before and after learning about ecosystems and food webs, the role of bacteria and other decomposers is often ignored, and the process of decomposition is viewed simply as disappearance.[10] The term "misconception" is not exactly appropriate to describe missing bits of knowledge, but it is nonetheless a useful practice to flag gaps that are common, and especially those that tend to remain after instruction on the topic.

Gaps may give rise to new misconceptions. For instance, even after studying chemistry, students may have little understanding of the particulate nature of matter, such as that when a substance changes phase from a liquid to a gas the molecules spread out. Asked to give a particle-level explanation of what happens when a substance is heated, students may infer that the molecules themselves change size, and draw diagrams showing them growing from small to large spheres.[11] The students may not have started out with a misconception of ballooning molecules but generated it on the fly because of their lack of an alternative explanation.

Misconceptions Can Result from Shortcomings of the Curriculum

Instructional materials can inadvertently create or reinforce misconceptions through misleading imagery, including problematic metaphors and analogies (as described in the previous chapter) or misleading graphics. For example, textbook illustrations of Earth's orbit around the sun often depict a highly exaggerated ellipse, which may reinforce the misconception that distance to the sun causes the seasons.[12] In reality, Earth's orbit is nearly circular, and Earth is closest to the sun when it is winter in the Northern Hemisphere. Another misconception associated with textbook visuals is that rivers can cause vertical but not horizontal erosion, which may be due to the prevalence of images of the Grand Canyon in earth science texts.[13] Curriculum materials also have confusing visuals, ambiguous terminology, and unclear explanations about causal mechanisms, leading to a plethora of misconceptions about environmental issues and other topics.[14]

Misconceptions can also arise from what is emphasized in or absent from the curriculum. Due to the heavy focus on Mendelian inheritance (in which traits are controlled by single genes) in introductory genetics courses, and the widespread use of the colloquial "gene for X (trait)," students, teachers, and publics have a deterministic view of genes. This neglects the role of interactions among genes, the role of the environment (nature versus nurture), and the ways that gene activity may be altered during an organism's lifetime through epigenetic mechanisms.[15] Genes are often viewed as acting directly, and there exists a lack of awareness of the role of proteins in traits and in disease. These fundamental genetics misconceptions in turn lead to misconceptions about technologies like gene editing and cloning, such as the belief that transferring genes between organisms will exactly replicate desired traits or that cloning could produce people with identical personalities (even though the personalities of identical twins differ).

Misconceptions Can Emerge as Learners Extend Ideas in New Ways

Misconceptions arise as a part of the learning process as ideas are applied and combined. Ideas may be overgeneralized, such as the way (as discussed in the previous chapter) students extend the Bohr model of the atom to reasoning about planetary systems. Likewise, learners generalize macroscopic properties to microscopic entities, inferring that water molecules are wet or gold molecules are golden.[16] These inferences may feel more intuitive than the reality that the properties of a substance depend on how its constituent particles are organized and interact, which explains why different phases of the same substance have different properties. Overgeneralization of ideas is also rampant in popular coverage of science, in which conclusions reached in one population or context are presented as applying universally.

Learned ideas may also be combined in unexpected ways. An example is the confusion of two environmental issues, the hole in the ozone layer and global warming, creating a chimera misconception along the lines of "the hole in the ozone layer is allowing more sunlight in, which causes global warming."[17] This fusion of two learned ideas is similar to the fusion of learned and experiential ideas that resulted in the aforementioned whimsical misconceptions about the shape of the Earth. These chimera misconceptions should not be thought of as monsters to be slain. They are dynamic, shape-shifting creatures that arise from active sensemaking on the part of the learner; therefore, communicating in a way that supports active sensemaking is also the secret to taming them.

Learning, therefore, is not only the acquisition of knowledge; it is the organizing and restructuring of knowledge. The body of scholarship that focuses on what changes as we learn disciplinary concepts is known as **conceptual change** research. It has a rich history and clear applications to improving communication.

BUILDING BLOCKS, NETWORKS, TAPESTRIES, AND SCAFFOLDING KNOWLEDGE INTEGRATION

Learning of Science Has Been Compared with Learning in Science

Conceptual change research in the learning sciences is rooted in the work of psychologist Jean Piaget, who established what would become its central tenet – new knowledge and ways of thinking are built on prior ones, a view termed "constructivism."[18] Piaget, however, aimed to identify domain-independent explanations of learning. Modern conceptual change research is concerned with how learning occurs in specific domains.

Another major influence on conceptual change in the learning sciences was work in the history and philosophy of science on conceptual change in science. In *The Structure of Scientific Revolutions*, Thomas Kuhn argued that revolutions in scientific thought replace one set of theories and ways of thinking with another incommensurable set, for instance the way Copernican (heliocentric) astronomy replaced Ptolemaic (Earth-centric) astronomy.[19] Because children's ideas about the world can resemble past scientific theories, some viewed conceptual change in learning as a microcosm of conceptual change in science, which led to the proposition that both children and scientists would change their views when certain conditions were met.[20] Namely, they would need to be dissatisfied with their current understanding because they have encountered anomalies, and they would need an alternative conception that is intelligible, plausible, and fruitful. For example, learning about the tilt of the Earth will not automatically lead students to give up their prior conceptions about the seasons being caused by the distance to the sun. They would also need anomalous evidence, such as images of snowy Christmas scenes in the Northern Hemisphere juxtaposed against pictures of Australians celebrating Christmas on the beach at the height of summer.

Attention to the central role of addressing specific prior ideas represents an advance in thinking about conceptual learning. Yet the view of conceptual change as a revolution makes no room for prior ideas in the new understanding, which does not reflect the reality of the history of science or of individual learning.[21] It suggests that ideas can simply be uprooted; yet both scientists and children have many ways to deal with anomalous evidence that do not involve changing their current ideas.[22] (For instance, perhaps it is always hot in Australia because it is so far south.) Instead, prior ideas about the world, whether those of scientists or children, are often resources to be incorporated into the new understanding.[23] For example, students' prior idea that air pressure pushes downward can be refined into the normative understanding that air pressure pushes in from all sides, and their prior idea that passive objects do not exert forces can be refined into the physics concept that passive objects do no work.[24]

Individual conceptual learning only superficially resembles the progress of science. Students' ideas are far more fragmentary and context-dependent than scientific theories.[25] In contrast with theories that are applied consistently, students' ideas are often dynamically emergent structures; therefore, students need the opportunity to learn in multiple contexts.[26] Learners also differ from scientists in their goals, motivations, and self-efficacy, which influence engagement and persistence.[27] Learning is also contingent on a kind of Goldilocks principle of instruction, because the potential for learning is in a zone between what a learner is capable of alone and what the learner is capable of in the presence of a more competent other.[28] This learning zone – the so-called zone of proximal development – expands as mastery increases. Classroom experiences and communication efforts should build incrementally on a learner's current level of mastery.

Too often people's inability or unwillingness to change their "incorrect" views is blamed on ideology. Later chapters of this book explore the role of ideology on reasoning about socio-scientific issues, but the preceding discussion about misconceptions highlights politically neutral topics, such as photosynthesis, the role of microorganisms in ecosystems, forces in physics, the reasons we have seasons, and the phases of the moon, which can be challenging for people of all ages and backgrounds, including high-achieving graduates of the most prestigious institutions. Perhaps as you have read about these common misconceptions, you too realized that you have or had one or more of them. For me that realization has been simultaneously humbling and inspiring.

Conceptual Change Research Necessitates New Metaphors of Learning

In the overview of conceptual change research above, the metaphor of learning immediately shifted from acquisition to construction. Snapping together Lego bricks is one way to think about construction. Alternatively, imagine assembling intricate networked structures with another children's toy – the construction set with wooden rods and round connectors – Tinkertoys (see Figure 4.1). At the risk of mixing metaphors, I also admit a fondness for envisioning learning as weaving and re-weaving threads. Spool-knitting (corking) on a spool and weaving on a trivet-sized loom were, along with building things, activities that occupied me as a kid. Most everyone has relevant sensory experiences that provide an embodied understanding of these metaphors. The weaving metaphor and the assembling metaphor both illuminate the challenge of learning, but like all metaphors, they have limitations. Learning is more dynamic and context-specific than either suggests – the pattern of the tapestry is

Figure 4.1. A Conceptual Tinkertoy Image of Scaffolded Knowledge Integration (SKI)

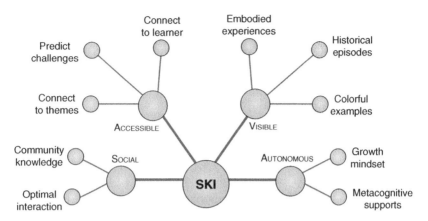

constantly changing, and the construction project is less like a geodesic dome and more like the painstaking and epic creation of Antoni Gaudi's church of the Sagrada Familia. Despite the metaphors' shortcomings, they do function as a call for communicators to scaffold learning, or more specifically, to scaffold knowledge integration.

The Role of the Communicator Is "Scaffolder" of Knowledge Integration

The education research group in which I completed my doctorate developed a theoretical framework for teaching and learning called **Scaffolded Knowledge Integration (SKI)**. It derives from conceptual change research and extensive testing in formal and informal education environments.[29] While much of the work on SKI was conducted in a K–12 setting, the principles are broadly applicable to other communication contexts. The four principles of SKI are straightforwardly stated yet rich in practice:

1. Make science (or your topic) accessible.
2. Make science visible.
3. Facilitate learning from others.
4. Promote autonomous, lifelong learning.

Scaffolding learners' knowledge integration requires a specialized type of knowledge that is beyond disciplinary knowledge. It is knowing what kinds of misconceptions learners may have about specific subject matter, knowing the best ways to introduce difficult concepts, and the ability to meet learners where they are conceptually at any given moment. This knowledge of how to reach people when communicating disciplinary content is known as **pedagogical content knowledge**.[30] The following sections provide tips on how you can use pedagogical content knowledge to implement the SKI principles.

MAKE THE TOPIC ACCESSIBLE

Making concepts accessible involves connecting to learners' current understanding, predicting and negotiating challenges, and linking to relevant crosscutting themes:

- *Connect to learners.* For example, when young pupils learn subtraction, they often learn "buggy algorithms."[31] When taking the difference of two digits in a column, they may consistently take the smaller away from the larger, regardless of which digit is on top. A teacher with insufficient pedagogical content knowledge will simply mark their answers wrong. A teacher with strong pedagogical content knowledge can home in on the individual's reasoning pattern and tailor feedback accordingly. In short, making the topic accessible requires learner-centric communication approaches.
- *Predict and negotiate challenges.* In retrospect, it seems obvious why people would blend understandings about the greenhouse effect and the hole in the ozone layer. Both phenomena involve Earth's atmosphere, solar radiation (of different wavelengths), and humans releasing gases into the environment. Communication about these phenomena should therefore point out their similarities and differences. To respect and refine learners' initial conceptions linking these phenomena, it could also be worthwhile to introduce the emerging science on the actual chemical and atmospheric links between them.[32]
- *Link to crosscutting themes.* Many concepts only make sense in the context of broader themes, such as patterns, relationships across scales, stability and change, direct and indirect causation, and central control versus emergent behavior. Crosscutting themes are

apparent to experts but need to be made explicit to those unfamiliar with a discipline.

MAKE THE TOPIC VISIBLE

How to design images and multimedia with the audience in mind was the focus of Chapter 2. Making the topic visible also includes offering different entry points for diverse learners, such as through hands-on experiences, stories from the history of science, and compelling examples:

- *Hands-on experiences can promote an embodied understanding.* I had trouble grasping the phases of the moon until I spent time manipulating a golf ball moon around a tennis ball Earth in the beam of a flashlight sun. Without the experience of manipulating the three-dimensional objects, I could not visualize how the full, half, crescent, and new moon could be related to the angles between the Earth, moon, and sun. What about when misconceptions arise due to the very experiences we have manipulating things in the world? Simulations can help; for example, an interactive computer simulation of a frictionless world helped students understand and retain the physics concept that objects in motion stay in motion.[33]

- *Episodes from the history of science that have parallels to students' misconceptions can make concepts more tangible.* For example, in the 1640s, Johannes van Helmont conducted an experiment in which he planted a five-pound willow sapling in a pot and found that after five years the tree had grown to 169 pounds, but the weight of the soil had barely changed at all.[34] The finding conflicts with the notion that plants grow by consuming the soil. Note that when using historical examples, diligence and fact checking is needed because inaccuracies about the history of science are widespread, even in textbooks. For instance, contrary to a popular misconception about misconceptions, Columbus and his contemporaries did not think the Earth was flat.[35]

- *Compelling (and colorful) examples make underlying concepts salient.* A true-blue rose has proven so challenging to engineer that it has been called the Holy Grail of Horticulture. Although hundreds of rose varieties have names associated with blue, such as Shocking

Blue, Blue Moon, and Blue Bayou, they are not really blue.[36] Roses engineered to produce the blue pigment delphinidin are more mauve than blue because of the absence of molecules known as co-pigments that stack together with delphinidin to form a bluer complex and because of the high acidity in rose petals. (The pigment is redder in a more acidic environment, just as purple cabbage is redder in vinegar.) The dearth of Valentine's blue thus highlights the complex relationship between genes and traits.

FACILITATE LEARNING FROM OTHERS

Learning is inherently social (even when you are alone with a book, you are learning from others). One way that communicators can facilitate learning from others is by drawing on cultural "funds of knowledge." Also, in group settings, it is useful to optimize the context by designing for social learning:

- *Draw on the intellectual resources – funds of knowledge – students bring from their families and communities.*[37] A curriculum that values and draws on these funds of knowledge promotes rightful presence in the sciences for students who might otherwise feel excluded from these disciplines.[38] For instance, some Indigenous populations have culturally distinct ways of thinking about agency that are consistent with insights into plant communication and kin altruism that were unknown until recently in the greater scientific community.[39]
- *Design for social learning.* Demonstrations to groups are common in formal and informal education settings, but research shows that unless audiences are given the opportunity to make predictions, demonstrations do not result in learning gains.[40] In a thoughtfully designed demonstration dubbed a benchmark lesson, audience members make and justify predictions about a phenomenon, such as whether an object is lighter, heavier, or weighs the same in a vacuum. They note the different possibilities and then watch a demonstration (e.g., a weight is suspended on a spring scale in a jar and the air is pumped out) and discuss the outcome.[41]

PROMOTE AUTONOMOUS, LIFELONG LEARNING

People's beliefs in their ability to learn and the skills to assess and regulate their own learning are essential in the classroom and beyond:

- *Foster a growth mindset.* Instruction that fosters a growth mindset of learning can narrow or eliminate the performance gap that arises when self-doubt or imposter syndrome leads individuals to question themselves.[42] Fostering a growth mindset includes treating setbacks as opportunities to learn, accompanying critical feedback with an explicit statement about the belief in students to reach a high standard, and sharing stories from diverse successful students who initially questioned whether they belonged. To avoid sending unintended messages, these interventions should never be treated as remedial, nor should they single out particular individuals or groups, as doing so will only emphasize the stress of negative stereotypes. (This applies to inviting people to communication workshops as well.)
- *Think about thinking.* The skills of assessing and regulating one's own thinking (or thinking about thinking) are subsumed under the heading "metacognition." These skills are usually first experienced in social settings but then become internalized.[43] Carefully designed prompts that model discipline-relevant metacognitive reflection can greatly improve how much students learn from science inquiry activities.[44] Explicit instruction on how to study and assess one's own understanding improves performance in college science courses.[45] Reflection prompts and direct instruction of metacognitive strategies can benefit all learners while reducing the achievement gap.

The SKI principles provide a broad view of how communicators can create conditions that support learning. A thread that runs through this discussion about implementing the SKI principles is story: helping learners construct logic stories, stories that learners tell themselves about their belonging, stories that students bring from their families and cultures, and thinking skills that shape the learning of new stories. The final section of this chapter places the spotlight on story and how to tell concise, logically cohesive stories that connect with audiences.

STORYTELLING AS FISHING, MATRYOSHKA DOLLS, AND TOPIARY

Humans use story to make sense of happenings in their lives and in the social and natural world.[46] Compared with disconnected facts, stories facilitate comprehension and recall.[47] People who perform seemingly impossible feats of memory, such as recalling the order of cards in a randomly shuffled deck, do so by creating elaborate stories about the items to be memorized.[48] Plenty of books and workshops tell scientists they need to become better storytellers.[49] Yet the advice on story seems to be driven by an acquisition metaphor for learning (if we entertain them, they will accumulate the facts we deliver), rather than a construction metaphor that prioritizes scaffolding learning. Here the goal is to bring the focus on logic and learning back into the conversation about story.

In one of the rare photographs I have of myself as a child, I am (barely age three) standing on a concrete embankment holding a fishing rod. Bowl haircut tousled by the breeze, squinting along the line to the water below, I am intently adjusting the reel handle. Going fishing with my grandpa to a flood-control-dam lake was a delight of my childhood summers. I loved the relative cool of the early morning that preceded the hot, humid summer days, the earthy smell of the lakeshore as the waves gently lapped against it, the kinesthetic grace of casting, the satisfying sound of the reel unwinding and the sinker dropping into the water with a ploop, and the exhilarating anticipation of watching the bobber. I also loved the time with my grandpa and the wonderful aroma and deliciousness of the fillets of bluegill and perch that my grandma fried up in a light batter after we returned home with our catch.

One day, when I was just a bit older than I am in the photograph, I hooked a really, really, really big one fishing off that embankment. Fiercely grasping my rod, filled with the joyous excitement that everyone was going to see what a great fisher I was, I reeled that fish in slow and steady like a pro. Grandpa was right there, ready to scoop my catch into the net – but disaster struck when the fish was halfway up the wall – the line broke and the big one fell with a sploosh back into the water. By the time we got home I looked like a raccoon from rubbing my crying eyes with my grubby little fists. In my heart, I feel for my inconsolable child self, but I must admit that the story of the big one that got away is better than the story of the big one we ate with ketchup.

Give Them a Nibble before You Try to Reel Them In

In all those magical hours staring out at my bobber waiting for a nibble, it never occurred to me that fishing was a lesson in communication with anyone other than the fish, until Nick Spitzer, neurobiologist and advisor to our Research Communications Program, used the comparison to describe his strategy for gauging a questioner's interest. Rather than launching into a long spiel when someone is asking about his work to be polite at a cocktail party, his strategy is to dole out a tantalizing nibble to see if they are hungry for more. If they are, he gives them a little more and a little more, entering a conversation. When he talked about the strategy of "reeling them in," Nick gestured with both hands, as if holding a fishing rod and winding his line. His fishing comparison is not the idiom to "take the bait hook, line, and sinker" – the goal is not gullibility or excessive enthusiasm on the part of the audience – instead it is avoiding the naïveté and overzealousness on the part of the speaker. Nick also uses a chemistry-inspired comparison of "titrating" out a little at a time. Both the chemistry and the fishing comparisons are reminders about the importance of considering the audience's response and letting it shape where you go next.

As I adopted it in my coaching and teaching, Nick's metaphorical description of how he invites a conversation about his research spawned the additional "Fishing Lessons for Storytellers." Memorable anecdotes and other kinds of stories are said to have four elements: setting, characters, plot, and a moral or solution to offer.[50] Fishing lessons about setting, characters, and plot are summarized in the box. Fishing stories also provide plenty of moral lessons, but communication about research is not usually intended to offer a moral lesson and only sometimes offers a solution. It should be purposeful, however, and the first fishing lesson for storytellers is to consider the audience, context, and goals when entering the story. Have you ever gotten distracted during a presentation just because you could not figure out where it was going? Let the audience in on the purpose of the story before too long, or at least foreshadow where you are heading. To the lessons about purposefulness, setting, characters, and plot, a fifth lesson focuses on the dynamic or shifting relationship between storytellers and audiences – that is, the importance of thinking in terms of progressions of stories and the skill of crafting stories of different sizes.

FISHING LESSONS FOR STORYTELLING

1. *Opening: Use the right hook.* As a kid, I mostly used earthworms as bait, but I knew how to secure a doughball to catch carp using a hook jerry-rigged with a pen spring. For fly fishers, tying flies is an artform in which they take great pride. Likewise, the art of telling stories about research begins with finding the right story and entry point for each audience, context, and goal.

2. *Setting: Take us there.* The setting of a fish tale may be tranquil like my childhood memory, remote and rugged, or a terrifying experience on a small fishing vessel in a storm. Each research lab or field setting is also unique. When telling a story, set the scene using as many of the five senses as you can.

3. *Characters: Make us empathize.* Connection with characters in a story requires that their motivations be apparent. Reach back in time to get in touch with what first motivated your protagonist to pursue a career path or research question. Also invite the audience in by highlighting the satisfying research catches and the big ones that got away.

4. *Plot: Identify the conflict.* Fishing may be human versus fish, human versus elements, or it can be a context in which other conflicts play out (such as the coming of age and family relationships in the film *CODA*). Good research stories do not all revolve around a huge conflict, but like the joy of watching the bobber on the lake, the plot should be enough to keep the audience in interested anticipation.

5. *Book jacket blurb: Give them a nibble before you try to reel them in.* The fishing story I told in two paragraphs could be summarized in a sentence or expanded into a book. It is helpful to have a tackle box full of stories of different sizes to describe your work (or to use the metaphor used in the main text, a Matryoshka nested doll of stories).

Develop a Matryoshka-Nested-Doll Set of Stories

Preparing to be an effective communicator involves crafting alternative explanations and stories to keep in your back pocket. A metaphorical way of thinking about crafting stories of different sizes is nested wooden figurines or Matryoshka dolls. Like the dolls, each story can stand alone, or the set of stories can be assembled from smaller to larger in an interaction. Whether you are a researcher explaining your work or a writer pitching an article to an editor, you need a "baby Matryoshka doll" one-liner and the next size up, the short synopsis paragraph. These are stories about research stories, like a book jacket blurb is a story about the story in a book. Beyond the brief synopsis, common research story lengths are 2–3-minute website videos, 5-slide big-picture presentations, 10–20-minute TED-style talks, and keynotes of 45 minutes to an hour (not to mention written stories of various lengths). Pick the formats most relevant to your audiences, contexts, and goals and develop a set of stories of different sizes as needed. The sections below provide tips on crafting one-liners and short synopses that encapsulate your work. They also provide pointers on crafting longer stories that help support learning by incorporating key take-home messages, building a gap-free logic structure, streamlining the plot, and considering learning progressions.

Regardless of the size of your story, avoid the temptation to try to cram all the exciting aspects of your work or discipline into one talk; save something for another day or for the Q&A. Sometimes a Q&A starts with a bit of awkwardness while audience members are thinking and deciding if they want to be the first to ask a question. At this moment, your heart can start to sink. Not to worry – a moment of silence is helpful to allow your audience to process (and to type into the chat if you are in a virtual space). Take the time to have a sip of water or check in with your breathing. If no questions have appeared, that is okay. Sometimes you just need help getting things started. This is where your preparation in thinking about the story from the audience's point of view comes in handy. You can get the Q&A rolling with, "A question I often hear is …" The point of developing all these tools is to have them in your back pocket so that you can relax and be responsive to the audience in the moment.

Design One Line to Encapsulate Your Research

Your itty bitty Matryoshka doll, that first nibble, is something tinier than a tweet, an "**encapsulate one-liner**" that can logically summarize your research story:

I'm investigating a perplexing protein involved in the disease _____.

My research applies the phenomenon that makes the sky blue and sunsets red.

I'm studying the intricate architecture of the _____.

I work on a proof that has been tormenting mathematicians for 200 years.

Captivating one-liners and stories of any length are easy for those who work on charismatic megafauna, such as dolphins and elephants, or anything that is directly applicable to problems facing humanity. Those who do foundational or fundamental research get frustrated when communication trainers rely on easy examples or push them to overinflate the claims about the potential societal applications of their work. This is a pet peeve of mine too! My graduate research investigated the developmental cues responsible for the stereotypical innervation patterns of a single neuromuscular junction in the body segments in *Drosophila melanogaster* larvae. Yes, in short, I studied nerves in maggots. I grew surprisingly fond of my maggots, but I digress. It is indeed possible to create accessible one-line summaries of fundamental research. The little wrigglers are handy for investigating the mysterious guidance systems used by developing nerves to rendezvous with their target muscles.

The one-liners above exemplify four strategies:

- *Connecting to a societal problem.* Much research in the life sciences is at least peripherally related to diseases, and research in other fields may be related to issues in the natural or built environment. In such cases, variations on the first one-liner may work.
- *Relating to a familiar phenomenon.* In other cases, research can be linked to something that people are familiar with in other settings. For instance, the second one-liner could work for someone who uses Rayleigh light scattering to study materials.
- *Inherent interest of the research.* Another strategy (exemplified by the third one-liner and my maggot nerves one-liner) is to appeal to people's sense of wonder and natural curiosity about how things

work, whether it is the intricate architecture of the trachea, the orchestration of cell communication in embryonic development, the interdependency of relationships in the natural world, or the beauty of a supernova.

- *Highlighting the humanity in the work.* Highly theoretical or mathematical projects may be difficult to encapsulate in lay language, but puzzles and long-standing problems are relatable, especially if a researcher alludes to some of the emotions that arise in the process. At its core, after all, research is a human story.

It is also helpful to develop encapsulate one-liners to describe any potentially challenging concepts that arise when you discuss your research. For example, the word "protein" may call to mind steak or power powder for smoothies, and even for researcher colleagues, "protein" has multiple meanings. Is your protein a lock to open a door (receptor), a matchmaker (enzyme), a relay runner (signaling molecule), a beast of burden (transport molecule), or … ? So if you use the first one-liner, be prepared to offer a brief follow up or add a clarifying phrase. It will make conversations and interviews go more smoothly if you have thought through your initial and follow-up encapsulate one-liners in advance.

Create an Essence Synopsis that Explains Your Work in a Nutshell

> My research aims to end the scourge of malaria. Malaria, which is transmitted by mosquitoes, is a leading cause of death, disability, and economic loss around the world. Many approaches tackle its transmission, such as pesticides and bed nets, but these approaches are insufficient. So my laboratory is developing new genetic tools to sterilize mosquitoes that transmit the disease.

In many communication settings, an elevator pitch is the longest story you get to tell. Using the term "elevator pitch" in communication workshops tends to make people rush unfeelingly through it; thus, I like to think of it as an **essence synopsis** instead. Things are distilled down to their essence, but an essence is not pitched. An essence is shared with care. As concisely as possible, your essence synopsis should introduce

Figure 4.2. Logic Structure of the Essence Synopsis

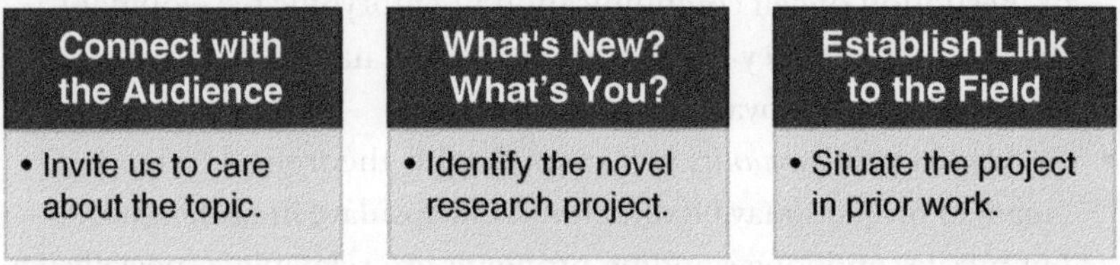

Connect with the Audience	What's New? What's You?	Establish Link to the Field
• Invite us to care about the topic.	• Identify the novel research project.	• Situate the project in prior work.

the problem with the relevant background and make the case for your research. The above example does not go on about all the horrors of malaria without introducing the actual research (the potential nonscientist pitfall), and it does not start off with "Our lab uses the genetic technique CRISPR to …" (the potential scientist pitfall). The essence should grab your audience *and* say where you fit in.

In graduate school, one of my committee members (physics education researcher Andrea diSessa) would ask students, "What's new? What's you?" These two seemingly simple questions have stuck with me and influence how I teach communication. In my experience, communication trainers and journalists who have not studied science tend to push researchers to speak more about the application of their work than the work itself. They may encourage sweeping statements that make researchers squeamish, implying that they alone are going to cure a disease or save an endangered species, when hundreds or even thousands of researchers around the world are working on various aspects of the same problem. A good synopsis is not an oversimplification. It is a neat logic structure that connects the "What's new? What's you?" to the extant body of work and to the audience (Figure 4.2).

The logic structure is three seamlessly interconnected parts: (1) Identify what you are working on; (2) state how prior work led to your question or approach; and (3) think about why you care about this work and tell the audience in a way that piques their interest. Be as concise as you can (this should be shorter than an abstract, perhaps 15–20 words for each part). Combine these answers, preferably in the order 3, 2, 1. Remember that providing the "who cares" is a balancing act between getting too technical and focusing on the big picture to the exclusion of your actual research. In thinking about how to make an adroit transition between what has been done and what you are doing, common "What's new? What's you?" themes are new instruments (such as more sensitive telescopes or microscopes or faster lasers), new techniques or approaches (such as gene editing or computational methods), and new insights (such as a newly recognized interdisciplinary connection or relationship between phenomena). It is your response to "What is the one thing that is going to allow you to break new ground?"

A second synopsis also answers the three questions above, but in a different order:

> I work on a proof that has been tormenting mathematicians for 200 years. Recently, I made a breakthrough in graph theory that I am applying to this old conundrum. If the new approach is successful, mathematicians will be dancing in the streets.

It sums up the prior research, states the "What's new? What's you?" and then provides the answer to "Who cares?" using a bit of humor. This research may very well have practical applications, but our (fictional) mathematician does not work on those applications, which are difficult to explain without background details. Note that for non-mathematicians, graph theory is hidden jargon (because here a graph refers to a mathematical structure, not data plotted on axes), so our mathematician may want to add a phrase defining it or at least be prepared to clarify when the shared laugh about mathematicians dancing in the streets gives the listener confidence to request more details about the work.

For Longer Stories, Incorporate a "Tantalize One-Liner" and a "Take-Home One-Liner"

> She thought she must be having a stroke, but it was the rocks in her head.

> Miniscule stones in our ears act as accelerometers.

The first sentence above is what I would call a **tantalize one-liner**. It grabs your attention. In this case, it does so by creating cognitive conflict that makes you want to know more. The second sentence is a **take-home one-liner** from a longer story that might begin with something like the following paragraph, which is inspired by a friend's experience that landed her in urgent care:

> The whole room was spinning. She thought she must be having a stroke, but it was the rocks in her head. We all have rocks in our heads. To be more precise, the rocks are in our ears and are known as "otoliths" (literally ear stones). These miniscule stones in our ears act as accelerometers. They help us sense gravity and motion, and if they get knocked out of place, they can turn our world upside down.

The tantalize one-liner introduces your story (though you can also embellish to set the scene, as I have above). In interactive settings, the tantalize one-liner can be in the form of a question that brings out the audience's prior conceptions. The take-home one-liner is a memorable message for your audience. When you are communicating with policymakers, potential funders, or even potential collaborators, your "ask" may be your take-home one-liner. If your time with them is short, use your essence synopsis to set the stage by piquing their interest in the problem and the innovativeness of your solution's approach. Follow with a take-home one-liner that is explicit about how their involvement could be beneficial and makes clear your request (e.g., for a meeting, an introduction to someone in their network, or an invitation to submit a proposal).

An encapsulate one-liner can also be useful in a longer story. For example, if the paragraph above is leading into a talk or article on fundamental research about otoliths, such as their chemical composition or how they are formed, the encapsulate one-liner could be the transition from the attention-grabbing introduction of otoliths to the cutting-edge research that will be the focus of the communication.

In crafting and using the one-liners, think of them as support beams for the knowledge structure. One additional one-liner to plan is your last line – the last chance you have to reinforce the learner's knowledge structure. You can choose from several options: (1) Revisit your tantalize one-liner (i.e., connect the end to the beginning); (2) use, repeat, or rephrase your take-home one-liner; (3) sum up a personal or philosophical lesson you have learned; (4) look to the future or next steps for the work; or (5) relate the work to something in popular culture that makes people think and smile as they exit. The last line can come naturally as you write your piece or practice your talk, but avoid a throwaway last line, such as, "That's my last slide." Craft your last line with the aim of helping learners remember your overall message.

Talk of messaging can sometimes feel unsavory to scientists, but Descartes' "I think, therefore I am" was the take-home one-liner from a longer passage in which he philosophized about how to prove anything can be known for certain. The whole passage did, not make it into popular knowledge, but the main concept did, thanks to the take-home one-liner. A popular guide to academic writing, *They Say/I Say*, points out that while this succinct distillation does not capture the nuances of the rest of the passage, it had the power to stick with readers and took on a life of its own.[51] A take-home one-liner is reductive, but it has legs. It is thus useful in both academic and popular communication. Another way to think about the take-home one-liner is to imagine what line you might like to be emphasized as its own graphic element – a pull quote – like the ones I have included here.

A take-home one-liner is reductive, but it has legs.

Beware of Gaps in Logic

A challenge of telling stories is avoiding gaps in logic – specifically, gaps between the information the audience needs and the information you make explicit. When you take someone on a journey, gaps in your story are like crevasses on a glacier. Both can swiftly and tragically claim your companion. Even the smallest gap in logic can leave audiences puzzling such that they miss what you say next and become hopelessly lost – all while trying to maintain a neutral expression, because they blame themselves for tuning out. Specialists are so steeped in their disciplines that they unknowingly leave gaps in logic when they are speaking about their work. Consider the following examples, which arose in workshops/seminars with our researchers:

When you take someone on a journey, gaps in your story are like crevasses on a glacier. Both can swiftly and tragically claim your companion.

- When discussing research on cell proliferation, a biologist was puzzled to be asked why cells in our bodies are dividing. The missing link (cells die and are replaced) was immediately apparent to me, and when I articulated it, both the researcher and the questioner had "aha" moments. The researcher recognized the tiny piece of unarticulated knowledge that led to the confusion, and the questioner related it to the experience of using a loofa sponge to slough away dead skin cells.

- In the context of discussions about strategies to control malaria by targeting female mosquitoes, audience confusion led the researchers to realize that they had failed to mention that only female mosquitoes bite, and they bite because protein in the blood meal is required for egg development.
- After a technical talk on the genetics that control mouthpart development in two *Drosophila* species, a fellow geneticist asked the speaker why the mouthparts of the two species differed. While this piece of information was not essential to understanding the technical talk, it is notable that even a disciplinary colleague found the information gap a puzzling distraction.

In each example, supplying the missing information could be done with a linking phrase or sentence. It did not require a lengthy tangent. The real skill comes in possessing the adequate pedagogical content knowledge to clearly understand the progression of logic needed for the audience to understand your research. In addition to avoiding problematic omissions of information, help audiences connect the dots by using the voice or visual signaling techniques discussed in Chapter 2 (e.g., billboarding words that mark important transitions or contrasts).

Keep the Plot a Happy Medium

Crafting logic stories is akin to turning bushy junipers into artful topiary. Logic stories support the audience by making connections visible. Avoid endless lists of details (like a messy pile of cuttings) and avoid heavy-handed turns and tangents (like horticulture by an overzealous landscaper). In his book *Houston, We Have a Narrative*, Randy Olson refers, respectively, to these two extremes of undesirable story structures as AAA (And, And, And) and DHY (Despite, However, Yet).[52] As a happy medium of plot structure, Olson advocates for an ABT or ABS (And, But, Therefore/So) story structure. Beware of the AAA lack of plot and the DHY unruly plot, which do not support knowledge integration, but do not be limited by the ABT template:

Crafting logic stories is akin to turning bushy junipers into artful topiary.

> Templates are useful mnemonic devices **and** you may find them helpful, **but** they can be overly constraining. **Therefore**, use them as guides, not as rules.

Figure 4.3. Building Your Repertoire of Nested Stories

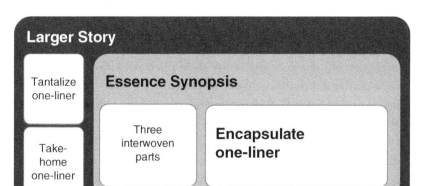

In the essence synopsis section, the first (malaria) example used the ABS template, but the second (mathematical proof) worked better without that constraint. In both cases, however, an adroit transition from the prior work to the "What's new? What's you?" provides the link that takes the audience on a journey without losing them to tedium or confusion. The difference between crisp, concise communication and AAA or DHY story structures is careful planning and ruthless editing. Brainstorming one-liners onto sticky notes and experimenting with their organization can help optimize the logic structure. The one-liners are units of thought that can serve as steppingstones to organize your thinking (Figure 4.3). Writing an article or practicing an oral presentation is not a product of the thinking process, it *is* a thinking process. It is normal for the first draft to contain irrelevant details, missteps in logic, or have confusing twists and turns. Most good writers spend far more of their time editing than writing. Try reading your written work aloud to determine whether what you have written can be modified to better help the reader follow your logic structure. Likewise, when practicing oral presentations, experiment with altering the tempo and emphasis. Feedback from a colleague or someone in the intended audience can also help you turn a bushy juniper story structure into artful topiary.

Spiral Learners through Complexity

A quick online search turns up all sorts of sets of nested dolls, from simple monochromatic ones to intricately detailed hand-painted ones.

Like the dolls, your repertoire of stories may not only need to range in size but also in complexity. At times, such as in a business pitch when you have mixed audiences of researchers and those without a science background, you may need to interweave stories of different levels of complexity. For instance, for a five-slide pitch deck to a mixed audience of potential funders, you could begin each slide by providing a one-liner suitable for all audience members, including those unfamiliar with the field, and follow that with a synopsis of the details desired by those with more knowledge of the field. By juxtaposing levels of explanations and moving back and forth between them, you can manage different levels of complexity within the same setting. Perhaps as an adult you have rewatched a cartoon that entertained you as a kid, and it hit you that the script contains innuendo and cultural references that completely flew over the head of your child self. Artfully done, juxtaposition of complexity can feel seamless.

Some settings, such as educational ones, call for transitioning to greater levels of complexity over time. A tiered approach to telling stories is a microcosm of what is known in education as the **spiral curriculum**. The spiral curriculum, based on the work of psychologist Jerome Bruner, is the idea that students should revisit important topics multiple times over their educational trajectories at increasing levels of complexity.[53] An example is photosynthesis, a topic of cutting-edge research in plant genetics and molecular biology that nonetheless can be introduced in basic ways in elementary school. In a spiral curriculum, learners are given the opportunity to master each successive level of understanding before building on it. For topics in the K–12 curriculum, learning progressions have been developed to map out how concepts can be presented in increasing levels of complexity in successive grades.[54] Think about how your own topic can be introduced at different levels of depth in a series of interactions with an audience over time or with audiences at different points along a learning trajectory.

"WHEN ALL IS SAID AND DONE"

Your tantalizing one-liner motivates your audience to join you. Your logic story helps audiences construct an edifice of understanding. Your take-home one liner can be a crossbeam to support a more robust knowledge structure. Your research on people's prior conceptions, your attention to how previous audiences have made sense of your work, and your give-and-take with the current audience tell you where more scaffolding is needed and where restructuring can help learners interlink new and existing knowledge. Yet, "When All Is Said and Done," the logic story of the communicator and the logic story of the audience are never one and the same. That can feel frustrating, but it is the inevitable outcome of our ability to think independently and inventively, and without creative thinking, scientific progress (the topic of the next chapter) would not be possible. So before turning the page to explore another kind of story, the story of science and scientists, consider the underwater sculptures of artist Jason deCaires Taylor that become more fascinating as they engage in a conversation with the sea. It is this last metaphor that reminds us learning is ongoing, organic, and beautiful.

5

The Hidden Climb Revealed: Giving Voice to People and Process

My canine companion and I make our way down a steep ravine toward the ocean, searching for a way to reach the top of the adjacent cliff. As the terrain becomes unnavigable, we backtrack, make a failed attempt to scale an unstable surface, and backtrack again, scrutinizing the landscape. We finally claw our way up the least hostile section, four legs ably assisting two legs on the steepest part. Stepping onto level ground, I lift my gaze to behold the endless expanse of blue rolling against cliffs tawny in the early morning sunlight. The beauty worthy of the toil sparks in me exhilaration with a hint of self-satisfaction. I can almost hear the plucking of harp strings. The feeling is abruptly cut short when movement catches my eye – hikers coming from the opposite direction along a wide, stable trail to the same cliff we had labored to summit! For a moment, I feel deflated, but then I remember the quotation below. The aptness of it to my morning efforts makes me laugh, and I return to enjoying the view:

> I am fain to compare myself with a wanderer on the mountains, who, not knowing the path, climbs slowly and painfully upwards, and often has to retrace his steps because he can go no farther … till at length when he reaches the summit he finds to his shame that there is a royal way by which he might have ascended, had he only the wits to find the right approach to it. In my works, I naturally said nothing about my mistakes to the reader, but only

described the made tracks by which he may now reach the same heights without difficulty.[1]

Written by famous physicist, physician, and philosopher Hermann von Helmholtz in 1891, the mountain climbing metaphor draws attention to the discrepancy between the process of scientific discovery as it unfolds in reality and the way researchers report on their discoveries in scientific publications. Although the "royal way" makes a readable recipe for colleagues, it obscures the tale of the voyage into uncharted territory and the voyager's struggles and triumphs. In doing so, it leaves room for problematic myths about discovery and discoverers.

CHAPTER LEARNING OBJECTIVES: HIDDEN CLIMB

Knowledge: How do popular portrayals of discovery and discoverers mislead, and why should you care?

Skills: Reveal the humanity and the untold stories in the retelling of the research journey.

Habits of Mind: Reflect on your (or the field's) implicit motivations and assumptions.

GETTING PAST MYTHS AND BLACK BOXES IN PORTRAYALS OF SCIENCE AND SCIENTISTS

The treatment of discovery is murky in the classroom, the media, and popular culture. Generations of curriculum reform efforts have targeted the teaching of scientific inquiry.[2] Philosopher and psychologist John Dewey advocated for the inclusion of scientific inquiry in the K–12 curriculum at the turn of the twentieth century, but calls for reform reached the public and political imagination during the Cold War after the Soviets launched the first Sputnik satellite.[3] The alarm was amplified by findings that both high school and college students had unfavorable images of science careers and failed to recognize the intellectual activity of scientific research as rewarding in itself.[4] Yet, more than a century later, textbooks still present an oversimplified and inaccurate view of the process of scientific discovery, including the myth that there exists a single formulaic scientific method.[5] Likewise, in science journalism, the process of science is glossed over and, when it is presented, it is greatly oversimplified.[6]

In fiction, portrayals of scientists have changed over time, but stereotypes still abound. A common horror movie trope in the 1930s and 1940s was a good man corrupted by his obsession with science or an evil man using science as a means to satisfy his desires.[7] This "mad, bad, dangerous scientist" is personified by the most well-known fictional exemplar, Dr. Frankenstein. Another common stereotype is the scientist who is neither mad nor bad, but inadvertently unleashes unforeseen dangers.[8] Yet another is the naïve scientist easily manipulated by powerful interests.[9] Fictional scientists are more likely, compared with other professions, to be portrayed as violent or victims of violence.[10] Scientist stereotypes are also employed for comedic effect, such as the nutty professor or the socially awkward nerd.

Although twenty-first-century fiction is less likely to portray scientists as objects of fear or mockery, and more likely to portray them as well-intentioned and altruistic, even heroic, clichés like the geek stereotype remain, and scientists are still largely portrayed as white and male.[11] Scientist characters work alone in basement laboratories or other secret locations. Their research is in fictional scientific fields or real fields in a fictional state of development.[12] They are often unrelatably intellectually gifted individuals, and their breakthroughs occur by genius or accident.[13]

For all these reasons and more, students, teachers, and broader audiences have little understanding of the real-life scientific discovery process.[14] Also, most young people lack contemporary role models in science.[15] Improving understanding of discovery and discoverers has the potential to enhance societal conversations about science-related issues, because knowledge of the scientific process increases acceptance of scientific claims.[16] Therefore, to better foster appreciation for the beauty of science as a cultural endeavor, to inspire students to study science, and to support personal and policy decisions, science communication should open the black box of scientific discovery – or to return to the metaphor that opened this chapter, reveal the hidden climb. Specifically, in ways suitable for the audience, context, and goals of the communication, it should strive to do the following:

1. Give voice to and humanize the climber(s).
2. Highlight the inherently collective aspect of science.

3. Depict the research journey accurately and accessibly.
4. Explore the role of values in motivating and conceptualizing the work.

This chapter explores each of these aspects of the hidden scientific climb and provides recommendations for peeling back the layers of the discovery process. The focus is then expanded to the intersection of science and society more broadly, including tips for bridging the cultures of science and policymaking.

Give Voice to and Humanize the Climber(s)

To label the process by which scientific discovery is transformed from an exploratory journey to a series of logical arguments, philosopher of science Hans Reichenbach coined the term "rational reconstruction."[17] Rational reconstruction is a way of making scientific papers efficiently comprehensible to colleagues. It reflects the need to make practicable the task of keeping up with the ever-burgeoning scientific literature, and it is a response to the tight length limitations on peer-reviewed publications, especially in the most prestigious journals (for example, 2,500–4,500 words in *Science* and *Nature*). Other than in the most technical communication, however, the climber needs more of a voice.

APPROACH THE RETELLING WITH "BEGINNER'S MIND" AND HEART

Beginner's mind is a concept from Buddhist philosophy that means meeting the world as if experiencing it for the first time. For example, if someone were walking into the lab for the first time, what would they see, hear, and smell? When I first started working in a fly lab, the yeasty smell of the food was overpowering, but it faded into the background over time, as did the hum of the incubators, the mechanical clinking of the shake tables, and the rows of dissecting microscopes on the long black counters covered in tattered white absorbent paper. Describing the setting with beginner's mind invites the audience into the climber's world the way novelists invite a reader into the world of their protagonist.

Recapture the emotional highs and lows of the scientific journey and allow the audience to be moved by what moves you. This may entail a bit of a character study. What ignited your passion for science in the first place? Do you remember the thrill of your first significant discovery, the surprise of a mistaken prediction, or the sense of awe and wonder you had while exploring nature with your first mentor? Whether you see research as a mountain climb or as sleuthing or as assembling the pieces of a jigsaw puzzle, reconnecting with the emotions can help the audience connect with science and scientists. Sharing what you feel in your heart (along with your evidence) has the potential to both inspire public action and advance science. An example is Rachel Carson's *Silent Spring*. Although not initially well-received in the scientific community, this touchstone of environmental writing had a profound impact on research, legislation, and the public imagination because it reached people's hearts.[18]

SHOWCASE INDIVIDUAL DIVERSITY AND PERSONAL OR PROFESSIONAL CHALLENGES

Sharing details that help portray scientists as whole people with multifaceted lives can make it easier for young people to get past stereotypes and imagine themselves in a scientific career. When stories of researchers' intellectual or personal struggles are incorporated into lessons about scientific discoveries, students are more motivated to learn science, and the positive impact is greatest for students who are underperforming academically.[19] Personal loss, negotiating cultural barriers, impostor syndrome, balancing work and family may seem peripheral to the discovery story, but these struggles have the power to inspire. Also, they may not be peripheral, because they may provide the motivation that drives the work or the unique perspective that shapes it. Some researchers have taken to creating a "CV of Failures" to document their professional setbacks to serve as encouragement to others.[20]

Highlight the Inherently Collective Aspect of Science

In contrast with images in popular culture, the production of scientific knowledge is a collective enterprise.[21] Community aspects of science include collaborations within and between laboratories, mentoring, formative conversations with colleagues, and peer review. Unfortunately, even undergraduates doing research may not truly grasp the collective nature of science.[22] Yet the variety of roles and the often-distributed nature of the work means everyone has a contribution to make in the research process.[23] This message is important for laboratory newcomers, who often begin with self-contained tasks that may seem removed from the final product but nonetheless allow them to gradually advance toward mastery and become enculturated – a learning process dubbed "legitimate peripheral participation."[24] In discussing the scientific community and the collective nature of the enterprise, strive to address misconceptions about diversity and about disagreements.

SHOWCASE DEMOGRAPHIC DIVERSITY TO OVERTURN STEREOTYPES

As in popular culture, scientists represented in textbooks are largely white and male.[25] On the draw-a-scientist-test, which is commonly used in educational settings to examine students' views of scientists, students' drawings typically depict white middle-aged men with glasses and a lab coat; however, their depictions become less stereotypical when they meet or learn about demographically diverse researchers.[26] Coverage of science and scientists in curriculum materials, the media, and popular culture should promote diversity with respect to age, gender, race and ethnicity, disability, and other demographic characteristics. Science writer Ed Yong, for example, has discussed coming to recognize the gender and racial imbalance in his stories and the steps he has taken to be more inclusive.[27] To help attract and retain minorities in science, dedicated mentors are vital, but so are small but sincere affirmations of an individual's identity as a scientist.[28]

In addition to showcasing diversity, curriculum materials and other communication about science should avoid sending the message that the only science is Western science. Indigenous cultures, for example, have amassed significant knowledge about many scientific topics, including medicinal plants; tides and currents; migratory habits of fish, birds, and mammals; and geological processes.[29] Indigenous peoples' songs and stories reflect long histories on the land and careful observations of patterns and deviations – for example, of cycles of glacial advance and retreat, flooding and drought. Such knowledge has given geologists testable hypotheses and can be successfully incorporated into a culturally congruent science curriculum.[30]

SHOW HOW DISAGREEMENTS ADVANCE DISCOVERY

The peer review process is central in science, but it does not represent the first (or last) vetting of scientific claims. Science has become increasingly abstract, tied to mathematical models and tools that provide indirect ways to study unobservable phenomena.[31] An anthropologist visiting a science laboratory is struck by how much of the discovery process entails researchers discussing findings with colleagues and gathering data or modifying conjectures to address the challenges they raise.[32] The way these disagreements shaped the work can be shared with audiences, as space and time permits, to counteract narratives that disagreements are a sign of something wrong. Communicators, particularly those who are not scientists, must take care to distinguish between disagreements over knowledge claims or evidence and those that involve disputes over the applications of scientific knowledge. Researchers can help by clarifying this distinction for their own work.

Depict the Research Journey Accurately and Accessibly

As Reichenbach and Helmholtz make clear, rational reconstruction of the research journey for publications is not a deliberate attempt to obscure or misrepresent the scientific record. Nonetheless, it has been fiercely criticized. Immunologist Peter Medawar asked, "Is the scientific paper a fraud?"[33] Philosopher of science Thomas Kuhn rejected rational reconstruction as systematically misleading, comparing it to images of a national culture portrayed in a tourist brochure.[34] These official records of science obscure the inherent craft of science that sociologist of science Karin Knorr-Cetina has described as the creation of knowledge through a form of artisanal tinkering.[35] Observing scientists, she noted that this was overwhelmingly the focus of their efforts. As with any artisanal tinkering, scientists often attempt procedures, run into snags, and either modify or abandon the procedures. Because it can take an infinite number of tiny "tinkers" to make a fussy procedure work, knowing when to cut one's losses is key to keeping a research project moving forward.

Portraying the research journey more accurately does not mean giving a boring list of procedural details in the style of "and then ... and then … and then." Instead, it is an invitation to tell a story of discovery using aspects of a particular research journey to illustrate big-picture concepts about scientific research. Consider the following:

- The creativity of discovery, including the diversity of thinking and the fact that different methods can be applied to solve the same problems, has been identified as a key aspect of science that needs to be better communicated to students, teachers, and others.[36]
- Although serendipitous findings are common in science, these are not the same as the popular culture version of "happy accidents"; instead, they are typically variations or anomalies that research- ers notice and follow up.[37] They can be introduced as examples of scientific thought in action, or what Louis Pasteur described as chance favoring the prepared mind.[38]
- A key insight from colleagues often shapes the research journey. For instance, pivotal in the elucidation of the structure of DNA, a chemist who shared an office with James Watson noticed that the textbook Watson was using gave the incorrect structures for the nucleic acids.[39] Anecdotes about receiving key insights can help emphasize the collaborative nature of discovery.
- Researchers rarely discuss the timescales of discoveries (that a sin- gle paper can represent years of work, for instance), but doing so and providing a bird's-eye view of the paths taken and abandoned would not only help nonscientists appreciate the craft of science, but also clarify why answering certain questions is painstaking and expensive.
- New technologies and procedures make it possible to answer ques- tions that could not previously be answered. These are often the results of fundamental scientific discoveries that become taken-for- granted tools in other disciplines.[40] They thus underscore the merit of fundamental research.

SUPPORT TEACHERS AND STUDENTS TO LEARN BOTH "WITH" AND "ABOUT" SCIENTIFIC INQUIRY

The implicit lessons about pedagogy in future teachers' college science classes, such as the all-too-common "cookbook" labs, conflict with the explicit reform-minded curriculum in teacher education courses. Most teachers, irrespective of their academic backgrounds, lack an under-standing of the nature of scientific discovery, unless they are exposed to interventions that give it explicit attention.[41] Even when students and teachers are engaged in inquiry, this does not automatically translate to an understanding of the process of scientific discovery.[42] Teachers should have the opportunity to learn *with* the scientific inquiry practices they are expected to teach, but they also need to learn *about* how actual scientific discoveries are made.[43] To learn *with* inquiry, they should experience the practices identified in the relevant science standards (such as those in the Next Generation Science Standards):[44]

1. Asking questions and defining problems
2. Developing and using models
3. Planning and carrying out investigations
4. Analyzing and interpreting data
5. Using mathematics and computational thinking
6. Constructing explanations and designing solutions
7. Engaging in argument from evidence
8. Obtaining, evaluating, and communicating information

To learn *about* how actual scientific discoveries are made, and to fully appreciate that the practices do not define a scientific method or cap-ture all the relevant aspects of the discovery process, they also need exposure to real stories of discovery.

PROVIDE A RECORD OF THE PATHS TAKEN AND ABANDONED FOR COLLEAGUES AND MENTEES

Supplementing the rational reconstruction could help fellow scien-tists too. For example, a record of the paths taken and abandoned could benefit science's so-called "replication crisis."[45] The failure of one laboratory to replicate a procedure that worked in another labo-ratory may raise fears of academic dishonesty, but unknown differ-ences may lead a procedure to fail in a new context. For example, in one case, an eight-month investigation to determine why a published chemical reaction was not working in other laboratories turned up two unknown essentials: proximity to the laboratory lights (because the reaction was photochemical) and a leaky magnetic stir bar, which

Figure 5.1. Peel Back the Layers of the Discovery Process

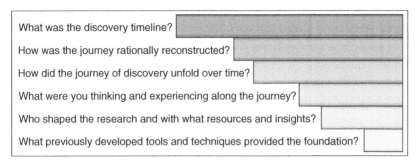

was serendipitously providing a metal catalyst.[46] Many failures are not documented anywhere but the laboratory notebooks of researchers who simply gave up and tried something else. Perhaps sharing them within the scientific community could tap into the benefits of crowd-sourcing to determine the reasons for the failures and save future climbers from the same fate.

Another potential benefit of making the "artisanal tinkering" or paths taken and abandoned transparent is for the morale of students in the science pipeline. Even graduate students have misconceptions about the process of science.[47] Graduate student attrition has remained consistently high, and graduate students leave even while holding prestigious fellowships.[48] The reasons for graduate student attrition are complex, but a student's sense that they are moving forward on their research project is among the most important factors.[49] If the scientific community were to regularly convey the many paths taken and abandoned, it could give students a healthier perspective on their own research setbacks, potentially fostering retention. See Figure 5.1 for some questions you could answer to provide your audience with a better sense of the path.

Explore the Role of Values in Motivating and Conceptualizing the Work

The definitions of "science" and "scientists" have been a source of debate since the terms were introduced.[50] Philosophers have struggled to find a straightforward way to demarcate science from nonscience. Karl Popper posited that, although scientific theories cannot be proven, they can be falsified.[51] Thomas Kuhn, however, argued that theories are not over-turned by one or even a few anomalous observations, but rather by a social consensus within the scientific community.[52] In short, no satisfac-tory single line can be drawn to demarcate science from nonscience, but boundaries between science and other intellectual activities can be drawn in narrower contexts, such as for a particular discipline or purpose.[53] The philosophical debate should therefore not be an impediment to discuss-ing the scientific process, but it should be a reminder to avoid overly broad statements, particularly a naïve view that science is free of values.

Sociologist Robert Merton identified four norms that distinguish the scientific endeavor: communalism, universalism, disinterestedness, and organized skepticism.[54] Communalism is the norm of sharing sci-entific knowledge openly in the scientific community. Universalism is the norm that scientific claims should be judged solely on their merit and that people from all social backgrounds can do science. Disinter-estedness is the norm of working for the common good rather than for personal gain. Organized skepticism is the norm of subjecting scien-tific claims to scrutiny. Scientists use careful documentation, controls, replication, peer review, and so on, but values are also inherent in the process. What counts as acceptable evidence in a field is a value – an epistemic value – but social, political, moral, or economic values also come into play in science, for instance in problem selection and choice of methods.[55]

COMMUNICATE THE ALTRUISTIC MOTIVATIONS THAT STUDENTS CAN RELATE TO

The book *Talking about Leaving: Why Undergraduates Leave the Sciences* dispels the notion that high attrition rates in science, mathematics, and engineering majors mainly weed out students who are not sufficiently capable.[56] The authors found that many high-achieving students, but disproportionately high-achieving women and underrepresented minorities, abandon the sciences because what they are learning feels disconnected from their lives and their desire to have a career through which they can have a direct, positive impact in their communities and beyond. Successful women of color in science mention altruistic goals as motivations to persevere in the face of setbacks.[57] Unfortunately, sci-entists are portrayed as so utterly consumed by a single-minded pursuit that they are lacking in humanity.[58] Researchers need to communicate their motivations, and journalists and others need to more accurately portray researchers' motivations.

ASK WHAT IMPLICIT VALUES AND ASSUMPTIONS MAY SHAPE THE WORK AND HOW

Ambivalent portrayals of science reflect complex societal attitudes, with great expectations tempered by worries about science getting out of control.[59] From the history of science, it is apparent that not all the values that drive science are inherently good. An example is the eugenics movement in the 1920s and 1930s, in which genetic principles were viewed as a way to improve the human race. Although eugenics is no longer mainstream, genetic determinism lives on in the discourse of scientists.[60] Researchers themselves may not be fully aware of how their implicit views shape their work. For example, an article about Indigenous sciences points out that standard depictions of ecosystems are devoid of humans or only show humans as observers.[61] The authors argue that a shift to the Indigenous perspective that humans

Standard depictions of ecosystems are devoid of humans or only show humans as observers.

are a part of (not apart from) nature could benefit research on climate change and sustainability. Conversations about values in science could thus increase transparency and improve research. Acknowledging the plurality of research approaches, and the composite picture they provide, may also make research more useful to policymakers.[62]

Allow the first half of this chapter to serve as encouragement to free yourself from the canonical Introduction, Methods, Results, and Discussion (IMRAD) rational reconstruction story structure when communicating with nontechnical audiences. Using the above discussion as your guide, brainstorm about the stories hidden behind IMRAD in your research or field. Reconnect with the diverse characters, unique settings, motivations, creative insights, setbacks, and triumphs along the discovery journey. The fresh perspective will help you reach new audiences in new ways and dispel myths, and it may even help you rekindle your own sense of awe and wonder about science.

SCIENCE, SOCIETY, AND THE DIRECTIONALITY OF COMMUNICATION

In the second half of this chapter, we return from our mountain adventures to the urban landscape – or to be more literal, to where the products of science intersect with society.

Informing Decisions Shifts the Dynamic between Communicators and Audiences

Directionality of communication can be placed along a continuum roughly segmented into five categories (Figure 5.2):

1. *Pure transmission.* The underlying assumption is that unidirectional communication from experts to nonexperts is effective.
2. *Transmission requires checking.* Experts need feedback from audiences to ensure that audiences comprehend without misinterpretation.
3. *Receptiveness to individual.* In informing an individual's decision-making, experts need to make room for the individual's personal values.
4. *Receptiveness to collective.* In informing decisions that affect society, experts need to make room for others' values.
5. *Expertise is distributed.* Communication must take into account not only others' values but also others' knowledge.

PURE TRANSMISSION / TRANSMISSION REQUIRES CHECKING

Pure transmission (or nearly pure) modes of communication are common in many education and communication settings (and, of course, written works). To be effective, however, *transmission requires checking*, which may be formative feedback during creation when the communication context does not permit real-time checking. Checking provides insight into people's conceptual knowledge of science; their understanding of the scientific process; the different ways they are interpreting terms, metaphors, analogies, and information graphics; and whether or not their interest is piqued.

Figure 5.2. Directionality of Communication

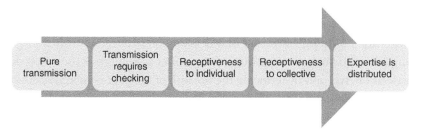

RECEPTIVENESS TO INDIVIDUAL

Receptiveness to individual values requires accepting that two people can look at the same evidence on a complex scientific issue but weigh the costs and benefits differently and come to different (evidence-based) decisions. Deciding whether to get a mammogram before age 50 is an example. Taking the test introduces a risk of a false positive and unneeded medical treatment. Not taking the test may mean failing to detect breast cancer. In considering the same scientific data in the context of similar personal risk factors, an individual's decision will depend on how much they are willing to take a chance on detecting something that is not there versus failing to detect something that is there. You can help inform complex personal decisions by letting the decision maker talk through the options, respecting the individual's autonomy, while listening to make sure that all the relevant evidence is on the table. In the mammography example, clinicians use decision aids to help people make an informed choice.[63]

RECEPTIVENESS TO COLLECTIVE

Receptiveness to collective is the view that, in making decisions that affect society, communicators need to be responsive to people's values. This is a step beyond listening to individuals who are making personal decisions, because it is possible to simultaneously believe that people have the right to make a "wrong" decision when it only affects the decision maker but do not have that right when it comes to decisions that affect others. In informing societal decisions, experts may see themselves as possessing the relevant facts and being able to sort through evidence unencumbered by values; however, judgments are inherent in most statements by scientists, with statements falling on a continuum from lower to higher levels of advocacy.[64] Although advocacy may be based on science, it involves shaping advice to favor one outcome over another or to narrow the scope of a decision, typically by reducing the breadth of the peer-reviewed science on which the statements are based.[65] It can be difficult to detect, even by those endeavoring to provide unbiased information. The receptiveness-to-collective view of communication entails recognizing that dialogues with diverse constituencies are needed to bring tacit assumptions (your own and society's) to the fore and to help reveal where decisions about science and technology have the potential to exacerbate inequities.

EXPERTISE IS DISTRIBUTED

The *expertise-is-distributed* view of science communication is the acceptance that not only are values diverse, but knowledge is diverse. Scientists can embarrass themselves when they assume that everyone without their knowledge has the same frame of reference – frame of reference fallacy.[66] Consider a communication debacle that illustrates the dangers of unidirectional science communication and its inherent assumptions about the nature of expertise. When the Chernobyl nuclear power plant in Ukraine exploded in 1986, Cumbria in northern England, known for its thousands of sheep farms, was particularly affected because heavy thunderstorms there coincided with the arrival of the radioactive cloud. The unsatisfactory response from national government experts was initial false assurances, followed by the implementation of a series of ever-changing restrictions on the movement and sale of sheep that ultimately lasted years.[67]

The trust-destroying debacle could have been avoided if the scientists had held an expertise-is-distributed view of communication and had solicited the farmers' craft knowledge. Without it, the scientific recommendations and restrictions ignored the pragmatic realities faced by sheep farmers, such as pasture conditions, buildup of disease, rates of finishing of lambs, and the need to ready ewes for the next breeding season. Even more damningly, the government scientists failed to account for the local geological conditions (known to the farmers), including variations in rates of water runoff, accumulation patterns across the landscape, and the dissimilarity in soil types between valleys and hills. From modeling based on the alkaline clay soils in the lowlands, the scientists concluded that the radioactive cesium would be quickly immobilized in the soil, halting incorporation into the vegetation. This optimistic prediction did not hold up in acidic upland soils, where cesium was not immobilized, and the vegetation continued to take it up and transfer it to the sheep.

Non-credentialed Persons Can Make Essential Contributions to Science

Craft knowledge, cultural knowledge, and local knowledge are imperative, and a whole range of citizen science initiatives have emerged to monitor and analyze natural phenomena and to advance locally relevant conservation goals.[68] The expertise-is-distributed view raises questions about the epistemic division of labor and the nature of expertise. In thinking about the ways those lacking credentials in a field could nonetheless contribute valuable expertise, a distinction between the different types of expertise is helpful. In their "Periodic Table of Expertises," Collins and Evans distinguish five increasingly deep "specialist expertises": beer-mat knowledge, popular understanding, primary source knowledge, interactional expertise, and contributory expertise.[69] Progressing to mastery of the primary literature may give people increasing confidence in their knowledge, but because papers only tell part of the discovery story, understanding the nuances of scientific findings and interpretations is only possible through interaction with the scientific community.

Contributory knowledge is what we usually think of as specialist expertise. Perhaps the most famous historical example of contributory expertise of non-credentialed persons is in the case of AIDS treatment activism by the group ACT UP. The members of the group, although lacking formal credentials, developed considerable interactional expertise and ultimately informed the design of the clinical trials of the drug AZT (and influenced broader conversations about the ethical design of clinical trials). ACT UP members not only argued that placebo-controlled trials were unethical for patients with a fatal disease like AIDS (because they would be a death sentence to those in the placebo group); they also provided the medical experts with key knowledge, such as the fact that trial participants would share medications across experimental and control groups, a practice that made placebo-controlled trials scientifically unsound.[70]

The Boundary between Science and Society Is a Liminal Space

In his often-cited work, physicist and novelist C.P. Snow wrote about the separation of the sciences and humanities and the loss of a common culture.[71] His criticism was aimed at the education system, not scientists, but scientists have been criticized for allegedly seeing themselves as separate from society.[72] In my own experience, this is not how scientists see themselves, but if we substitute "science" and "society" with "knowledge production" and "knowledge consumption," the boundary between them may be fuzzier than some scientists view it to be. One example is when societal influence on knowledge production moves upstream in **anticipatory governance**; a second example is when aspects of knowledge evaluation are shifted downstream by **civic epistemologies**.

The notion of anticipatory governance has been introduced as a way to not only broaden participation in decisions that affect society but to institutionalize a capacity for reflection and agile responsiveness, or "reflexiveness," well upstream of the decisions, perhaps even in time to shape the scientific research itself.[73] In contrast to science policy decisions that often take place behind closed doors in high-level state, national, or international meetings, anticipatory governance seeks the participation of diverse individuals and citizen groups. Anticipatory governance dialogues can help answer four questions about the decisions to be made: (1) What choices are available? (2) What are the values of those making the decisions? (3) What is the range of values within the complex social setting? (4) What outcomes can result from the interaction of scientific advances in the complex cultural, economic, environmental, and political setting?

With respect to the latter question, when faced with the same technological alternatives, societies with similar levels of socioeconomic development may nonetheless choose to go in different directions. Biotechnology – specifically, genetically engineered food – is an example where this has occurred.[74] Societal differences in regulation and uptake of technologies are due at least in part to tacit institutionalized practices – civic epistemologies – by which members of different societies assess the strength and rationality of knowledge claims.[75]

Models Are a Particular Challenge in Communicating to Inform Decision-Making

Historian of science Naomi Oreskes points out that models of complex nonrepetitive biological, ecological, geological, atmospheric, and hydrologic natural systems have little or no historic track record of success.[76] She acknowledges that such models can inform policy discussions with comparisons of potential outcomes of alternative courses of action. At the same time, she cautions researchers against making long-range deterministic predictions and falling victim to thinking that including more aspects of the system necessarily increases the accuracy of predictions – the **complexity paradox**. Table 5.1 highlights this and other potential misunderstandings about models, and how they can be addressed or avoided.

Speaking to legislators, offering expert testimony, preparing risk assessments, and participating in citizen forums are ways that scientists may have a voice in societal decision-making, but having effective conversations with policymakers involves more than simply returning from the scientific climb and changing clothes. The next section offers guidance on how scientists and other specialists can negotiate the challenges of the policymaking arena.

TIPS FOR DIALOGUES WITH POLICYMAKERS

"Policymaker" is a heterogeneous category, encompassing elected and nonelected officials at the local, state, and national level. Collections of people, with formal roles and informal influence, are involved in crafting and implementing policies, and interactions occur at three levels: individual (micro), groups and coalitions (meso), and institutions and cultures (macro).[77] Likewise, policy encompasses a broad array of government actions, including laws and regulations, voluntary agreements, financial incentives or penalties, education campaigns, provision of services, and allocation of funding.[78]

Table 5.1. Communicating about Models and Modeling

Aspect of Model	Avoiding Potential Misunderstandings
Type? (physical replica, visual simulation, numerical calculation)	For nonscientists, the word "model" is most likely to bring to mind something tangible that resembles the thing it represents. *Be specific. For example, is your model a physical model, a dynamic rendering on a computer screen, or a calculation with only a numerical output?*
Status? (historical, currently used, under development)	People may think of models as static once developed, and they may not understand the concept of model testing. *Indicate whether the model is being actively revised. Does your work use the model as a tool (e.g., an "off-the-shelf" model for simulation) or does your work inform the model design?*
Purpose? (teaching, synthesizing data, guiding observation, predicting the future)	Nonscientists may not think of models as being research tools and may tend to think of them as tools of communication. *Provide background on the purpose of the model. For example, does the model provide insight into a hidden biological or geological process?*
Forecasting? (predicting a future scenario well beyond the timeline of the data in the model)	Audiences may assume that numerical models have the purpose of forecasting future scenarios. They may also assume that models are correct if they make true predictions. *Distinguish the process of model testing and refinement from predicting beyond current data. Explain that false models can make true predictions (e.g., the Ptolemaic system).*
Complexity? (the number of parameters or factors in the model)	People may think that the more factors in the model, the better the model and its predictive power. *Address the potential "complexity paradox." On the one hand, a complex model is more realistic, but it may also be more uncertain because each additional factor raises new questions.*

It follows that communication with policymakers may be undertaken to achieve a variety of goals, such as the following:

- Attest to the importance of basic science or advocate for funding for your discipline, area of research, or a specific project.
- Provide scientific evidence that highlights a societal problem.
- Describe findings or technologies that may help solve a societal problem.
- Report on the efficacy of a policy or compare the efficacy of policies that have been implemented in different regions or time periods.
- Establish an ongoing relationship as a trusted advisor or as a boundary spanner between the science and policy communities.

Beyond the problems of jargon and the sheer volume of the scientific literature, cultural differences between the scientific community and the policymaking community can impede the use of science in policy decisions. If you are accustomed to being immersed in a scientific culture, it is easy to assume that those community norms and problem-solving approaches are the only ways to get things done, an assumption that can lead to major gaffes in the policy arena. The better you understand the policymaking context and the needs of policymakers, the more productive your conversations will be. Informed by findings of an extensive review of the literature on the barriers to evidence-based policymaking, seven features of the policymaking environment and their ensuing communication recommendations are detailed below:[79]

1. Compared to an academic laboratory with a principal investigator, influence on policy tends to be less top down.

    Implications for research communication: The government relations office at your institution or in your professional society may be able to provide background about the networks of individuals working on a particular policy. When you do reach out to the relevant individual(s), do not feel offended if a policymaker wants you to instead meet with staffers. It does not mean the policymaker is brushing you off. The staffers may be the ones with the relevant expertise. They may also have considerable influence on the policymaker's priorities and decisions.

2. Academics typically have a narrow research focus, but policymakers tackle many issues and must rely on others' expertise.

    Implications for research communication: Before meeting, do your homework to know the policymakers, the legislation they have sponsored, and the constituencies they represent. Be mindful that you do not automatically have the same status with a policymaker as you do at your home institution. To become a trusted advisor, you will need to work to establish a relationship. Ask the policymakers how you can be of help, listen carefully, offer to follow up with additional information as needed, and thank them for their time.

3. Policymakers rely on different kinds of evidence.

Implications for research communication: Make the peer-reviewed findings accessible in a jargon-free form with sufficient, but not extraneous, detail. Qualitative examples can be helpful. As appropriate, explain how the findings apply to the relevant local or situational context. Be aware of potentially relevant "grey literature," such as regulatory documents, expert testimony, or government reports about related policies tested in other regions or time periods. Be prepared to explain any real or apparent discrepancies.

4. Policymakers may not want to attend to the problem if a solution is not available.

Implications for research communication: If a viable solution exists, make that clear from the beginning. If no solution exists, make it clear how policymakers' attention to the problem might help in identifying a solution. A potential role for their constituents to help in finding a solution may be another reason for a policymaker to invest time or money in an issue.

5. Policymakers inherit programs, commitments, and rules.

Implications for research communication: Rather than merely critiquing existing policies, begin with a dialogue to understand the aims of the policymaker. Frame advice in response to the current situation, but seek to understand the history that has led up to it. Do you know what needs, constraints, and zeitgeist are behind a past policy and to what extent they still exist?

6. Crises, such as natural disasters and pandemics, serve as focusing events for policymakers, who need to be responsive to the moment.

Implications for research communication: Recognize that science and policy often must act on different timescales. Communicate the current state of the relevant science, including the source and magnitude of uncertainty, as well as the implications of the uncertainty for the policy decision.

7. Policymakers need to balance differing opinions, values, and needs.

Implications for research communication: Be aware of your own and others' values and be transparent about what tradeoffs are involved in a decision for which you are advocating. Set goals that are realistic given the size of the budget and number of competing priorities. Avoid the disconnect that can happen when scientists focus on only one aspect of a multifaceted political problem. Aspire for the scientific evidence to be considered fully, but do not expect it to be the exclusive consideration.

Regulatory decisions usually involve a bifurcated process, in which scientists synthesize and analyze the literature before the policymakers take over.[80] Values clearly come into play when science and technology are applied to societal problems, the second part of the regulatory process, but recognize how the first part involves subjective judgments as well. For example, a high standard of evidence may be required to claim that a drug works, but a lower standard of evidence may be acceptable to show that an environmental chemical causes harm.[81]

Communicating to support good deliberation for decision-making requires the skills to make information comprehensible without losing those details and nuances that make the information meaningful. Oversimplified popular science accounts can actually impede the goal of supporting deliberation. This is because of the tendency of people to overestimate their understanding when they read popular depictions of science, compared to when they read more substantive accounts.[82] Ignorance of one's ignorance is known as the Dunning-Kruger effect.[83] The common "keep it simple" communication advice can serve to fuel the Dunning-Kruger effect; better advice is "keep it clear." To explore what that means when communicating to inform decisions that involve comparing complex tradeoffs and uncertainties in the context of diverse values, we will trade in our mountaineering gear for a warp drive.

6

Negotiating Uncertainty and the Intricacies of Tradeoffs

Was the solution to "The Trouble with Tribbles" ethical?
Does artificial intelligence deserve rights? What about Lt. Commander Data?
Would you like genetically modified produce to have a GMO label?
Should non-native species be removed to save native species?
Is it appropriate to require doctors to get an annual flu vaccine?
How should greenhouse gases be regulated?

Tribbles, as Star Trek fans will know, are tiny fuzzball pets from the *Star Trek: The Original Series* episode "The Trouble with Tribbles." Their astounding rate of reproduction led to trouble on the *Enterprise* – at least until Spock and Chief Engineer Scott found a solution that, the viewer is left to assume, did not end well for either the tribbles or the Klingons. Lieutenant Commander Data is the very human-like android on *Star Trek: The Next Generation.* The question of his rights was the focus of the powerful "The Measure of a Man" episode. Fiction often raises enduring ethical questions, either grappling with them head on, as in "The Measure of a Man," or opening the can of worms (or tribbles, as the case may be) and leaving the grappling to the audience.

Art imitates life. The myriad health, science, and technology choices we make as individuals and societies (such as the choices highlighted in the non–Star Trek questions above) involve complex tradeoffs and uncertainties. Effective communication about these issues considers the full range of tradeoffs. Whether the decision is to be made collectively or will ultimately be left to the individual, you can inform the conversation by bringing what is missing to the table, by understanding and making room for others' values, and by developing transparent ways of discussing uncertainty. How communication can do these things to meaningfully inform the decision-making process is the focus of this chapter.

CHAPTER LEARNING OBJECTIVES: TRADEOFFS AND UNCERTAINTIES

Knowledge: How should potential costs, benefits, and uncertainties be identified and discussed?

Skills: Clarify complexity with humility, humanity, and room for multiple perspectives.

Habits of Mind: Cultivate awareness of value judgments made in assessments of tradeoffs.

THE SMORGASBORD OF TRADEOFFS AND THE HEKARAS CORRIDOR

Identify the Types of Tradeoffs and Help Get the Full Scope of Tradeoffs on the Table

A decision about the best treatment for a health condition involves comparing the pros and cons of alternative treatments. A decision about how to handle an environmental problem involves comparing the environmental pros and cons of the alternative remediation plans. In both these examples, the pros and cons appear to fall into the same category, human health in the first example and the environment in the second. Yet the reality is more complex. Environmental and health decisions typically involve economic calculations. The decision to remove non-native species will likely require an assessment of the economic costs and benefits of intervening. In making decisions about preventive health measures, individuals and governments may calculate potential economic costs of the intervention versus the disease. Some decisions, such as regulating greenhouse gases, must consider economic costs and benefits, as well as those to human health and the environment. Facilitating the assessment of tradeoffs entails listening to determine whether economic, environmental, or human health costs and benefits may be missing from the conversation, and respectfully introducing them as appropriate. Discussion may need to make room for well-being costs and benefits that go beyond standard measures of health, such as the psychological benefits of preserving natural beauty or protecting cultural heritage.

Ensure that the Proverbial Can Is Not Kicked Down the Road to Other Times, Places, and People

For many decisions, costs and benefits are not incurred simultaneously. They may accumulate over a lifetime, as is the case with many nutrition and lifestyle choices. They may be separated by more than a human lifespan, as is common in decisions that affect the environment. Very long-term tradeoffs therefore separate costs and benefits across generations. Shorter-term tradeoffs may also split the costs and benefits across individuals or populations. The affected individuals or ecosystems may be from different geographic regions, such as with respect to water usage by those higher in the watershed. They may be in different socioeconomic (or other demographic) groups, such as in decisions about urban development that lead to gentrification. Costs and benefits may also be distributed across populations separated by both geography and socioeconomic status, either within one country or between developed and developing nations.

As underscored in the *Star Trek: The Next Generation* "Tapestry" episode, in which the god-like being Q allows Captain Jean-Luc Picard to go back in time to alter a pivotal life decision, we are not especially good at predicting the knock-on effects of our actions. A strategy used to handle knock-on effects in formal risk assessment is **bounded rationality**, which addresses complexity by leaving out certain elements to more thoroughly address those that remain.[1] Consider the example of farm regulations to protect drinking water supplies. Reducing runoff of farm waste may protect the environment by preventing algal blooms in downstream rivers and lakes, thereby safeguarding the drinking water supply, but resulting in higher food production costs. The impact on food prices could be estimated by assuming that the costs incurred by farmers will be passed on to consumers; however, predicting how this cost may in turn alter consumers' nutritional intake, with potential resulting health implications, is likely to be beyond the scope of the assessment. Bounded rationality may cause local impacts to be emphasized over global impacts or more certain short-term effects to be emphasized over long-term ones.

Highlight Both Individual and Altruistic Reasons for Action

In the *Star Trek: The Next Generation* "The Forces of Nature" episode, two funkily dressed Hekaran scientists make the case that the fabric of space in the important Hekaran Corridor is being destroyed by the cumulative erosion caused by the warp drives of passing vessels. The Federation ultimately agrees to reduce the use of warp drive in the Corridor, but, in an example of "the tragedy of the commons," it is noted that compliance may not be universal.[2] Likewise with vaccination against an infectious disease, there exists a "paradox" between the interests of the individual and the interests of the community. Herd immunity reduces risk of infection among those who are not immune (including young children and the immunocompromised), and thus adds a benefit to the cost-benefit analysis of vaccination from the perspective of society. If herd immunity reaches a certain level, however, it is rational for an individual to "free ride," because a free rider gets the benefits of the vaccine through herd immunity without the risks of the vaccine.[3] Communication about tradeoffs must therefore distinguish between individual and societal benefits. Making altruistic reasons for actions explicit can encourage individuals to act in the interests of the common good.[4]

RESPECTING THE KLINGONS AND THE ROLE OF VALUES IN WEIGHING TRADEOFFS

Be Explicit about What "Currency" Is Being Used to Compare Incommensurables

Trading off environmental or human health with economics is comparing the incommensurable.[5] Although it is possible to assign a worth in dollars to a species or to the reduction in a person's joint pain, this "currency conversion" is arbitrary. It follows that identification and weighing of costs and benefits can never be a cut-and-dried objective process. For example, if a decision could lead to premature deaths (or the prevention of premature deaths), should the loss (or gain) be measured in terms of lives or in terms of life-years? Counting life-years is more transparent in certain contexts (such as a medication that can extend the lifespan by a year or two), but in other contexts (such as who should be given priority to receive an organ donation), counting life-years instead of lives can be criticized as devaluing the lives of older adults and creating a "senior discount." The value judgments made in the comparison of incommensurable costs and benefits should be articulated.

Be Cognizant of the Misalignment between Technical and Popular Risk Assessment

In introducing policies or approving new products, regulatory agencies conduct technical assessments of the potential costs and benefits, but sociological analyses reveal that these focus on only a subset of what people typically value.[6] Technical assessments of the possibility of loss or injury, **risk**, are based on two factors: the severity of the potential adverse event and the likelihood of its occurrence.[7] Public perception of risk is also influenced by severity and likelihood, but decades of research on risk perception demonstrates that people's views of risk are influenced by a much richer array of factors, including familiarity, control, understanding, naturalness, and equitability.[8]

FAMILIARITY

When a potential hazard is new or unfamiliar, perception of risk is increased.[9] In general, people are more willing to tolerate risk from established activities and technologies than from new ones.[10] This is logical in that more is known about how to protect oneself from a familiar risk, but this precautionary approach can result in the grandfathering in of old technologies while equally or less risky newer technologies are deemed unacceptable.[11]

CONTROL

A foundational article in the field of technical risk assessment differentiated between risks from voluntary and involuntary activities.[12] Voluntary activities are under the control of an individual, and thus exposure is governed by the individual's own value system, whereas (human-made) involuntary risks are under the control of an authoritative body, such as a government agency. For a given level of benefit, publics are more willing to tolerate voluntary than involuntary risks.[13]

UNDERSTANDING

When a risk is perceived as not well understood by scientists or by those exposed to the risk, it tends to be perceived as larger and less acceptable.[14] Nonetheless, more scientific knowledge does not necessarily reduce perceived risk, because research can draw attention to how much remains unknown. For example, in a replication of a study on how people rank risks, conducted nearly 40 years after the initial study, high school football jumped markedly along the scale from known to unknown risk.[15] Although more is known about head trauma today, in the decades since the original study, people (including scientists) have come to recognize substantial gaps in scientific understanding.

NATURALNESS

Public perception of risk is increased when the risks are human-made, particularly when they are due to human failure, compared to the risks from natural causes.[16] Tampering with nature is another aspect of how naturalness plays into risk perception; for example, it is a factor that explains part of the variance in perceptions of risk from nuclear power.[17] These views may be at least partly attributable to the underestimation of the potential for human error in past nuclear disasters.[18]

EQUITABILITY

Questions about equity in the distribution of risk may be raised when publics feel they are being unfairly burdened – the not-in-my-backyard (NIMBY) issue – or when concerned stakeholders assess that vulnerable groups are being burdened by more than their fair share of the risks.[19] For example, poor and minority communities tend to be disproportionately exposed to environmental hazards.[20]

To improve communication, expand on technical assessments of costs and benefits to make room for a broader array of considerations, such as familiarity, control, and understanding. Because people consider many factors other than severity and likelihood when reasoning about risk, comparisons made by communicators in good faith can backfire.[21] You may try to show people that they have accepted "similar" risks in the past, only to discover that your comparison is too crude to account for the nuanced ways people reason about risk.

Explore Alternative Problem Formulations to Reveal Implicit Value Judgments

The "Trolley Problem," commonly used in philosophy courses, involves two similar ethical dilemmas: (1) By flipping a switch you can save several people from a runaway trolley by sacrificing one person; and (2) you can save several people by sacrificing one person, but this time instead of flipping a switch, you have to push that person in front of the trolley. In both scenarios, the number of people sacrificed and saved is the same, and thus based on cold logic, people should respond identically to both scenarios. Of course, this is not what is observed. In the first scenario, most people say they would flip the switch. In the second scenario, most people say that they would not push the person onto the tracks.[22] The tradeoff of one life for several is deemed reasonable in one context but not in the other, which highlights the difference between **consequentialist** and **deontological** ethics. In consequentialism, only the outcomes matter (lives are saved by sacrificing one person), but in deontology, principles matter (it is wrong to push someone into harm's way). The alternative problem formulations bring different ethical considerations to the fore.

In the same vein, what if the word "removed" was replaced with the word "killed" in the question about native species at the beginning of the chapter: "*Should non-native species be killed to save native species?*" This is not a hypothetical example. In the Pacific Northwest, the larger, more aggressive, and voracious barred owl is moving into the habitat of the native spotted owl and threatening the extinction of the latter. Barred owls are being killed to save spotted owls.[23] Does your own view of the issue shift if, instead of "aggressive and voracious," barred owls are characterized as "highly adaptable"?

Consider minor edits to the other questions at the beginning of this chapter. Change "require" to "force" in the fifth question to stress the (lack of) freedom of choice: "*Is it appropriate to force doctors to get an annual flu vaccine?*" Highlight the economic considerations by adding them to the question about food labeling: "*Would you pay more to ensure that all genetically modified produce has a GMO label?*" Remove the implicit assumption inherent in the "How?" and ask "*Should greenhouse gases be regulated?*" The alternative formulations can spotlight alternative viewpoints.

Familiarize Yourself with the Different Dimensions through which People See the World

The portrayal of the Klingons in *Star Trek: The Original Series* is as antagonists deserving of the dangerous joke played on them in "The Trouble with Tribbles." Their portrayal shifts dramatically in the later Star Trek series, in which the Klingon Empire has become allied with the Federation. The audience is invited to learn about the rich history and culture of the Klingons, particularly through Worf, a main character on *Star Trek: The Next Generation* as well as *Star Trek: Deep Space 9*. We learn about Klingon customs and values, and while we (and even Worf himself) do not always relate to Klingon worldviews (or universe-views), we learn to respect them. Respect for difference and sincere efforts at understanding are at the heart of successful coalitions in the Star Trek universe.

To understand differences in culture back here on Earth, Dutch management researcher Geert Hofstede developed a framework, known as **Hofstede's cultural dimensions theory**, which identifies six dimensions along which cultures differ.[24] Consider how the Klingons or your own favorite science fiction culture falls along these dimensions:

1. *Power distance* – the extent to which the culture is egalitarian or embraces hierarchy
2. *Collectivism versus individualism* – the extent to which the emphasis is on group well-being or on attaining personal goals
3. *Uncertainty avoidance* – the extent to which uncertainty, ambiguity, and risk-taking is accepted or regulated through rules and regulations

Figure 6.1 Unbounding Rationality to Prepare for Dialogues on Complex Issues

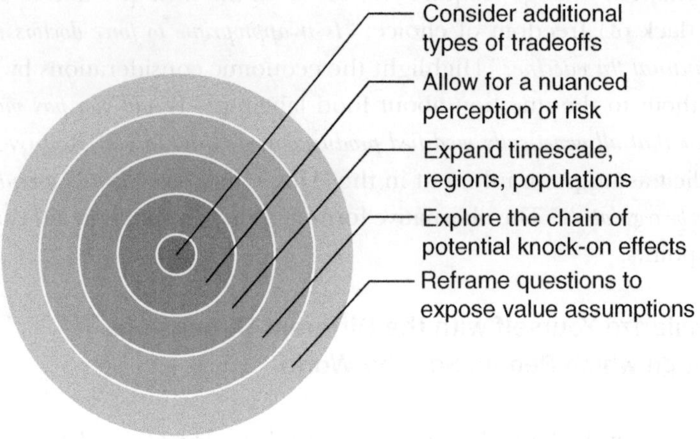

- Consider additional types of tradeoffs
- Allow for a nuanced perception of risk
- Expand timescale, regions, populations
- Explore the chain of potential knock-on effects
- Reframe questions to expose value assumptions

4. *Femininity versus masculinity* – the extent of fluidity in gender roles and whether the focus is on quality of life or material wealth
5. *Short-term versus long-term orientation* – the extent of focus on the present and quick results or on delaying gratification to achieve future goals
6. *Restraint versus indulgence* – the extent to which social norms regulate gratification of impulses and desires

The first two of these dimensions have received more study than the others, as part of a theory – cultural cognition – that has been used to (partly) explain how people make sense of environmental and health risks.[25] Hofstede's cultural dimensions have received criticism for treating cultures as static rather than as dynamic and painting them in broad strokes, ignoring differences such as influences of gender, age, and geography within countries.[26] Just as Worf does not speak for all Klingons, culture must not be equated with language or national identity. With that important caveat in mind, the dimensions are a thought-provoking way to think about the diversity of values that may influence people's actions and decisions. Figure 6.1 summarizes the steps in a holistic approach that sets the stage for making decisions about complex issues.

TALKING ABOUT WHAT WE KNOW ABOUT WHAT WE DON'T KNOW

It took over a generation for Star Trek fans to find out the ending of the tribble trouble story (with the thread having been picked up in *Star Trek: Deep Space 9*: "Trials and Tribble-ations"), and no one could have predicted it. Sure, time travel adds extra uncertainty to the Star Trek universe, but our universe can be pretty uncertain too. During the COVID-19 pandemic, uncertainty shook individuals, societies, and economic systems to their cores. Communication about uncertainty beyond technical audiences requires a special skill set for several reasons:

1. Representing uncertainty accurately is central to ethical communication.
2. Uncertainty is often inaccurately portrayed to publics, especially in the media.
3. Uncertainty takes different forms, some of which are difficult to identify.
4. Uncertainty comes in different magnitudes.
5. Uncertainty arises from many sources.

To provide a foundation to discuss uncertainty with diverse audiences, this section begins with a meta-level perspective and builds to practical guidelines in the form of a "documenting uncertainty framework."

Balance the Ethical Norms in Communication about Uncertainty

Ethical norms for communication of uncertainty in science have been established and include the following:

- Honesty
- Process transparency
- Specification of uncertainty about conclusions
- Precision
- Audience relevance[27]

Honesty is the primary norm and is a matter of not only avoiding deliberate misstatements, but also avoiding deliberately misleading incompleteness. It entails intellectual honesty with your audience as well as with yourself. With respect to the latter, researchers must give full consideration to legitimate criticisms of their methods, results, and conclusions.

The norms of **process transparency** and **specification of uncertainty about conclusions** refer to what should be communicated. Process transparency means explaining the process by which a conclusion was reached. Specification of uncertainty about conclusions means describing the source and degree of uncertainty in the conclusions, which may be a numerical value or a subjective best judgment. This is especially challenging when different experts have legitimately different predictions for future scenarios, particularly when a small but significant probability of a very damaging outcome exists.

Precision and **audience relevance** must be balanced against each other. Scientists endeavor to describe the world in precise terms, but this typically requires technical language and details confusing to non-technical audiences. To be intelligible to those outside their fields, researchers must strive to provide the pertinent details without assuming that the needs of all publics are the same. It is in this balancing act of precision versus audience relevance that the distinction between simplification and clarification is pivotal. Simplification removes unnecessary technical details, but clarification makes explicit the essential details that specialists in a discipline take for granted. For example, policymakers may need clarification about what factors are missing from a model (even when it is obvious to research colleagues).

Avoid the Common Pitfalls in Portrayals of Uncertainty

BY RESEARCHERS

False assurances, doomsday forecasts, and hyped promises portray uncertain outcomes as certain. "Incredible certitude" is common in predictions of policy outcomes; for example, the US Congressional Budget Office is required by Congress to make point predictions 10 years into the future about the federal debt implications of pending legislation, unaccompanied by measures of uncertainty.[28] The dangers of incredible certitude are elevated during a crisis, when honest and clear communication about uncertainty, and avoiding the downplaying of ambiguities, is key to building and maintaining public trust.[29] For example, early in the bovine spongiform encephalopathy (BSE) crisis in the United Kingdom, government authorities did not address the uncertainty at all; instead they attempted to assuage panic by confidently stating that BSE in cows could not transmit to humans.[30] The false assurances led to a long-lasting lack of trust in the regulatory authorities. In addition to maintaining trust, the open acknowledgement of uncertainty can fuel public support for future research to reduce uncertainty. In a health setting, the acknowledgement of uncertainty can help terminally ill patients maintain a positive outlook.[31]

Yet researchers may have legitimate concerns about being transparent about uncertainty. The existence of uncertainty has been used to legitimate the status quo, for example in the case of the application of the precautionary principle to new technologies.[32] Furthermore, those with vested interests can manipulate the boundary between certainty and uncertainty.[33] For example, the same cast of characters that propagated doubt about the causal relationship between smoking tobacco and increased risk of cancer (long after the scientific community was in agreement) were also the most vociferous in propagating doubt about the existence of anthropogenic climate change.[34] The possibility of manipulation may make communicators hesitant to communicate uncertainty, but inadequate communication of the real uncertainties, including those about the impacts of global warming at the local level and the uncertainties about the best course(s) of action, may have inadvertently fed the debate about the soundness of climate science.[35] Furthermore, when people are likely to encounter conflicting news stories about a topic, the stories may be deemed incoherent in the absence of an explanation for the uncertainty.[36] These findings underscore that it is in researchers' best interests to clearly communicate the uncertainties of their research to the media and place new findings in the context of prior work.

BY THE MEDIA

In covering complex scientific issues, journalists run the risk of making Type 1 (accepting false information by relying on an established view,

such as a government authority) and Type 2 (rejecting true information by placing too much credence in opposing voices) errors.[37] In the
interest of avoiding a Type 1 error, journalists may go out of their way
to present the views of maverick scientists, even when they do not find
those views credible.[38] The effect is to give audiences the impression
that scientists are more divided than they actually are.[39] Audiences may
devalue or discredit the information as a result.[40] In news stories about
contested science, weight-of-evidence reporting, which provides information about how experts and evidence are aligned along a continuum
of claims about an issue, helps audiences sort out the relative validity of
claims.[41] Over time, coverage of an issue may gradually shift from false
balance to weight of evidence, but the shift may lag the general scientific consensus on the issue.[42]

Journalists need to better distinguish between well-founded and
not-well-founded findings. Findings are more likely to be true when
the studies are larger, the effect sizes are larger, hypothesis testing is
selective (as opposed to high-throughput discovery-oriented research),
methods are standardized, conflicts of interest are absent, and the field
is not too hot and rushed.[43] In science coverage, two message features
help audiences recognize the tentativeness of findings: the avoidance
of purely optimistic framing and the inclusion of details about study
limitations.[44] Inclusion of information about gaps in knowledge or
about technical limitations of studies does not have negative effects
on the credibility of information.[45] In fact, publics are skeptical when
statements are presented as overly certain.[46] When conflicting evidence
exists about a topic, however, people have much more favorable attitudes when the information is disclosed in the form of study caveats –
that is the reasons for the uncertainty – than when presented as dueling
experts without sufficient context.[47]

Develop a Common Language to Identify and Describe Uncertainty

Scholars have defined the term **uncertainty** in different ways. In *Ignorance
and Uncertainty: Emerging Paradigms*, it is narrowly defined as a situation
in which we know what we do not know and have a numerical range of
possibility.[48] That book introduces two terms to express other aspects of
the unknown: indeterminacy and ignorance. **Indeterminacy** is defined as

the state of affairs in which we know what we do not know, but we do not have numerical estimates of the gap in knowledge. The third category is **ignorance**, defined as the situation in which we do not know what we do not know. These are the "unknown unknowns" made infamous in Donald Rumsfeld's speech about Iraq's weapons of mass destruction.[49]

The distinction between these types of knowledge gaps is crucial for scientists and for communicators who may overlook what cannot be measured. A critique of technology and policy risk assessments is that they focus on the unknowns that are easiest to analyze but omit the less obvious unknowns. This tendency has been called "lamp-posting," referring to the story of a drunk man searching for his keys under the street lamp, not because he lost them there, but because that is where there was sufficient light to see.[50] When unknown unknowns are very large, lamp-posting leads to overconfidence as risk assessors emphasize the quantifiable uncertainties to the exclusion of indeterminacy and ignorance.

With respect to language to communicate about unknowns, however, the term "indeterminacy" is jargon to most audiences and the term "ignorance" is hidden jargon with negative connotations. Also, the boundary between unknowns is blurry. In the real world, uncertainty comes in multiple gradations between statistical uncertainty and ignorance, and it also includes conflicting evidence.[51] Another problem with the terminology is that different scholars use different terms for the same forms of unknowns and the same terms for different forms of unknowns.[52] In *Rationality*, for example, uncertainty is narrowly defined as Rumsfeld's unknown unknowns.[53] Note the discrepancy with how uncertainty is defined, and unknown unknowns are termed, in *Ignorance and Uncertainty: Emerging Paradigms*. To help those communicating about research and its implications, the documenting uncertainty framework presented in this chapter provides a more precise and accessible way of communicating about uncertainty, and one that allows room for nuance. The framework uses uncertainty as the umbrella term for all unknowns, and it instead differentiates uncertainties by their magnitude and source.

Do Not Overlook the Magnitude of the Uncertainty

Uncertainty comes in degrees, but puzzlingly, prior research has often failed to explicitly identify the magnitude as an aspect of uncertainty.[54] Magnitude of the uncertainty has been confounded with the type of knowledge gap – that is, the continuum from statistical uncertainty to ignorance.[55] It is not necessarily the case, however, that statistical uncertainty is smaller than ignorance; for example, a situation may have few unknown unknowns, but many known parameters with large statistical uncertainty. Another overlooked aspect of magnitude is that the different types of uncertainty about a situation are not necessarily additive. One form of uncertainty may overlap with another. Uncertainty in two parameters may partly cancel each other out. Therefore, in documenting uncertainty, all the distinct forms of uncertainty should be itemized as well as evaluated as a whole.

Specify the Sources of the Uncertainty

Meta-level research about uncertainty tends to focus on single topics, such as climate change models or food hazards or health care.[56] As a result, each study presents distinct takes on uncertainty. An attempt to synthesize across the literature identified three "objects" of uncertainty: facts, numbers, and scientific hypotheses.[57] These distinctions are valuable, particularly for the paper's intended audience of other researchers; however, on their own they are too simplistic for communicating meaningful information for practical decision-making purposes. It is relevant to know the source of uncertainty, not simply that the uncertainty is about a fact, a number, or a scientific hypothesis. Various taxonomies of uncertainty have been developed, but their heavy use of hidden jargon, terms such as "vagueness," "fuzziness," "ambiguity," and "imprecision" make them unsuitable as tools to meaningfully categorize uncertainty for publics.[58] Nonetheless, this research provides a foundation on which to build. One of the taxonomies of uncertainty begins with a split into three branches: world, evidence, and decision maker. Despite interconnections between these categories (e.g., evidence is about the world, and decisions lead to actions on the world), this parsing has intuitive appeal and forms the backbone of the user-friendly documenting uncertainty framework presented here.

A DOCUMENTING UNCERTAINTY FRAMEWORK

The documenting uncertainty framework includes a checklist of the sources of uncertainty in three categories: (1) the world (the object of study), (2) the research (the study), and (3) the decision-making (the application of the study), each with a checklist of items. The framework also includes questions about the magnitude of the uncertainty, the potential for resolution of the uncertainty, and the nature of any disagreements about the research. The framework thus guides users to prepare for communication by thinking through the following questions: What is uncertain and why? How uncertain is it? When might it be more certain? Who is uncertain?

What Is Uncertain and Why?

SOURCES OF UNCERTAINTY ABOUT THE WORLD

Several sources of uncertainty exist about the world, which is broadly defined to include anything that is the focus of the research. One source of uncertainty is *variation across contexts*. Human aspirations, behaviors, and health vary across age, gender, and other demographic factors, and rules, customs, and habits vary across cultures and societies. Living things share many basic building blocks and organizing principles, but different species or strains of organisms can vary unexpectedly. Variation also characterizes the nonliving (abiotic) aspects of the world. Geography, such as topography and soil composition, as well as weather patterns and other conditions, vary by locale. Variation also occurs across historical time periods or geological eras. All this variation means that the conclusions of any research conducted in one context may not hold up in others.

Another aspect of uncertainty about the world is *divergence of immediate and long-term outcomes*. For example, small amounts of a chemical may not be immediately harmful to an organism or ecosystem, but bioaccumulation may lead to harmful effects in the longer term. In other cases, short-term harms or benefits may occur, but adaptation may diminish the long-term impacts. *Complexity due to indirect or multifactor causality* is a tricky source of uncertainty in issues including human health, genetic engineering, and climate change. It is difficult to tease apart the causal influence of genes and environmental factors, the interlinked networks of responses in ecosystems, and the complexity of climate feedbacks among landmasses, oceans, and the layers of the atmosphere. In addition to indirect causality, *randomness or chaotic behavior* is characteristic of some systems, such as weather and geological processes. Finally, the world has dark matter and other *unobservable or unstudiable phenomena*, which may become researchable as new scientific tools are developed.

SOURCES OF UNCERTAINTY ABOUT THE RESEARCH

The first aspect of uncertainty about research is *statistical variation due to instrumentation or methodology*. Examples are false negative or false positive rates of medical tests and sampling error in conducting surveys. Another cause of uncertainty about research is *incomplete data*, which includes preliminary studies with small samples or a small number of observations, studies that are more robust in terms of the number of observations but nonetheless are confined to one or a limited number of contexts, and studies with only short-term data when effects may be longer term. *Ambiguous data* can result from issues with study design, such as a longitudinal study in which data collection procedures have changed over time, or studies in which experimental observations perturb the subjects or phenomena under study. An example of this is the Hawthorne effect, in which humans change their behavior when they know (or just think) they are being studied.[59] Ambiguous data may also arise from research that is thoughtfully designed but nonetheless can only demonstrate correlation, not causation. *Conflicting data* can arise inexplicably or when a study is performed with even small context or procedure variations. Finally, mathematical and computational models have *model limitations*, arising from uncertainty associated with the factors that are part of the model as well as from possible missing factors or relationships between factors.

SOURCES OF UNCERTAINTY ABOUT THE DECISION-MAKING

Additional uncertainties crop up when the fruits of scientific research are to be applied to the world, in the form of advice, policies, or technologies. *Ethical questions about the best course of action* develop because societal decisions about science involve tradeoffs that may differentially benefit or burden different segments of society. Another source of uncertainty that arises during the decision-making process is the *identity and behavior of the decision maker(s)*. Researchers cannot usually control who the policymakers or other decision makers will be and how those individuals or collectives will use the products of science. Uncertainty may also arise because of a *mismatch between context of research and context of application.* Application of research often involves generalization beyond the context of the research study. Furthermore, the real world may have an *unpredictable response to implementation* of the decision. This can happen because the research is applied in a novel context, but also because a real-world phenomenon may be irreducibly complex. Finally, *technological surprises* in the form of unexpected breakthroughs or side effects may occur.[60]

How Uncertain Is It?

For each of the sources of uncertainty relevant to the research under consideration, both direct and indirect levels of uncertainty should be documented.[61] The *magnitude* of the uncertainty (direct uncertainty) should be noted as precisely as possible, either quantitatively or as a qualitative verbal statement. The *degree of confidence* or the uncertainty about the uncertainty (indirect uncertainty) should accompany the statement of magnitude, either as a confidence interval or as a qualitative statement. The magnitude and degree of confidence for each source of uncertainty may not be relevant to a particular audience, but be prepared to provide details as appropriate. At minimum, a *holistic evaluation* of uncertainty across sources should be shared in an audience-accessible manner.

When Might It Be More Certain?

For those applying information to personal or policy decisions, it is useful to know how the state of understanding may progress. Uncertainty may be unresolvable or aleatory; for example, it is not possible to precisely predict a future scenario that is influenced by random or chaotic behavior.[62] Alternatively, uncertainty may be epistemic, in which limited information is available about things that are at least theoretically knowable. Communicators should state whether *additional research* could resolve or reduce the uncertainty and whether the work is currently *feasible.* Audiences will also want to know *when* more could be known. Naturally, if a follow-up study is currently underway, the answer to the "when" question can be more precise than if the research is not currently feasible.

Who Is Uncertain?

When differences of opinion exist about research, audiences need to know who disagrees. Is the *disagreement* among scientists? Disagreements between scientists are a natural part of the scientific process, but even when the science itself is fairly settled, *decision makers* may disagree about how to apply the science. *Stakeholders* may deliberately play up or play down uncertainty.

The documenting uncertainty framework (Table 6.1) provides a structure and vocabulary for conversations about uncertainty and a systematic way for communicators to take stock of the uncertainty. For nonexperts writing about a study, it provides insight into what questions they may need to ask the researchers. For the researchers themselves, it is an opportunity to reflect on what the audience needs to know. It is also a reminder why it is unhelpful and patronizing to tell people, "There is nothing to worry about." When I hear this, it raises my hackles. Closed mindedness inhibits communication and, for that matter, science. If, after examining the evidence and taking stock of the uncertainty, you are not worried, make your thinking visible instead of telling people what they should think. Say what course of action you prefer and why. What uncertainty information ultimately needs to be communicated to a particular audience depends on the type of decision to be made, whether it involves identifying a threshold for action (such as evacuating from a flood zone), selecting among fixed options (such as raw materials for dam construction), or designing options (such as new approaches for conserving water resources) by imagining what is possible.[63] For any decision to be made in the face of uncertainty, effective communication not only entails providing the relevant information but also establishing trust.

CLARIFY COMPLEXITY WITH HUMILITY, HUMANITY, AND PERSPECTIVE-TAKING

When communicators are trusted, communication is relatively easy, and good communication can help prevent errors that lead to misuse, accidents, and other unintended consequences. In the absence of trust, however, communication is likely to fall on deaf ears. The challenge of

Table 6.1. Documenting Uncertainty Framework

SPECIFY THE SOURCES OF UNCERTAINTY *(What and Why?)*

World *(The object of study)*
- ◊ Variation across contexts
  - ○ Individuals or societies
  - ○ Strains or species
  - ○ Geography or conditions
  - ○ Time or era
- ◊ Divergence of immediate and long-term outcomes
- ◊ Complexity due to indirect or multifactor causality
- ◊ Randomness or chaotic behavior
- ◊ Unobservable or unstudiable phenomena

Research *(The study)*
- ◊ Statistical variation due to instrumentation or methodology
- ◊ Incomplete data
  - ○ Small sample or few observations
  - ○ Limited context(s) studied
  - ○ No or insufficient long-term tracking
- ◊ Ambiguous data
  - ○ Issues with study design
  - ○ Data show correlation but do not prove causation
- ◊ Conflicting data
  - ○ Inexplicable replication failures
  - ○ Variation across study contexts
- ◊ Model limitations
  - ○ Factor (parameter) variability
  - ○ Possible missing factors or relationships

Decision-Making *(The application of the study)*
- ◊ Ethical questions about best course of action
- ◊ The identity and behavior of the decision maker(s)
- ◊ Mismatch between context of research and context of application
- ◊ Unpredictable response to implementation
- ◊ Technological surprises

DETERMINE THE MAGNITUDE OF THE UNCERTAINTY *(How?)*
- ◊ Magnitude as numerical value or verbal statement?
- ◊ Degree of confidence in quantity or estimate?
- ◊ Holistic evaluation of uncertainty across sources?

PROJECT PROGRESS ON STATE OF UNDERSTANDING *(When?)*
- ◊ Could additional research resolve or reduce the uncertainty?
- ◊ Is the research currently feasible? If not, why not?
- ◊ When could more be known?

PROVIDE INSIGHT INTO DISAGREEMENTS *(Who?)*
- ◊ Disagreement among scientists?
- ◊ Disagreement among decision makers or others?
- ◊ Stakeholders playing up or playing down the uncertainty?

---

establishing and maintaining trust is that it tends to be created slowly over time, but it can be destroyed relatively quickly by a single mishap. This has been dubbed "the asymmetry principle," and it results from the fact that trust-destroying events are typically more dramatic, visible, and likely to receive news coverage than trust-building ones.[64] Inaccurately conveying tradeoffs or uncertainties can lead to a trust-destroying event. An example is the 1997 Red River Flood in Minnesota and North Dakota that caused more than a billion dollars in damages. The National Weather Service was blamed for making inaccurate predictions about the extreme flooding event, but the crux of the failure was not inaccurate predictions – it was unclear communication of the uncertainty to local decision makers.[65]

TRUST-BUILDING PRINCIPLES FOR COMMUNICATION
TO INFORM DECISION-MAKING

1. *Clarifying complexity* is central to effective science communication.
2. *Humility* is paramount when assessing tradeoffs and uncertainty.
3. *Humanity* needs to be acknowledged and discussed transparently.
4. *Perspective-taking* makes room for diverse stakeholders' viewpoints.

Clarify Complexity

Clarifying complexity is a thread throughout this book and is central to effective communication, whether the audience is nonscientists or colleagues in your field of research. The skill lies in being able to identify what needs clarification (why do Romulans look like Vulcans?), how much clarification is needed (state they are related or give the details of their history?) and how to provide it (by selecting among your many creative options). In informing decisions, clear communication is not only a matter of being understood, but also (as the Red River Flood example illustrates) about being trusted. Along with the ability to clarify complexity, building trust and fostering inclusive communication requires humility, humanity, and perspective-taking.

Cultivate Humility

Humility is paramount because decisions are made on the basis of incomplete information. To better govern risk and to avoid trust-destroying debacles, Harvard Kennedy School of Government's Sheila Jasanoff has advocated for methods and institutionalized habits of thought that can help political leaders, regulators, and societies come to terms with and manage uncertainty – what she calls "technologies of humility."[66] She argues that humility requires new forms of engagement between decision makers, experts, and publics, specifically, the opportunity for dialogues that allow for a wide range of knowledge and skills to be brought to the governance process. After all, ethical uncertainty about the best course of action is a distinct form of uncertainty that necessitates explicit consideration.[67] To cultivate humility, channel the warmth and wisdom (and listening skills) of Guinan, the El-Aurian bartender portrayed by Whoopi Goldberg on *Star Trek: The Next Generation.*

In envisioning new forms of engaging with stakeholders, note that dialogue and decision-making are distinct processes. From top down to bottom up, decisions may be made in one of the following four ways.[68] **Command decisions** are made by a leader without discussion and can be suitable when the stakes are low and the leadership already has all the relevant information. **Consult decisions** are also made by someone in charge, but after gathering and considering input from others. **Vote decisions** allow team members or constituents to select one option from multiple options or to narrow down a large number of options to further consider the most popular ones. **Consensus decisions** involve dialoguing until everyone agrees on one option. Because consensus decisions take time, they are most appropriate for high-stakes issues. All these forms of decision-making have their place, but dialogues should never be used as a charade when the decision has already been made. It follows that humility entails transparency about how the final decision will be made and by whom.

Acknowledge Humanity

Be candid about what judgments play a role in each step of the decision-making process by being able to answer the following questions:

• Who enumerated the costs and benefits?
• Who assigned costs and benefits a worth and with what "currency system"?
• Who decided on the boundaries of the assessment?
• Who framed the problem?
• Who has been left out of the conversation?

Not only may viewpoints differ between different individuals within a society (like the unalike Ferengi brothers Quark and Rom on *Star Trek: Deep Space 9*), societal viewpoints change over time. The consequentialist ethical system known as utilitarianism – a moral perspective that emphasizes the greater good and the idea that the ends justify the means – long dominated views about medical research; however, modern guidance for the use of human subjects emphasizes informed consent.[69] Although doing the greatest good seems like a noble aim, utilitarianism has been used to justify medical research that cruelly disenfranchised human beings and in which less privileged groups have borne more than their fair share of the costs, while the affluent have reaped more than their fair share of the benefits.[70] The humanity principle thus invites tough questions about social justice.

Engage in Perspective-Taking

All the "who questions" raised by the considerations of the human elements in decision-making raise corresponding "what questions," as follows:

• What potential costs and benefits are missing from consideration?
• What are the alternative ways of assigning worth to the costs and benefits?
• What has been left out of the formal (bounded) assessment?
• What are the alternative ways to frame the problem?

- What are the potential inequalities in terms of how costs and benefits are divided across generations, locations, or demographics?

Researchers, especially those doing fundamental research, may need more encouragement to participate in conversations about ethical, legal, and social issues relevant to their fields.[71] Decisions, particularly those about complex socio-scientific issues, are design problems. Perspective-taking discussions are to inform a decision (whether a consult, vote, or consensus decision), not to evaluate value systems. We try to see the world from the warrior-honor perspective of the Klingons or the wealth-honor perspective of the Ferengi. When discussed in the abstract, value systems may seem irreconcilable, but in the context of a specific design decision, with the tradeoffs well articulated, the pragmatic task of deciding what can be traded off may very well converge on a workable solution that everyone can get behind.

Decision science is an approach that seeks to clarify costs, benefits, and uncertainties well enough that people can make informed decisions that reflect their own values.[72] It involves making predictions about the choices that fully informed individuals would make and then examining how people actually behave under those circumstances. This body of research must be read with a critical eye, but it has nonetheless shed valuable light on the reasoning shortcuts – heuristics – that we all use to make decisions in the face of unclear information. The next chapter explores this body of research and draws from it to provide guidance on the most effective ways to communicate about tradeoffs and uncertainties, including how to present numerical data. Turning the page will also blast us off from one science fiction universe to another.

How (Not) to Trigger Audiences' Decision-Making Survival Tactics

There are 27 sheep and 15 goats on a ship. How old is the captain?

This may sound like a satire of math word problems, but most elementary school students would answer it. Their likely response is also the answer to "the ultimate question of life, the universe, and everything" in Douglas Adams' *The Hitchhiker's Guide to the Galaxy*. This class of nonsense mathematics questions – so-called age-of-the-captain problems – has led to great consternation since it was discovered that students are seemingly oblivious to their nonsensicalness.[1] We could bemoan the state of the universe and then search for a cup of tea, but like in *The Hitchhiker's Guide*, things are not what they seem.

First, the mathematical operation students perform depends on the reasonableness of the answer. In the above instantiation of the problem, addition gives a reasonable answer for age, but when it does not, they may instead subtract, divide, or multiply, which demonstrates that they are engaging in sensemaking to solve the problem.[2] Moreover, changing the circumstances under which children receive this kind of problem completely changes the way they approach it. When told that a student wrote the problem and a textbook writer would like their feedback about it, nearly all identify its flaw.[3] Some even offer suggestions for improvement, for instance by incorporating an explicit statement that age is equivalent to the number of animals, or by stipulating that the person had acquired one animal annually since birth.

Children's seemingly nonsensical approach to age-of-the-captain problems is in actuality a sensible response to the trap of being asked by an adult to solve a nonsensical problem. The topic of this chapter is an aspect of reasoning that has likewise been treated as a shortcoming of the reasoner but is also often a survival tactic activated by confusing or flawed communication.

CHAPTER LEARNING OBJECTIVES: HEURISTICS

Knowledge: What kinds of shortcuts in reasoning do people use and under what conditions?

Skills: Provide relevant context and intelligible statistical information to support reasoning.

Habits of Mind: Recognize the adaptive benefits of intuition and emotion in decision-making.

TWO SYSTEMS OR NOT TWO SYSTEMS? THAT IS THE QUESTION

We Reason Systematically, Heuristically, or Both

The previous chapter focused on how to get costs, benefits, and uncertainties on the table in a way that allows people to engage in a systematic analysis of tradeoffs to make a decision. It was noted that even the most systematic analysis differs from a pie-in-the-sky ideal objective route to a decision, because perfectly rational beings can weigh tradeoffs differently, and practical limitations on how much information can be taken into account means that rationality is bounded. This chapter introduces yet another caveat of decision-making: the use of reasoning shortcuts called heuristics.[4]

Heuristic processing and systematic processing have been described as two systems of reasoning, also referred to as System 1 and System 2, where the former is quick, intuitive, and emotional and the latter is slower, methodical, and logical.[5] Heuristic processing involves reducing the scope of the information considered or simplifying the weighting of evidence.[6] Yet systematic and heuristic processing are not mutually exclusive systems, because these two forms of reasoning can co-occur and can mutually influence each other.[7] Individuals' motivations play a role in which processing mode is used, but even when people are motivated to process information systematically, heuristics may be used.[8] Heuristic processing can be used spontaneously and unconsciously, but it can also be used in a controlled and conscious manner.[9] Moreover, considerable evidence disputes the distinction between logical and emotional thinking.

Feelings Provide Information that Supports Decision-Making

Decision-making has traditionally been viewed as an "either-or" endeavor – either it is purely cognitive and rational, or it is tainted by emotion-driven mental shortcuts. In reality, emotion can play the supervisor on the construction site of rational thought. The most compelling evidence for this comes from the work of neurologist Antonio Damasio.[10] Damasio studied people who sustained brain damage that left their IQ and performance on cognitive tests intact but whose decision-making ability was nonetheless terribly compromised.

One striking example is a patient, "Elliot," who underwent surgery to remove a rapidly growing tumor that was pressing against the frontal lobes of his brain. Elliot had been a model husband and father and a successful businessperson, but after the brain damage his personal and professional life fell apart as he struggled with everyday decisions. He could still perform many distinct actions and retained his knowledge base, but faced with more complex tasks that involved categorizing, sorting, or choosing between options he would get stuck on steps at which he had to make a decision, such as which principle of categorization (e.g., chronological, alphabetical, pertinence) should be applied. His inability to complete the assignment made him appear lazy; instead, he was working hard on unnecessary details while losing sight of the overall purpose of the task.

Given a battery of cognitive tests, he passed them with flying colors, including tests of memory and intellect and tasks that involved performing moral reasoning, predicting the outcomes of social situations, and spontaneously considering the consequences of the different options. Yet after coming up with a variety of valid options, Elliot stated that he would not know what to do. Thus, the defect in Elliot's decision-making was in the later stages of reasoning near the point of choice. He could get all the options on the table, but then he could not settle on one of them.

Alongside the changes in Elliot's decision-making behavior were changes in his ability to experience emotion. He spoke detachedly about his personal tragedies. Those who knew him said that after the surgery he was uncharacteristically calm. Elliot himself articulated that situations and topics that had once elicited strong emotions no longer had the same effect. This is consistent with Elliot's injuries, which disrupted the circuitry between the higher regions of the brain and the amygdala, which serves as a clearinghouse for the positive and negative emotional associations that we accumulate over our lives. Elliot and other patients with similar symptoms and brain damage (including the famous case of Phineas Gage, who survived an accident in which an iron rod tore through the front of his skull and brain) led Damasio to conclude that input from the emotional regions of the brain streamlines the process of sorting through options in decision-making.

Emotions support rational decision-making by helping us deal with an overwhelming set of possibilities. A negative feeling a person experiences, even fleetingly, when an option comes to mind can act as an alarm to immediately reject that bad option. In contrast, a positive gut reaction focuses attention on the option that generated the feeling. These automated cues can narrow down the number of alternatives, increasing the efficiency of the decision-making process. Damasio called these feelings that serve as cues **somatic markers** (somatic from the Greek word "soma" meaning "body," and marker because they serve to mark the image that has come to mind). Somatic markers are feelings that past learning has connected to predicting future outcomes. In short, logic and emotion are integrated, not separate approaches to decision-making. Moreover, neuroanatomy and neuroimaging studies demonstrate that no region of the brain is purely responsible for emotion or purely responsible for cognition.[11] Cognition involves regions of the brain that are involved in emotion, and emotion involves regions of the brain that are involved in cognition.

Heuristics Can Be Both Efficient and Effective

Heuristic processing has been presented as a tradeoff between mental effort and accuracy.[12] In other words, in an ideal world we would use systematic processing for every decision, but if we did, our movement through the world would be slower than molasses in January. The assumption that relying on heuristics always sacrifices accuracy turns out to be incorrect: Heuristics improve reasoning in many contexts, particularly when attending to more information distracts a reasoner from what is most important. An example is the use of the recognition heuristic to infer which of two cities has the larger population. When students in another country were asked whether Detroit or Milwaukee was the larger city, nearly all got the right answer. They had heard of Detroit, but not Milwaukee, so they correctly guessed that Detroit was more populous, but only two-thirds of American students guessed correctly. They had more information, which distracted them from their gut feeling.[13]

Gut feelings and simple rules of thumb are forms of unconscious intelligence that take advantage of the evolved capacities of the brain and are driven by underlying reasons of which we are not fully aware. Psychologist Gerd Gigerenzer has argued that some purported examples of flawed reasoning identified in laboratory studies are in fact examples of unconscious intelligence.[14] The fact that people reason differently when the outcome of a surgery is presented as a "90 per cent chance of surviving" than when it is presented as a "10 per cent chance of dying" could reflect a lack of understanding of probability, but this apparent quirk in reasoning illustrates the distinction between attending to the numbers only – logical rationality – and considering the numbers as well as the social cues – ecological rationality. People use their social intelligence, in this case a relevance heuristic, to fill in a missing point of reference – namely, how patients fare without the surgery. In the real world, the speaker's choice of frame is relevant. If more patients will survive with the surgery, speakers would typically choose the survival frame, but if more patients would survive without the surgery, they would choose the death frame.[15] The supposedly neutral framing thus contains social cues that convey an implicit recommendation.

Heuristics Can Also Lead Everyone (Including Experts) Astray

Your intuition about the expression "molasses in January" (and the annoyance at getting that last glob out of the jar to make a fragrant batch of molasses spice cookies) likely makes it difficult to imagine a rushing flood of the sticky stuff destroying everything in its path. It seems like something from Douglas Adams' *Hitchhiker's Guide* series. Yet it is exactly what happened in the Boston Molasses Disaster on January 15, 1919, when a tank containing over 2 million gallons of molasses burst.[16] The colossal wave, moving 35 miles per hour, killed 21 people, injured another 150, killed 20 horses, and flattened multiple buildings. This dramatic counterintuitive example illustrates how going with our gut can sometimes lead us astray.

Likewise, our bodily sensations, emotions, moods, and attitudes – collectively referred to as **affect** – are useful sources of information when they arise from the target of judgment, but they can mislead when they arise from something incidental.[17] For example, when in a good mood after a conversation with a dear friend, we may miss subtle signals about a problematic situation that would otherwise draw our attention to it and lead us to consider it more systematically. Affect can also blur our assessment of risks and benefits. Benefits are not only weighed against risks in cost-benefit analyses; they can also directly influence the evaluation of risks. When the perceived benefits of an activity or technology are high, the perceived risks are lower, and vice versa. Affect explains why risks and benefits are negatively correlated in people's minds, even though they are usually positively correlated in reality.[18] Particularly salient risks generate negative affect that overshadows our assessment of the benefits.

A program of research that investigates mental shortcuts and quirks of reasoning – the heuristics and biases approach – has demonstrated countless ways that processes of intuitive judgment can bias decision-making processes.[19] These play out in day-to-day decision-making, including the decisions of experts. A foundational study, conducted with mathematical psychologists, demonstrated that their intuitions about statistics were not statistically accurate.[20] Although the statisticians had the skills to compute the correct answer (System 2 processing), when they instead relied on their impressions (System 1 processing) they placed unwarranted confidence in small samples. These biases can lead researchers to select inadequate sample sizes to test their hypotheses.[21]

In law and medicine, statistical biases can be a matter of life and death.[22] Positive HIV tests have led to suicides in low-risk populations (blood donors), and an undercover investigation discovered that a majority of AIDS counselors incorrectly informed low-risk clients that false-positive HIV tests do not occur.[23] Medical professionals often fall victim to this **illusion of certainty**, even when they are given the relevant statistics to calculate the actual probability. An example is a study that asked gynecologists to estimate the chances a woman had breast cancer given a positive (flagged) mammography result. Even when the doctors were provided with the prevalence of breast cancer, the test sensitivity, and the rate of false positives, they grossly overestimated the probability of a woman having cancer by nearly an order of magnitude. The problem is so widespread that it has been dubbed "collective statistical illiteracy."[24]

To provide a sense of the scope of heuristics and biases (statistical and otherwise) in everyday decision-making, Table 7.1 presents a list of 10 that have been found to play a role in reasoning about childhood vaccination.[25]

Table 7.1. Heuristics Applied in Decision-Making about Childhood Vaccines

Ambiguity avoidance	Delayed and uncertain outcomes lead to more negative perceptions of risk, especially when the benefits are not readily apparent.[26] Consequently, parents may be more willing to accept a known risk from a disease than a seemingly unknown risk from a vaccine.[27]
Apparent paradox of infection	When vaccination rates are high, more vaccinated than unvaccinated individuals may catch the disease (leading people to conclude the vaccine is not working), even though the vaccine is highly effective.[28] This paradox is because the small proportion of the large number of people vaccinated can outnumber the large proportion of the small number of those unvaccinated.
Availability	Estimates of the likelihood of an event occurring are based on how salient and imaginable it is.[29] Vivid and emotional descriptions of adverse vaccine reactions can therefore lead to overestimates of the risk.[30]
Confirmation bias	New evidence is unconsciously interpreted to fit existing beliefs.[31] The bias is especially problematic in internet searches, because search terms determine the results.[32]
Correlation as causation	Temporal association leads to "after therefore because of" – post hoc ergo propter hoc – reasoning. This leads to vaccination being blamed for diseases with idiopathic origin that become apparent in early childhood.[33]
Naturalness bias	Things considered "natural" are seen as safer and superior, leading some parents to believe it is better for their children to develop immunity from the disease than from the vaccine.[34]
Omission bias	The potential consequences of not taking an action (omission) may be implicitly preferred over potential consequences of taking an action (commission), leading some to avoid making the decision to vaccinate.[35]

(Continued)

Table 7.1. (*Continued*)

Optimistic bias	The ability to control personal risks is often viewed unrealistically positively.[36] This bias may lead parents to conclude that statistics about disease risks do not apply to their children.[37]
Overgeneralization	Because information that applies in one circumstance or context is commonly applied in others, a side effect of one vaccine or vaccine batch may be thought of as a side effect of vaccination in general.[38]
Risk aversion	People are particularly sensitive to potential losses as compared to potential gains or neutral outcomes.[39] Thus, advising parents that 98 per cent of children have no adverse reaction may better alleviate concerns than saying the risk of an adverse reaction is 2 per cent.

FROM VOGON SLAPSTICKS TO MAKING THE UNINTUITIVE INTUITIVE

Research on heuristics and biases in human judgment and research on scientific misconceptions are distinct disciplinary traditions with almost no citations in common, the former rooted in behavioral economics and the latter in educational psychology. From the point of view of extracting lessons to improve communication, a quick comparison of these research findings is useful. Many of the misconceptions discussed in Chapter 4 are readily articulated and consciously held. Although students may not recognize that the snow globe Earth is a misconception, they can describe it in words or draw a picture of it. In contrast, the heuristics and biases discussed in this chapter may not be consciously held or readily expressed, and as tempting as it may be to conclude someone has applied heuristics based on the outcome of that individual's reasoning (e.g., the decision to forgo vaccination), the reasoning process cannot be inferred from the decision made.[40]

(As a side note, some of the knowledge elements mentioned in Chapter 4 are heuristic-like, most notably those that provide an intuitive understanding of causality in physics.[41] In the education research literature, these knowledge elements are known as *phenomenological primitives* or p-prims, so called because they are primitive elements of cognition about mechanisms that originate in the experience of everyday phenomena. P-prims have been identified in other disciplines, including chemistry and biology, to explain features of the living and material world.[42] In education, the term "heuristic" is most closely associated with the mathematician George Polya and refers to practical strategies for solving mathematics problems, such as decomposing a problem into smaller elements or working backward from the goal.[43])

Like telling my dog that chasing and pouncing on butterfly shadows is futile (though irresistibly adorable), merely telling people about heuristics and biases does not help them recognize them in themselves.[44] Even when people acknowledge the potential for a specific bias, such as the way a positive or negative mood can bias assessment of risk, they deny that their own assessment was biased by their (experimentally manipulated) mood.[45] The direct education approach can be successful, however, when it teaches people about the invisibility of these heuristic processes. For example, in one study, those who read an article titled "Unaware of Our Unawareness" avoided the biases to which those who had not read the article fell prey.[46] Education is also effective when it provides people with accurate but intuitive ways of making sense of complex information.[47]

Communicating effectively means creating a terrain that does not trigger unproductive mental shortcuts – a terrain quite unlike that of the planet Vogon in the 2005 movie adaptation of the *The Hitchhiker's Guide to the Galaxy*, where sign-post-like "slapsticks" shot up from the ground to slam in the face anyone who engaged in thought. To escape, the characters had to stop thinking and make a run for it. Here on Earth the communication environment can be similarly hostile to thinking, forcing people to make a (cognitive) run for it that is not in their best interests. Effective communication provides a fertile ground to support informed, deliberative decision-making. The following are recommendations for doing so in general and in communicating numerical information (see Figure 7.1).

Make Key Information Salient, Individually Relevant, and Mechanistically Intuitive

INCREASE SALIENCE THROUGH IMAGINABILITY, EASE OF PROCESSING, AND EMOTIONAL IMPACT

Reasoning shortcuts such as availability, ambiguity avoidance, and omission bias prioritize certain information to the exclusion of other, potentially vital, information. To broaden the scope of what is considered,

Figure 7.1. Quick Tips for Supporting Reasoning

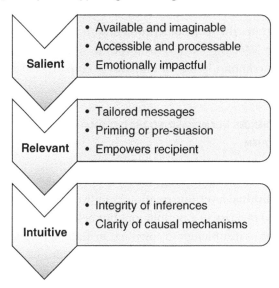

communication may need to be tailored to draw attention to what is missing by making it more imaginable, easier to process, or emotionally impactful. For example, when symptoms are easier to imagine (severe headaches) instead of abstract (a malfunctioning nervous system), the perceived likelihood of catching a disease is greater.[48] When information is easier to access or process, even due to simple techniques such as increasing font readability, it is more believable.[49]

Emotional impact elevates information, which is why personal stories, such as those in a successful "Tips from Former Smokers" campaign, are influential.[50] The importance of emotional impact is consistent with Damasio's somatic marker model. Exactly how somatic markers function in the decision-making process is an active area of research, but it involves an initial activation in which a positive or negative emotion becomes associated with representations (such as images of cigarettes) or actions (such as the act of lighting a cigarette), such that later encounters with them reactivate the emotion.[51]

Perhaps counterintuitively, but due to the greater emotional connection, stories about individual victims can have greater power to influence decision-making than statistics about large numbers of victims.[52] Statistics and case studies provide complementary information – how things play out on average and at the individual level, respectively. Also, some people are more drawn to stories and others to numerical information.[53] Thus, a useful strategy is to juxtapose statistical information that demonstrates the scope of a problem with a story that gives an issue a face. When selecting stories, however, do not assume that all audiences have a common sense of empathy – empathy fallacy – because responses to narratives are not uniform.[54]

PRE-SUADE AUDIENCES BY EMPHASIZING THE INFORMATION'S RELEVANCE TO THEM

People interpret media messages as conveying societal-level information, not individual-level information.[55] Individuals may acknowledge the likelihood of a risk in a population, but believe their own risk is different.[56] It is thus insufficient to convince an audience a message is true, because it leaves room for optimistic (or pessimistic) bias if individuals remain unconvinced the message applies to them. It is for this reason that advertisers speak directly to the audience by using the pronoun "you" instead of the more generic "people" or "they." Tailoring messages – for example, for a target demographic group or interest group – is another way to increase perceived message relevance. Priming audiences to pay attention by emphasizing up front the personal relevance of a message is a form of what psychologist Robert Cialdini calls pre-suasion.[57] Because people may shield themselves from emotionally unwelcome information – the ostrich effect – pre-suasion should not only emphasize the personal relevance, but also empower the audience by emphasizing their ability to act on the information.[58]

PROVIDE AN INTUITIVE REASONING FRAMEWORK FOR SCIENTIFIC MECHANISMS

Exaggerated causal claims (based on correlation) and overgeneralization (such as from animals to humans) are common in academic press releases and make their way into the news media from the flawed press releases.[59] It is no wonder that audiences are susceptible to overgeneralization and confuse correlation and causation. In addition to addressing these misleading tendencies in journalistic coverage of science, research communication must do more to help audiences develop mental models for understanding causation in science.

Intending to simplify, communicators may gloss over fundamental aspects of mechanism, such as relationships across scales, indirect causation, emergent behavior, and feedback loops, but topics as diverse as pain amplification, anger management, and climate change cannot be understood in a meaningful way without insight into mechanism. In feedback loops, for example, incremental changes can build on each other in a drastic amplification. Yet counterintuitively (and relevant to mitigation), flipping the direction of just one of the incremental changes can morph a self-reinforcing amplification into a steady-state oscillation.

An embodied demonstration of feedback loops can promote an intuitive understanding applicable to any phenomenon involving them.[60] A group of people stands in a circle holding hands, and each one is a "positive signal." The first person lifts one hand by two inches to trigger the positive feedback loop. Upon receiving a positive signal from their downstream neighbor, each person builds on that signal (by two inches), such that the signal is amplified as it continues around the circle, eventually reaching the limit of the system (height, in this case). Repeating the demonstration, but this time introducing just one negative signal, blocks the amplification. Communicators can draw on demonstration, visualizations, or analogies to help audiences gain an intuitive understanding of complex causal mechanisms.

Beware of Confounds and Confusions that Lead to Statistical Lies

There are many ways to deliberately or inadvertently lie with statistics (Figure 7.2). Below are some of the more common pitfalls to watch out for, including base-rate fallacy, lead-time bias, Simpson's Paradox, undefined single-event probability, and relative comparisons.

SUPPORT REASONING ABOUT BASE RATES AND CONDITIONAL PROBABILITY

Being misled by the apparent paradox of infection (see the list of heuristics applied in decision-making about childhood vaccines in Table 7.1) is an example of the base-rate fallacy. Another example is the illusion of certainty that people who get a positive test result on an asymptomatic

Figure 7.2. Statistical Lies

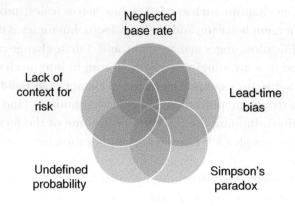

Neglected base rate

Lack of context for risk

Lead-time bias

Undefined probability

Simpson's paradox

screening for a rare disease must have the disease. In the case of the apparent paradox of infection, instead of comparing what percentage of the infected are vaccinated and unvaccinated, compare the percentage of vaccinated people who get infected to the percentage of unvaccinated people who get infected. In other words, the informative comparison is the probability of getting infected given that you are vaccinated versus the probability of getting infected if you are not vaccinated. The problem of base rate is thus a problem of conditional probability. Although conditional probability can be calculated using Bayes' rule, use of counts (natural frequencies) has been shown to improve inferences from statistics, as in the following example.[61]

In the case of a diagnostic test, three pieces of information are needed to calculate the chance that a patient has the disease given that they test positive for it:

- In the population, how many have the disease? (**prevalence**)
- Among those who have the disease, how well does the test detect it? (**sensitivity**)
- Among those who do not have the disease, how often will the test say that they do? (**false positive**)

Gerd Gigerenzer and colleagues have shown that frequency trees make it intuitive, because unlike with conditional probabilities, each level of the tree sums to the total population (see Figure 7.3).[62]

Figure 7.3. Trees to Dispel the Illusion of Certainty in Diagnoses

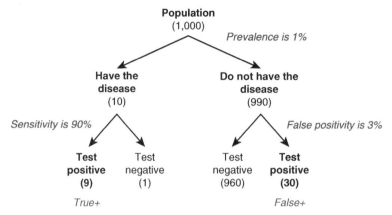

Note: The tree visually dispels the illusion of certainty about a positive test result. It is readily apparent that, despite the low false positivity rate, the false positives outnumber the true positives in routine testing for a rare disease.

REDUCE LEAD-TIME BIAS

Evidence of progress in the war on cancer is often presented in terms of five-year survival rates, but this is misleading because survival rates can be improved in a desirable way or a detrimental way. The desirable way is to advance treatments that reduce death. The detrimental way is to diagnose the disease earlier without increasing the lifespan – a confound referred to as **lead-time bias**. For example, if an old-fashioned test diagnoses a group of men with prostate cancer at age 71 and all have died by age 75, the five-year survival rate is zero, but if a new-fangled more sensitive test picks up the disease by age 70, but all those diagnosed still die at age 75, the five-year survival rate is 100 per cent, even though no lives or life years have been saved (Figure 7.4). Besides being statistically misleading, the earlier diagnosis may also lead to overtreatment.

A study that examined the correlation between five-year survival, mortality, and incidence rates for the 20 most common solid tumor types found strong evidence for lead-time bias.[63] Over time, the five-year survival rates have increased for all tumor types, but this change was positively correlated with incidence rates, not mortality rates, suggesting that diagnostic procedures have become more sensitive without a corresponding impact on lifespan. Therefore, to avoid lying with statistics, survival rates should be presented alongside annual population mortality data.

Figure 7.4. The Lie of Lead-Time Bias

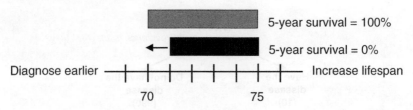

5-year survival = 100%

5-year survival = 0%

Diagnose earlier   Increase lifespan

70   75

UNAMALGAMATE TO SORT OUT SIMPSON'S PARADOX

Could Hospital A be a better place to get a surgery than Hospital B if Hospital A's surgery mortality rate is worse? Could Airline A be a better bet than Airline B for an on-time arrival if Airline B has fewer overall flight delays? In both cases, the answer is "yes" if a hidden variable is confounding data that should be examined by subgroup instead of being amalgamated. In these examples, the confounding variables are that the condition of the patients arriving at Hospital A is worse than that of the patients arriving at Hospital B, and that Airline A has more flights out of airports that are prone to weather delays than does Airline B.

Re-examining the data after separating patients by pre-operative health would reveal that, compared to Hospital B, Hospital A has lower surgery mortality for patients arriving in good condition, as well as lower surgery mortality for patients arriving in poor condition. Separating the flight delay data by city would show that Airline A outperforms Airline B in each city. The apparent reversal of a trend that occurs when amalgamated data are unamalgamated is known as Simpson's paradox, and it occurs in a variety of real-life settings.[64] The trend reversal seems utterly paradoxical, but it is just a dramatic reminder that making causal inferences from observational data requires expert knowledge to identify potential confounds.[65] In terms of communicating about the paradox, a three-way table, such as Table 7.2, which shows the death rates for two treatments with confound of age, can allow an audience to contemplate the effect "in action." Overall, the mortality appears to be worse for Treatment 1; yet it is clear from the age-segregated data that Treatment 1 is more effective (lower mortality rate) for both age groups.

Table 7.2. Simpson's Paradox in Action

| Treatment | Under 50 Years | | Over 50 Years | | Overall |
	# Treated	Mortality	# Treated	Mortality	Mortality
1	80	**25%** = 20	20	**10%** = 2	**22%**
2	20	**30%** = 6	80	**15%** = 12	**18%**
	Treatment 1 is better.		*Treatment 1 is better.*		*Treatment 2 is better.*

DEFINE THE OBJECT OF A PROBABILITY STATEMENT

What does "30 per cent chance of rain" mean? Specifically, to which (if any) of the following does it refer?

1. *Time* – It may rain for about a third of the day, but not all day.
2. *Area* – About a third of the geographic region will get rain.
3. *Forecasters* – Three in ten meteorologists predict rain.

Research demonstrates that people understand the numerical probability but not the event to which it refers.[66] The choices above are the most common interpretations of precipitation forecasts by publics.[67] The ambiguity arises from giving a single-event probability without specifying what single event it refers to. In this case, none of the above choices is accurate; the precipitation forecast refers to the chance of detectable rain at any point in the area covered by the forecast at any time over the period of the forecast.

A similar ambiguity occurs in communication about medical risks. The failure to specify what the probability refers to is common in medical communication.[68] When patients are told they have a 30 per cent chance of experiencing a side effect, many understand it to mean they will have a side effect 30 per cent of the time they are on the medication, instead of that 3 in 10 patients experience a side effect. The misunderstanding is because doctors are thinking in terms of groups of patients, but patients are thinking in terms of their individual case. To avoid ambiguity, be sure to define the object of a probability statement.

PROVIDE ABSOLUTE (NOT JUST RELATIVE) RISK

Health reporting in the news media usually fails to quantify risks and benefits, and when numbers are presented they are often in the form of relative rather than absolute comparisons.[69] This highly misleading practice has led to demonstrable harm, such as a "contraceptive pill scare," in which the relative risk of a potentially life-threatening side effect was twofold or 100 per cent greater for one type of pill than another, a panic-inducing statistic that appeared quite different in the context of the absolute risk (1 in 7,000 compared to 2 in 7,000).[70] Relative risks and benefits are attention grabbing, but presenting them without the absolute risks is just another way to lie with statistics.

Adopt the Best Practices for Verbal and Visual Communication of Data

When reasoning about data, people may see what they want to see, but clear communication can reduce this eye-of-the-beholder effect. For example, when the average of a dataset is communicated but the actual shape of a data distribution is not, audiences are forced to make judgments about the distribution's shape. A numerical value may reflect a uniform data distribution, in which data points across a range are equally likely; a bell curve distribution, in which data points are clustered around the midpoint; or a skewed data distribution, in which numbers at one end of the range are most likely. People imagine the shape to suit their prior views of an issue. Those less accepting of climate change imagine the shape of a temperature distribution to be uniform or skewed to smaller values, whereas those who are accepting of climate change imagine the data as normally distributed or skewed toward larger values.[71] Showing the actual distribution erases the bias. Table 7.3 presents a list of 10 dos and don'ts to promote clarity in communication about data.

ETHICS, ETHOS, AND EPISTEMIC GOALS

Subverting Heuristics "for People's Own Good" Raises Ethical Questions

Heuristics and biases can be exploited to influence people's decision-making. Not only can they be exploited, they are exploited (most obviously in marketing and advertising). An example is when an advertiser labels a product with a high price and then marks it down, or states that

Table 7.3. Dos and Don'ts in Data Communication

Practices to AVOID	Practices to ADOPT
Comparing inconsistent numerical formats (e.g., frequencies to percentages).	Be consistent (e.g., compare percentages to percentages and frequencies to frequencies).
Making the audience perform the calculations or using different denominators in comparisons.	Do the calculations and make comparisons obvious (e.g., by expressing numbers with denominators in base 10).
Presenting numbers as decimals or exponents or expecting audiences to intuitively grasp very large or small scales.	Round numbers. Use comparisons to help with numbers outside of a human scale (e.g., equivalent to one drop of water in an Olympic-sized swimming pool).
Logarithmic plots or complex, unfamiliar graphical forms (especially under time constraints).	Use familiar ways of displaying data. When unfamiliar displays are needed, take the time to orient the audience.
Stating statistical significance without stating meaningfulness (e.g., qualifying or quantifying effect size).	Provide expert judgment on the meaningfulness of a result (e.g., the effect is small but important across the population).
Data displays or statements that conceal important trends.	Consider showing the shape of a distribution and stating the range in addition to the average or median.
Expecting people to understand unfamiliar units (e.g., that light-year is a measure of distance, not time) or using units not easily tied to people's actions.	Explain what an unfamiliar unit measures (e.g., distance, density). Provide relevant units when possible (e.g., the financial costs of the energy consumed).
Inadvertently give short shrift to small probabilities, especially those that are cumulative.	State small risks as how many (e.g., 1 in 100,000 people) rather than how likely (0.001% risk). Small, cumulative risks can be expressed over an appropriate timescale (e.g., a decade or lifetime).
Expect audiences to reason about losses the same way they reason about gains (e.g., 1% have side effects versus 99% have no side effects).	Express numbers to draw attention to what is important or provide both loss and gain information (e.g., 70% recycled plastic and 30% nonrecycled plastic).
Presenting numbers without adequate context.	Provide relevant contextual information (e.g., compared to other technologies, historical trends, other geographical regions, populations, or to a baseline or threshold).

you might expect to pay $300 for this set of widgets that are yours for three easy payments of just $19.99. This strategy takes advantage of the tendency for people to become "anchored" to an initial number, however irrelevant, and fail to adequately adjust from it – known as the anchoring and adjustment heuristic.[72] If framing to get around people's heuristics is used manipulatively, does it have a place in ethical communication?

As discussed in the previous chapter, part of communicating ethically is making information intelligible to audiences. This intelligibility requirement could be interpreted in "weaker" or "stronger" ways. The former is making statements using language that is comprehensible to nonspecialists. The latter means also taking heuristics and biases into consideration when shaping messages. Some argue for the weaker version of the intelligibility requirement, noting that the stronger version can easily slide into manipulation.[73] Others have argued for communicating and setting up choices in a way that overcomes people's cognitive biases to steer them toward the choices they would make if they were acting without those biases.[74] This steering or "nudging" approach is referred to as "libertarian paternalism."[75] It is paternalistic because it nudges people toward certain choices but libertarian because it does not take any choices away.

Paternalistic nudges can benefit individuals, for instance setting up retirement contribution choice architecture to lead people to save more for retirement.[76] Nudges can also be used to promote a public good, such as increasing rates of organ donation. Some countries require explicit consent to become a donor – that is, they have opt-in policies – but in other countries everyone is considered a potential donor unless they opt out. Rates of organ donation are much higher in countries with opt-out policies. The difference is attributed to the aversion to making the choice, a conclusion supported by the finding that when one US state adopted a policy of asking people to choose to opt in or out, a quarter of them left the question blank.[77] The nudge of an opt-out organ donation policy helps address the shortage of available organs, but it raises the issue of informed consent if not everyone knows about the policy or how to opt out.

A major criticism of libertarian paternalism is that it assumes the choice architect is acting without unconscious bias or conflicting interest, an untenable assumption. Doctors, for example, could be viewed as benevolent choice architects, but they may practice defensive medicine by ordering unnecessary tests.[78] Choice architecture is, of course, a reality. When people do need to select options, it makes sense to present the alternatives in a way that supports healthy choices; however, rather than assuming this can be done by a benevolent choice architect, the design should be informed by input from groups that reflect the diversity of the end user.

Moreover, nudges are not a replacement for effective communication. Both can be used synergistically to help people make better decisions. People can even learn to change their own choice ecosystem to remove weak points and nudge themselves to change their own habits.[79]

Figure 7.5. The Essential Elements of Trust

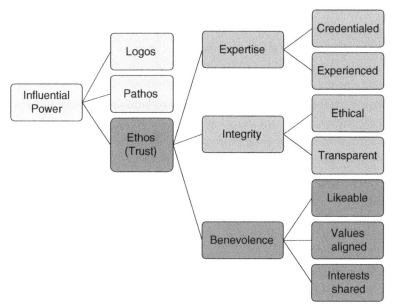

Note: Trust is accepted vulnerability. Having the appropriate expertise and acting with integrity are only two of the three pillars of trust. Experts often forget the third pillar, benevolence. Benevolence requires not only goodwill but also an understanding of the needs and values of those being asked to trust.

In thinking about nudging and educating, ethical gray areas arise. Ethical communication aims to reach the audience, promote good deliberation, and advance altruistic or democratic goals, but an ethical gray area arises when good deliberation is at odds with the common good (or the altruistic goals for the audience).[80] The appropriate course of action may vary, but this tension must be acknowledged when it arises.

Trust Is an Essential Heuristic in Science Communication

The influential power of communication is determined by three interacting elements: its content (arguments and evidence), its emotional impact, and the extent to which it inspires trust in the source – these elements were identified by Aristotle as logos, pathos, and ethos, respectively (Figure 7.5).[81] Trust is accepted vulnerability based on the confidence that the trusted will not take advantage of the vulnerability.[82] Trust is thus relational and an anticipatory emotion on the part of the truster.[83] Trust in knowledge – epistemic trust – is the foundation for effective communication about science, health, and the environment. More specifically, epistemic trust involves relying on the knowledge of the more knowledgeable with an awareness of the risk of being misinformed. In the context of epistemic trust, trustworthiness of a source is rooted in the perception of the source's pertinent expertise, integrity, and benevolence.[84]

For a professional with the relevant credentials (education, experience, certifications, institutional affiliations), the first of these three components of trust tends to be more readily established than the other two. Ethical conduct and transparency, such as the willingness to disclose a flaw in your own work, help establish your integrity. Establishing benevolence entails demonstrating that you are acting in the best interests of the other (or society more generally), not in your own best interests. An audience can believe that the experts are knowledgeable and conducted their work with integrity but still not trust in how their values shape their recommendations. In the context of the COVID-19 pandemic, some social groups believed in the knowledge but not the values of the public health authorities, while others believed in their values but not their knowledge.[85] Trust not only varies by source but also by topic. A source may be seen as equally knowledgeable about two topics, but only trusted on one of the topics according to how their values are seen to align.[86]

An important aspect of establishing shared values to build trust is to recognize another's good intentions. For instance, when discussing childhood vaccinations with health professionals, dialogue, cooperative decision-making, and the acknowledgement that the parents want to act in the best interests of their children builds trust.[87] Also, the greater the likeability of the source, the more their arguments will be accepted over those of a less likeable source.[88] Studies of the implementation of health and wellness programs consistently demonstrate that collaborative, nonhierarchical relationships among providers, researchers, and community members enhance impact and promote sustainability.[89] For the most part, however, with the exception of their health care providers, people in industrialized societies do not know or interact with the individuals or organizations that control their health and safety.[90] Because people tend to distrust authority when they are upset, these organizations must work to establish trust well in advance of a crisis.[91] Even when trust is necessary because of an epistemic division of labor, trust is a heuristic and a leap of faith.

Navigating Communication in the Context of Directional Motivation Requires Additional Knowledge, Skills, and Habits of Mind

Consider what statistical bias could be playing a role in the following statement:

> I am truly grateful that I received my diagnosis in the United States, where my chances of survival are almost double what they would be under socialized medicine in England!

This is a paraphrasing of a statement made by a famous American politician.[92] How critically you consider such a claim may depend on your stance on socialized medicine. With the added information about the source of the claim, you likely factored in your views about American politicians. If I specify that the claim was made by a conservative politician, your political leanings may come into play. The claim is tainted by lead-time bias, but it is not clear that the claim was made as a deliberate attempt to mislead. Nonetheless, the fact that it is consistent with political ideology suggests that if the politician did not intend to mislead, he did succumb to confirmation bias.

Heuristics are widely used, even by those who are not motivated by any particular ideology, but motivation to reason in a particular direction – directional goals – may trigger the use of heuristics that shift reasoning in that direction. This is true of any of the heuristics discussed in this chapter, including statistical heuristics, such as accounting for the base rate.[93] All can be applied in a way that casts one position in a favorable light while casting doubt on the alternatives. Individual and group values may be at odds and individuals may reason in accordance with their own values, by using group affiliation as a heuristic or by taking a middle ground in which they express abstract agreement with a group policy but decide not to act in accordance.[94] Motivational biases, whether they result from group affiliation or individual values, are much more difficult to "correct" than nonmotivational biases.[95] Attempting to correct them can backfire. The next chapter continues to build our communicator's guide to the galaxy, delving into the complex relationships between individual values and group affiliations and providing strategies to avoid communication backfires.

Navigating Communication in the Context of Dire
Motivation Requires Additional Knowledge, Skills,
and Habits of Mind

8

Obvious but Wrong: The Perils of the Backfire Effect and Tips to Prevent It

Remember when you were a child and an adult told you not to do something that you would have never thought of doing, and suddenly the previously unimagined bit of naughtiness became irresistibly appealing? Children who grow up on a glacial landscape like I did are sent outside to play in subfreezing temperatures with the peculiar bit of parental advice, "Don't lick the metal railing because your tongue will stick." To this budding scientist, that became a research question in need of an experiment.

Spit freezes. Spit freezes rapidly. And when it does, the spit-flooded hills and dales of your tongue get caught up in the rapid liquid-to-solid phase change and find themselves firmly stuck to the frosty metal you were told not to lick. In your (literally) tongue-tied state, you first feel stupid and then you feel scared – scared of skinning your tongue and of getting in trouble for your idiotic insolence.

Happily, the taste buds and I survived to tell the tale that introduces the theme of this chapter, the backfire effect. Communication that has the opposite effect of what was intended has backfired. Backfires occur for many reasons in communication about science and contemporary issues. Unlike my puerile rebellion, they are not always deliberate reactions to authority. Often, they are not conscious decisions at all.

People's values, tied to their worldviews, cultural affiliations, and individual identities, play an important and complex role in how we make sense of issues and whether a communicator's efforts will backfire.

This chapter explores what is known about the influence of these factors, the phenomenon of motivated reasoning, the backfire effect, and evidence-based strategies for minimizing backfires. This research is full of surprises and a grasp of it is a communicator's superpower.

CHAPTER LEARNING OBJECTIVES: BACKFIRE EFFECT

Knowledge: What is the backfire effect and what are the many possible causes of backfires?

Skills: Be proactive to avoid or reduce the cognitive and ideological triggers of backfires.

Habits of Mind: Avoid broad conclusions about group affiliation and seek shared identities.

RETHINKING GROUPTHINK

Research confirms that identification with a political party influences attitudes, viewpoints, and behaviors.[1] Political differences were dramatically displayed during the COVID-19 pandemic, but growing ideological divides long preceded it.[2] Although some research suggests conservatives and liberals differ in personality dispositions and patterns of brain activity, this is an unsatisfactory explanation for political polarization.[3] Conservatives are not more likely than liberals to rely on heuristics or intuitive reasoning.[4] Furthermore, while conservatives react more negatively to "conservative-dissonant science" (climate change or human evolution), liberals react more negatively to "liberal-dissonant science" (hydraulic fracking of natural gas or nuclear power), and both groups react the same way to ideologically neutral claims about astronomy and geology.[5] In other words, neither conservatives nor liberals have one-size-fits-all reasoning patterns – the context matters.

Furthermore, polarized reasoning on an issue may arise only after groups have political skin in the game. This is the case for embryonic stem cell research. Before the 2004 presidential election in the United States, partisanship was not a predictor of support for embryonic stem cell research.[6] Some leaders within the Republican Party supported funding, and others opposed it. Only after that election, in which the elites and campaign strategists turned embryonic stem cell research into a wedge issue, did the partisan divide emerge. In other words, the politicization of the issue preceded the reasoning divide.

Cultural Cognition Can Explain the Relationship between Polarization and Politicization

Members of a community that holds certain values will reason, usually unconsciously, in a way that protects those values when they are threatened – a phenomenon dubbed "cultural cognition."[7] Group loyalty can be sufficiently motivating that when people's values clash with those of their party, they may change their views to align them with those of the party, thus "choosing party over policy."[8] Why subjugate one's own views to go along with the group? A key reason is that partisanship involves emotional and identity attachment to one's party.[9] An individual is thus motivated to make sense of issues in a way that preserves that identity and feeling of connection to the group.

Another reason is that voters in representative democracies rarely get to directly choose policy alternatives. Instead, political parties offer a *prix fixe* menu.[10] In selecting a party, a voter gains a coordinated set of choices, and following the party can thus become an informational shortcut.[11] In the situation in which voters do get to choose a policy directly, their position on the policy can itself become a strongly held identity, as was observed with respect to Brexit. Not quite two years after the referendum to leave the European Union, with their prime minister struggling to work out a separation deal before the looming exit deadline, one in five British citizens did not identify with a political party, but only one in 16 British citizens did not have a definite Brexit identity.[12]

Polarization Can Become a Vicious Cycle

Ideology leads to motivated reasoning, which can occur at any stage of the reasoning process, from forming initial impressions, developing attitudes and beliefs, seeking and evaluating arguments and evidence, and comparing the pros and cons to arrive at a decision.[13] The tendency to seek attitude-confirming information is especially problematic in internet searches because results are determined by the search terms used.[14] Even when someone is presented with both confirming and disconfirming evidence on an issue, assimilation may be biased because individuals with strong prior opinions may subject disconfirming arguments and evidence to critical evaluation while accepting confirming information at face value.[15]

During the process of rationalizing the accepting and discounting of arguments and evidence, an individual's position may actually become more polarized, as the individual becomes more attuned to the weaknesses in the opposing arguments and evidence, but not in the attitudinally congruent arguments and evidence.[16] This biased process of accepting supporting information and discounting disconfirming information explains counterintuitive findings about the relationship between knowledge and polarization.[17] Under conditions of motivated reasoning, being more science literate can provide fodder to support one's position, as well as to better rationalize the discounting of the other side's arguments.

The key take-home message is that the more communication emphasizes ideological differences, the more it ups the ante, leading to more motivated reasoning and a vicious cycle in which people's views become increasingly entrenched, thus further amplifying partisan differences. This chapter offers strategies to break the cycle, starting with reminding ourselves why, beneath our divides (with a nod to Depeche Mode here), people are people.

We Are All Complex Mixes of Identities

Americans tend to be more religious than citizens of other wealthy nations.[18] Discussions of American politics often lump religious beliefs in with political beliefs, but this is misleading. More than half of Americans say religion is very important in their lives, and approximately another one-quarter say it is somewhat important.[19] While conservatives are more religious than liberals on average, party affiliation does not predict belief. Over three-quarters of Democrats, independents, and Republicans are certain or fairly certain in their belief in God (range 76–90 per cent).

The distinction between political ideology and religious beliefs is a reminder that we are all a mix of different identities. These identities may be tied up with group affiliations, such as race, ethnicity, national or regional origin, socioeconomic background, military service, gender, sexuality, disability, generation, or even being fans of a particular sports team. Other identities, such as occupation, being a parent, pastimes, and hobbies, may feel like individual identities but can become group identities when we are in the presence of those who share them. Still other identities are typically individualistic, such as having a concept of ourselves as humorous, health-conscious, or frugal. We have seen how identity can lead to ideological reasoning, but identity can also be an opportunity for connection.

BEFORE YOU READ THE NEXT SECTION …

How do you predict political affiliation, religion, and education or science knowledge influence people's views of anthropogenic climate change, evolution, vaccination, and genetically engineered food?

Identities Do Not Always Have the Influence You Might Predict

As tempting as it may be to paint groups of "others" with broad strokes, the influence of identities varies considerably on an issue-by-issue basis. The Pew Research Center examined the role of age, gender, race/ethnicity, political affiliation, religion, and education/science knowledge on public views of 22 science-related issues.[20] *Age* was a strong factor on several issues; for example, older adults were more likely than younger adults to consider childhood vaccines safe and something that should be mandatory for all children. *Gender* was a strong factor on only one issue, use of animals in research, which is favored by a majority of men and opposed by a majority of women. *Race and ethnicity* are strong factors on a handful of issues, including access to drug treatments before they are fully tested, which a majority of white individuals favor and a majority of African Americans oppose. The strength of the influence of *political party, religion* (religious affiliation/church attendance), and *knowledge* (educational attainment and/or science knowledge as measured on a short test of science facts) on views of four scientific issues is shown in Table 8.1.

Table 8.1. Influence of Party, Religion, and Knowledge on Views of Scientific Issues

	Strong	Medium	Weak
Earth is warming due to human activity.	Party	Knowledge	Religion
Humans have evolved due to natural processes.	Religion	Party Knowledge	–
Childhood vaccines are safe.	–	–	Party Knowledge
It is safe to eat genetically modified foods.	Knowledge	–	Party Religion

Political party was a strong factor for only one of the four issues, anthropogenic global climate change. Those who identify as Democrats were significantly more likely to say that scientists generally agree climate change is due to human activity than were Republicans. At the time of this survey, party did not influence reasoning about vaccination – a reminder that partisan divides around COVID-19 vaccination emerged from the ideological divides on the handling of the pandemic, not pre-existing party-aligned views on vaccination.

Religion was only a strong factor in predicting responses to the human evolution question. Religion was a weak factor with respect to views on climate change and genetically modified foods. (Unfortunately, religion details were not available for the vaccine question.) It is interesting to note that the difference in responses about evolution is not strongly influenced by knowledge. Although less than half of Americans agree with the statement, "*Human beings, as we know them today, developed from earlier species of animals,*" when the statement is prefaced by "*According to the theory of evolution,*" the percentage of Americans who rate the statement as true jumps to nearly three-quarters.[21]

Educational attainment and science knowledge was only a strong factor with respect to genetically modified food. Those with greater scientific knowledge were more likely to say these foods are safe to eat. On the safety of vaccines, in contrast, education and science knowledge played a weak role. Education and science knowledge played a moderate role on anthropogenic global climate change. On average, those with more education were more likely to say that scientists generally agree the Earth is getting warmer due to human activity. Those with a degree in a scientific field were not more likely than those with degrees in other fields to see scientists as agreeing about climate change, but respondents with low scores on the science facts test were a few percentage points less likely than those with higher scores to see scientists as agreeing.

Although this is just a brief overview of one survey done at one time point in one country, the patterns it reveals are instructive.

THE DEFICIT MODEL FAILS TO PREDICT THE REASONING PATTERNS

Scientific knowledge plays a role in people's reasoning – except when it doesn't! The role of education and scientific knowledge on people's reasoning is unpredictable. Although the measure of scientific knowledge used is limited (no in-depth examination of knowledge on specific issues), the data do not support the view that knowledge is the sole or even the main factor in whether people accept the scientific consensus on an issue.

NO ANTI-SCIENCE GROUP EMERGES

Blanket statements about particular populations being opposed to scientific advances are not supported by the data, as no factor was a strong predictor of reasoning on all, or even a majority of, the issues. Over the course of history, many scholars have depicted religious teachings as being at odds with science; however, a close examination of the doctrine of the major religious traditions in the United States reveals almost no knowledge conflict between science and religion.[22]

IDEOLOGY IS NOT THE ONLY REASON FOR GROUP DIFFERENCES

The age-related differences in reasoning about vaccination are presumably not due to ideological commitments to one's generation. A more plausible explanation is that older adults are more likely to have personal experiences with diseases that childhood vaccinations prevent, such as measles, mumps, and rubella. This would make the arguments in favor of vaccination more vivid and compelling. Similarly, the racial differences on whether drug treatments should be made available before they are fully tested likely reflect the breaches of trust that occurred during the unethical Tuskegee Syphilis study. The four-decades-long study (1932 to

1972) used inadequate and deceptive consent procedures to study the course of disease progression in African American men over time and failed to provide treatment even when treatment was available.[23]

COMMUNICATION STRATEGIES NEED TAILORING BY ISSUE AND AUDIENCE

Cultural affiliations with groups that espouse particular worldviews can be strongly influential, but only on a subset of issues. On other issues, personal or group histories come to the fore. In short, this research shows that reasoning about contemporary scientific issues is based on a complex mix of knowledge and values. It is thus crucial to know how these diverse and nuanced factors can make communication go awry or even backfire.

BACKFIRES AND BOOMERANGS – A COMMUNICATOR'S WORST NIGHTMARE

The backfire effect, also referred to as the boomerang effect, is the situation in which an attempt to inform, persuade, or correct misinformation causes those receiving the communication to adhere even more strongly to their original views. Backfires thus make communication not just unproductive but counterproductive. The backfire effect entered the political science and communication literatures relatively recently through a widely cited study demonstrating backfires to mock news articles that addressed misconceptions about policies of the second Bush administration.[24] Yet the phenomenon has deep roots in the psychology literature on resistance to persuasion. Moreover, the observation that people approach information with the aim of preserving their original viewpoint dates at least as far back as philosopher of science Francis Bacon in the 1600s.[25]

Resistance to persuasion is obviously essential in daily life in response to advertisers, peer pressure, and other unhealthy influences. It can involve any of several approaches: tuning out the message, bringing to mind others who share a view, dismissing the trustworthiness of the information source, rebutting the arguments in the message, calling to mind attitude-consistent arguments, reacting with anger, and selectively processing information to favor a point of view.[26] These approaches are termed, respectively, selective exposure, social validation, source derogation, counterarguing, support arguing, negative affect, and message distortion. These strategies that are adaptive in some contexts can lead to psychological reactance, in which attempts to promote adaptive behaviors, such as a reduction in alcohol consumption among heavy drinkers, backfire.[27]

The existence of the backfire effect – broadly defined here to include both knowledge backfires and behavioral backfires – is well documented with a substantial interdisciplinary research base. The backfire effect has different flavors, and the next section inventories the range of conditions under which the backfire effect has been observed to occur. The rest of the chapter is devoted to an in-depth discussion of how to minimize the backfire effect for each of these flavors of backfires.

Clashes with Cultural Affiliations

As we have already seen, when members of a group that espouses a particular ideology encounter information that challenges that ideology, they may reason in a way that preserves their relationship to the group by dismissing the information. Importantly, however, not all the views held more strongly by one group than another are subject to ideological backfire. Both conservatives and liberals typically overestimate, by about 10 times, the percentage of the US federal budget spent on nondefense research and development.[28] It has hovered around 1 to 2 per cent for the past decade. Although conservatives tend to be less supportive of federal funding for research than liberals in general, no backfire effect occurred when conservatives were corrected about actual expenditures. The correction generated support for increased research and development funding among both liberals and conservatives, presumably because for neither group was the information a challenge to core group values. In a nutshell, backfires occur not because information runs counter to one's beliefs but because the information has unwelcome ideological implications.[29]

Threats to Autonomy

Group identity is not the only value that people may seek to defend if they feel it is being threatened. As we saw during the COVID-19 pandemic, most people strongly value personal freedom and will behave in a way that protects it, even when the perceived threat is indirect. This is a problem with persuasive health campaigns, including on nonpartisan issues, such as limiting one's alcohol intake.[30] Particularly when a message is strongly worded, people react in a way that is at odds with message intent. This is thought to occur both because the authoritative tone of the message induces anger and because when someone who values a commodity or behavior thinks about it being taken away or forbidden, its value to them increases. Note that threats to autonomy are distinct from fear appeals. Appealing to fear has been found to have a modest positive effect on changing behavior in health campaigns.[31] If a fear appeal appears to threaten a person's autonomy, the fear appeal can backfire, but so can autonomy-threatening messages that do not appeal to fear.

Incompatibility with Self-Concept

We each view ourselves in certain ways – doting parent, health nut, independent-minded, sociable, bookworm – and often take pride in our self-concepts. When these are challenged, people tend to react in ways that protect their views of themselves. For example, reading a message advocating the acceptance of genetically modified foods increased negative attitudes toward these foods among individuals who said that an important aspect of how they define themselves is purity, health, and consciousness of their diet.[32] Attitudinal backfires did not occur in response to the message among those who did not have a strong dietary self-concept. The response to clashes with self-concept may be mediated by a brain system dubbed "the interpreter," which creates stories around our experiences and actions to maintain a view of oneself that remains coherent over time.[33]

Normalizing the Problem

Efforts that aim to change behavior may inadvertently normalize the behavior if they send the message that everyone is doing it, thus establishing it as a social norm. Inadvertent normalization has caused backfires in various contexts: anti-littering posters that stressed the extent of littering caused people to litter more; energy use reduction messages caused low consumers of energy to use more energy when they learned how their usage compared to others; and the D.A.R.E. "just say no to drugs" program may have inadvertently conveyed the message that everyone is doing drugs, thus encouraging some kids to want to try drugs to fit in.[34]

Mismatched Argument Strength

In day-to-day life we are typically exposed to a range of claims about a given issue, some of which are weak and some of which are strong. Even when your audience is not motivated by ideology, putting forth a weak argument can backfire. When two opposing claims that are approximately equal strength compete against each other, they tend to cancel each other out; that is, recipients are pulled toward a middle position.[35] In contrast, when weak claims for one position compete against strong claims for another, audiences can be pushed further in the direction of the strong claims than if they had only been exposed to the strong claim.[36] This backfire occurs because the strength difference in the opposing claims can convince a reasoner that the side putting forth the weak argument has an indefensible position.

Hidden Unintended Messages

Messages that attempt to inform or persuade may seem to the communicator to be a single unified message, while the audience receives an amalgam of messages. Whether the message succeeds in convincing the audience as intended, or it backfires instead, depends on which of the messages is accorded priority in the receiver's mind.[37] A possible hidden message is "This message does not apply to me because I do not identify with the individuals depicted or cannot envision myself in the scenario depicted." Another hidden message is that the behavior the message is intended to reduce has desirable side effects, specifically ones that would not have been salient in the receiver's mind prior to encountering the message. One such message, which came through in anti-drug campaigns, is that drug users are thin. Ironically, this inadvertent hidden message of drug campaigns in the 1980s went on to become a fashion advertising meme in the 1990s dubbed "heroin chic."[38]

Superficial Myth Debunking

A popular presentation format in science and health communication is "truth or fiction" or "myth or fact," in which a misconception is stated and then followed by a passage that debunks it. Unfortunately, as logical as this approach seems to be, it often backfires. For instance, one study examined the effects of a flyer "Flu Vaccine Facts & Myths" developed by the US Centers for Disease Control.[39] Immediately after reading the flyer, people remembered nearly all the facts as true and nearly all the myths as false, and the flyer improved people's attitudes toward getting the flu vaccine. Just 30 minutes later, however, people were beginning to recall some of the myths as truths. They also reported less favorable attitudes to flu vaccination and lower intention to get vaccinated compared to people who had read no flyer at all. The backfire effect occurs in this context because, as people forget the specific details of the information they read, they increasingly rely on the familiarity of information to establish its truth.[40] The myth–fact presentation format indiscriminately makes the myths more familiar. Also, the more frequently false claims are repeated, the more likely people are to attribute them to a credible source.[41]

PRACTICAL STRATEGIES TO TAKE THE "COUNTER" OUT OF COUNTERPRODUCTIVE

All these potential pitfalls, along with the finding that backfires can occur even when reasoning is not motivated by ideology, can leave you feeling downright gloomy. If communication is going to backfire, why not just call in sick and stay at home to play with the dog? Better no communication than communication that backfires! Fortunately, for each of the backfire-prone contexts described above there exist research-driven strategies that can help you reach your audiences and avoid backfires. These strategies are summarized in Table 8.2 and detailed below.

Minimize Clashes with Cultural Affiliations

DE-EMPHASIZE DIFFERENCES AND REMOVE CUES THAT MAY INCREASE POLARIZATION

Because people engage in protective cognition in response to information that appears to threaten their group identity, strive to set the stage for people to process information in the least polarized manner possible. Reducing polarization will make it more likely the content of

Table 8.2. Recommendations for Avoiding Backfires

Context of Backfire	Relevant Evidence-Based Strategies
Clashes with cultural affiliations	– Reduce the salience of group differences. – Keep to specifics and spotlight solutions. – Work with an ally who is a member of the group. – Appeal to another of your audience's identities. – Make it safe to go against the group.
Threats to autonomy	– Avoid coercive language. – Emphasize the audience's ultimate agency.
Incompatibility with self-concept	– Craft communication to be self-affirming to the audience. – Minimize threats to self-esteem.
Normalizing the problem	– Focus on the desired behavior rather than overemphasizing the problematic one. – Identify respected early adopters to shift norms.
Mismatched argument strength	– Select potent arguments that resonate with your target audience. – Tailor argument frames according to your goals.
Hidden unintended messages	– Scrutinize for factors that may distract or alienate your target audience.
Superficial myth debunking	– Provide the facts without repeating the misconceptions. – If debunking, aim for depth and understanding of cause. – Give warnings or information inoculations.

the argument will win out. One of the factors that helps determine an individual's support for a policy is the extent to which one believes others in one's group will support it.[42] This mediating factor (inferences about other people's evaluations) can amplify the effect of even small polarizing clues. An individual may assess a policy and agree that it is sound and consistent with group values, but then reject it because the mere presence of a polarizing word, such as "tax" for a conservative or "deregulation" for a liberal, leads the individual to conclude that the group will not support the policy.

People generally underestimate both Democrats' and Republicans' beliefs in climate change, but both groups underestimate Republicans' beliefs in climate change to a much larger degree.[43] The media also tends to overemphasize the partisan divide on climate change. The result is an increase in salience of group differences on the issue, which results in a vicious cycle feeding the partisan divide. Voters and policymakers thus reactively oppose policies from the other party, even when they support the same policy if it is put forth by their own party. The solution is two-fold: (1) Correct the perceptions about party position; and (2) decouple identity concerns from policy evaluation. Key to accomplishing the latter, by reducing both real and perceived threats to group identity, is replacing culturally loaded language with more neutral language.

FOCUS THE DISCUSSION ON THE RELEVANT QUESTION AND POTENTIAL SOLUTIONS

Broad issues – such as capital punishment – are often more intermeshed with ideological baggage than specific issues – such as the guilt of a defendant.[44] Therefore, try to avoid broad, theoretical discussions that may turn into ideological clashes. Instead, keep discussions on the specific situation and goal. Another reason to keep discussions focused is that people take a "head in the sand" approach when faced with an issue they feel is too complex for them to understand.[45] Consider whether you need to agree on all aspects of the problem to converge on a solution. A potential solution may be ideologically consistent even when the problem is not – for example, when the solution to an environmental problem valorizes human ingenuity.[46] Furthermore, individuals may be more likely to take an issue seriously when they know a potential solution exists.[47]

FORM AN ALLIANCE WITH A TRUSTED MEMBER OF A GROUP TO IMPROVE DIALOGUE

When potentially threatening information is supplied by a culturally similar communicator, a level of interpersonal trust allows people to be more open-minded about the information.[48] A communicator who is a member of a religious congregation, political party, or community organization can draw on that identity to relate to other members of that group. Therefore, if your goal is to reach a group of which you are not a member, collaborate with a respected member or leader within it. The "Scientists in Congregations/Synagogues" initiative is an example of this approach.[49] Scientists have worked with evangelical leaders using the language of "Creation Care" to encourage action on climate science by relating scientific research to values of social justice and commitment to preserving God's creation.[50] This strategy to reduce backfires has a beneficial side effect: Communicating about science within churches and other community organizations is a way to reach a much broader swath of the population than the segment that typically attends museums or regularly listens to science news, which has traditionally been small, mostly affluent, and white.[51]

APPEAL TO AN IDENTITY THAT WILL BE RECEPTIVE TO THE ISSUE UNDER DISCUSSION

We all have a variety of identities. When one identity interacts with another, the identity that is the most salient in a particular context trumps the influence of the other identities. This is highlighted by a study that examined the importance of voters' status as parents. It determined that when they were thinking about their children, voters were willing to oppose policies favored by their party.[52] Thus a viable strategy to get past ideological backfire is to tap into another of your audience's identities. For example, party identity may not be a gateway to a conversation about environmental regulations with a rural conservative, but appealing to that same individual's identity as a hunter, fisher, or steward of the family land can open a meaningful dialogue on the topic.[53]

Another example is that although American political independents tend to lean Democratic or Republican on many issues, the personal importance of their independent identity has a considerable influence on how they engage with politics.[54] Tapping into the independent identity can thus encourage an audience to be more skeptical of attempts at partisan influence. Promisingly in terms of applying this strategy in divisive US politics, the percentage of American voters not affiliated with a political party is growing.[55] Tapping into a "good citizen" identity can also reduce partisan influence. When people are primed to think about their civic duty, they seek more information and reason more evenhandedly.[56] Finally, if your goal is to encourage an individual to join a group that is engaging in desirable behaviors, such as a community group spearheading local conservation projects, it is important to highlight not only the shared values and identity, but also individuals' sense of efficacy that they are capable of doing what the community does.[57]

MAKE IT SAFE TO GO AGAINST THE GROUP

When encouraging people to go against the ideological commitments of one of their group identities, consider how to minimize the threat to the group relationship. One way to do so is by making it possible to take the desired action while maintaining anonymity. During the surge of the delta variant of COVID-19, some individuals in vaccine-hesitant communities sought the vaccine wearing disguises to prevent others from recognizing them.[58] Although it is not fair that anyone should feel the need to conceal a health choice for fear of being ostracized from their communities, most of us can relate to the reality of keeping secrets from family or friends just to keep the peace. Life is short; arguing is exhausting. In your communication efforts, do whatever you can to minimize any risks for people who wish to go against their groups, without passing judgment on their group affiliations (or their unwillingness to sport their "I'm vaccinated" sticker in public).

Reduce Threats to Autonomy

SELECT NONCOERCIVE LANGUAGE

Because overly coercive attempts at attitude change often backfire, it is possible to reduce the backfire effect by using less dogmatic language. This benefit of toning down the language was demonstrated in a comparison of alcohol-prevention materials aimed at college students.[59] Versions of the materials presented the same facts about the risks of alcohol consumption but either concluded with noncoercive language such as "you may wish to consider" and "we believe these conclusions are reasonable" or concluded with coercive language such as "make it obvious" and "any reasonable person must acknowledge these conclusions." Compared to the noncoercive message, the coercive message was rated more negatively, resulted in greater self-reported intent to consume alcohol, and greater alcohol consumption (as measured surreptitiously at a "beer taste test" that was a later part of the study). The difference in the effects of the coercive and noncoercive messages was largest among heavy drinkers. Furthermore, among heavy drinkers, messages advocating controlled drinking were more effective than messages advocating abstaining from alcohol. Avoiding toughly worded health campaigns is thus especially prudent when targeting high-risk populations.

DIRECTLY EMPHASIZE THE AUDIENCE'S FREEDOM OF CHOICE

Another study showed that although the use of coercive language such as "ought," "must," and "should," instead of "could," "may," and "might" led to backfires to health messages, the negative impact of the controlling language could be reversed by ending the message with an affirmation of the reader's autonomy.[60] Therefore, a second strategy to reduce the back-fire effect resulting from threats to autonomy is to state directly that the receiver of the message has the final choice of what actions to take. Inter-estingly, in fear appeals, emphasizing that the recommended action is doable by the message recipient makes the appeal most persuasive.[61] The distinction between fear appeals and threats to autonomy was pointed out above, but it is noteworthy that, in both cases, empowering the recipi-ent of the message increases the effectiveness of communication.

Increase Compatibility with Self-Concept

EMPHASIZE ALIGNMENT WITH HOW INDIVIDUALS VIEW THEMSELVES

If the perceived incompatibility with self-concept is due to a miscon-ception, the misconception can be respectfully addressed. The *Science, Evolution, and Creationism* publication takes this approach.[62] Although some people believe evolution is incompatible with their faith, the publication points out that their religious leaders may accept all or nearly all tenets of evolutionary theory. Another relevant resource is *The Clergy Letter Project*, a compilation of statements from clergy within various religious denominations attesting to the compatibility of their faith and science, including the science of evolution.[63] Con-sider sharing any personal stories you have of reconciling your faith or other identities with science. This approach is similar to identify-ing oneself as a member of a group to reduce clashes due to cultural affiliations, but it also applies when the self-concept is more abstract than belonging to a group – for instance, the interaction of the self-concept of being "natural" or "healthy" with someone's willingness to accept preventive health interventions like vaccines.

USE AFFIRMATION TO MINIMIZE THREATS TO SELF-ESTEEM

When the threat to self-esteem or self-concept is real, a different approach to minimizing the backfire effect is warranted. One such approach, demonstrated in a study aimed at discouraging tanning, involves self-affirmation. Ultraviolet photography, which reveals sun damage that is invisible to the unaided eye, has been used as an individualized intervention to discourage deliberate sun exposure. With high-risk populations (those who value tanning) this health intervention backfires: Individuals who receive photos showing their sun-damaged skin increase their sun exposure.[64] The backfire effect was completely eliminated when, prior to receiving their ultraviolet photo, these same populations engaged in a self-affirmation activity – completing a survey that asked them to rate how much they valued a range of personal strengths, such as "I value my ability to think clearly." With the affirmation, instead of the photo intervention backfiring it had the desired effect of reducing people's subsequent sun exposure. This dramatic reversal is attributed to the fact that with the self-affirmation, people no longer had to engage in a defensive reaction to maintain a positive self-concept. Therefore, in a communication situation that may challenge an aspect of your audience members' self-concept, provide them with the opportunity to recall other things that contribute to their self-esteem.

Do Not Normalize the Problem

EMPHASIZE THE DESIRABLE BEHAVIOR

Drawing attention to common behaviors can encourage their adoption. Beware – this works equally well for desirable and undesirable behaviors. If an undesired behavior is widespread, it is best to put the focus on what is desirable, rather than calling attention to the prevalence of the undesirable behavior. Also, because people tend to underestimate others' willingness to sacrifice for the collective good (compared with their own), when asking individuals to support policies that require cooperation, it is helpful to have them reflect on their own willingness to cooperate as a point of reference.[65]

POINT OUT ESTEEMED EARLY ADOPTERS

A strategy to promote shifts in behavioral norms is to recognize "early adopters," especially those who are respected members of a community. Research on diffusion of innovations finds that adoption of new technologies, such as solar panels, often spreads along lines of social affiliations and group membership.[66]

Match Argument Strength

CHOOSE ARGUMENT FRAMES MOST COMPELLING TO YOUR AUDIENCE

What counts as a strong argument is highly dependent on the target audience. Furthermore, how an issue is framed plays an even greater role than evidence in what arguments people find convincing.[67] Frames give more weight to certain factors than others. For example, global climate change can be framed as an imminent environmental catastrophe or a public health threat. The environmental-catastrophe frame has led to backfires among conservatives.[68] The public health frame, which emphasizes the potential impact of climate change on infectious diseases, asthma, heat stroke, and other medical issues, elicits more bipartisan support for climate action.[69] In another comparison of frames on the same issue, the more health-related "air pollution" frame generated more support for carbon emissions mitigation than the frames of "climate change," "global warming," and "carbon pollution."[70] Air pollution was the most compelling frame among liberals and conservatives, but the advantage of the air pollution frame over the other frames was especially pronounced among conservatives.

Another framing variation involves local or personal relevance. For example, when climate change victims are socially distant (farmers abroad), but not when climate change victims are locals, there is a backfire effect among conservatives, resulting in decreased support for climate change mitigation.[71] The impact of ocean acidification (caused by atmospheric carbon dioxide dissolving in the oceans) on the shellfish industry in one's local district has proven to be an effective frame among conservatives, and coverage of climate change using this frame has contributed to policy action.[72] In short, to avoid the backfire effect that occurs as a result of mismatched argument strength, select the most audience-relevant arguments.

CHOOSE ARGUMENT FRAMES CONSISTENT WITH YOUR GOALS

In selecting frames, also attend to the goals for communication. Is the scale of how the problem is framed consistent with the scale of the proposed solution? In calling attention to a problem, the focus can be placed on a particular case or episode, such as the story of one hapless polar bear stuck on an ice floe or one extreme weather event, or the focus can be on general trends or themes, such as what is happening to the overall polar bear population or the trends in extreme weather events. When arguing for policy changes, thematic framing is stronger because the scale helps highlight the need for collective action.[73]

Avoid Unintended Messages

SELECT CHARACTERS AND SCENARIOS THAT RESONATE

Entertainment education using narrative is a common format for campaigns to create awareness and change behavior on health and social issues, especially to target children and teens. This format has a long history: In the 1930s, the film *Reefer Madness* (previously called *Tell Your Children*) kicked off an era of short social guidance films produced by government and private agencies.[74] *Reefer Madness* and other films of the era have gone on to become cult classics, relished on social media due to their hilarious and exaggerated treatment of marijuana use and other social ills. Although today it is difficult to imagine anyone using such an over-the-top style for anything but satire, young people are also highly sensitive to subtle messages and are likely to react negatively to pressure from authority.[75] A modern anti-tobacco campaign "Talk to Your Kids," underwritten by a multinational tobacco corporation, may have deliberately exploited this knowledge to induce a backfire against the ads.[76]

When appropriately designed, narrative can make a message more persuasive than a similar non-narrative message, and the elements of the story format can reduce the backfire effect.[77] One mechanism by which this occurs is through the reduction of perceived invulnerability due to identification with the characters. The message must walk the fine line of being persuasive without triggering an audience reaction against its persuasive intent. Choosing the right characters (ones with whom your audience will identify) and ensuring that their appearance and behavior are not sending undesired messages may require input from a pilot group of target audience members.

Strategically Address Myths

IF THE CONTEXT NECESSITATES BREVITY, PROVIDE FACTS WITHOUT REPEATING MISCONCEPTIONS

Attempting to debunk myths by negation strengthens myth recall because the act of negating information activates that information in the brain.[78] When the brain encodes a sentence such as "GMOs are not Frankenfoods," the connection between GMOs and Frankenfoods is strengthened, and later we are steered wrong due to the reasoning shortcut of inferring veracity from familiarity – the familiarity heuristic. Therefore, when the communication context precludes deeper exploration of a myth to help the audience understand why it is wrong, it is more effective to present the facts without repeating the myths. The effectiveness of this approach was demonstrated using a facts-only version of the previously mentioned vaccine flyer. Unlike the "Flu Vaccine Facts & Myths" version that led to the backfire effect, the facts-only version had the desired effect. Both immediately after reading the facts-only version and after a delay, people reported more favorable attitudes toward flu vaccination and higher intentions of getting vaccinated than people who read no flyer.[79] The strategy of not repeating myths to avoid backfires also applies to affirmative phrasing (GMOs are safe) versus negative phrasing (GMOs are not dangerous) of statements. The affirmative phrasing gets around the idiosyncratic encoding and retrieval of negative statements from memory.

WHEN DIRECTLY ADDRESSING MISCONCEPTIONS, AIM FOR DEPTH AND UNDERSTANDING

Addressing myths directly is only effective when you have time to do more than state and negate. Decades of research on textbooks that directly address students' misconceptions – refutation texts – demonstrates that they are more likely to reduce misconceptions and help students come to a scientifically accurate understanding than traditional expository science textbooks.[80] Compared to fiction-and-fact flyers, a refutation text's treatment of a misconception, such as "Earth is closer to the sun when it is summertime in the Northern Hemisphere," aims for depth and understanding of causal mechanisms while addressing the specific shortcomings of the misconception – for example, pointing out that when it is summer in the Northern Hemisphere it is winter in the Southern Hemisphere and vice versa. The deeper exploration of the misconceptions allows people to form judgments about information when they receive it, and these judgments are stored along with the information.

The direct approach to addressing misconceptions is also more effective when people are given a reason to process information deeply. For example, in one study, people read an information sheet about a new cancer test, and half were told beforehand that the experimenters would ask their opinion of the content.[81] Those who did not expect to be asked about the content misremembered myths as truths more frequently. In addition, as they misremembered the information, their attitudes to the cancer test shifted to align with the misremembered information. In contrast, people who were encouraged to form an opinion about the content as they were reading it rarely misremembered myths as truths. Interestingly, even when they did this, misremembered information was much less likely to influence their attitudes.

GIVE PRE-EXPOSURE WARNINGS (INFORMATION INOCULATIONS) ABOUT MISINFORMATION

Warnings prior to misinformation exposure are far more effective than corrections after exposure, as illustrated by a study of people's responses to conflicting information about carbon nanotubes – tiny graphite tubes used to convert sunlight into electricity.[82] People were presented with scientific evidence as well as an unsupported counter-factual claim. The study included conditions in which the unsubstantiated information came with a post-exposure correction, a pre-exposure warning, or an initial expectation of accountability (the need to justify their reasoning) and a post-exposure correction. Although the warning and the correction were worded the same, they did not have the same effect. When given a warning before being exposed to an unsubstantiated claim, people ignored the claim in favor of the scientific evidence. The correction did not help people ignore the claim unless they had been given an expectation of accountability. In that case, reasoning was similar to the pre-exposure warning condition. Pre-bunking and accountability motivation encourage people to attend to the quality of the arguments and evidence as they are being presented, so they are less likely to be misled by misinformation.

An evocative term for pre-exposure warning is "information inoculation." The concept of information inoculation long precedes the age of social media, or even the internet.[83] Nowadays, of course, fake news leaves people across party lines confused about basic facts.[84] The ubiquity of misinformation raises the question of how to distinguish between inoculation against future exposure to misinformation and debunking misinformation previously encountered. Unlike the study about carbon nanotubes, to which the majority of the participants would come with "virgin ears" about the topic, this would not be the reality for the pressing issues of our time. To avoid backfires, therefore, inoculation cannot take the form of state and negate.

One inoculation option is to use a short general message. For example, a study on responses to messages about global climate change tested the inoculation "Some politically motivated groups are using misleading tactics to try to convince the public that there is a lot of disagreement among scientists."[85] A second inoculation option, for when the situation affords more time, is to directly address a myth. For example, the study also tested an example of a real global warming petition that included fraudulent signatories like Charles Darwin. Both inoculation strategies were effective, although the second was more effective than the first. It is also possible to inoculate people by teaching them about the misleading argumentation strategies or logical fallacies they will encounter.[86]

An active inoculation option, a game in which participants generate fake news articles about a politically charged issue from the perspective of denier, alarmist, clickbait monger, or conspiracy theorist, is ideal for a formal education setting.[87] A randomized study with high school students demonstrated that playing the game decreased the persuasiveness and perceived reliability of fake news articles. An in-depth activity like the fake news game not only serves as an inoculation against specific misinformation, it provides learners with the opportunity to explore the varied motivations of those who promulgate it.

Much communication, from fact sheets to videos to podcasts to books, are simply put out into the world, separated from the creator. But they are nonetheless entering into a conversation, just as the sea engages in a kind of conversation with Jason deCaires Taylor's hauntingly beautiful underwater sculptures. The evidence-based strategies presented in this chapter and throughout the book help a communicator design with the audience-scape in mind, the way deCaires Taylor designs with the sea-scape in mind. The real face-to-face (in-person or virtual) conversation, however, calls for an additional set of communication competencies,

Figure 8.1. Quick Tip Summary on Avoiding Backfires

Avoiding backfires to unwelcome information	Avoiding backfires to any type of information

• *Cultural clashes*
  • Highlight similarities and use neutral language
  • Focus on solutions and specifics
  • Collaborate with a group member
  • Connect through a shared identity
  • Make independence safe and confidential
• *Autonomy*
  • Select less dogmatic phrasings
  • Confirm liberty of choice
• *Self-concept*
  • Emphasize alignment with self-concept
  • Reduce threats to self-esteem
	• *Normalization*
	  • Point out desired behavior
	  • Identify culturally relevant adopters
	• *Argument strength*
	  • Choose audience-relevant arguments
	  • Choose goal-consistent arguments
	• *Hidden messages*
	  • Review from audience perspective
	• *Addressing myths*
	  • Apply facts-only approach
	  • If addressing falsehoods, treat them in depth
	  • Provide information inoculations

focused on the establishment of mutual trust. If they feel that they do not have the skills to succeed, scientists tend not to prioritize communication that seeks to build trust.[88] Trust has been a theme throughout the book, and the next chapter adds a missing piece. With the steady equanimity of the underwater sculpture gardens at the back of our minds, we turn to the physical, physiological, and psychological underpinnings of empathetic, trust-building communication.

Figure 8.1 summarizes the tips for avoiding backfires to both unwelcome information and any type of information.

9

Crucial Conversations, Trust, and the Dark Matter of Communication

When my dog dragged me into the rabbit-infested scrub brush one drizzly winter morning, I was not amused. We were a couple of miles from home on a nine-mile loop to the beach and I was aching for breakfast, a hot shower, and dry clothes. I loped along behind but decelerated and began to grumble when it seemed we were going in circles, presumably stalking bunnies. The response to my reluctance was an intense canine gaze. The message was clear: "I know something important. Trust me." So I shut up and followed the zigzagging. When my canine companion finally stopped and pointed to what she needed me to see, I vowed to never doubt her again.

It was my neighbors' scared, starving, shivering foster dog crouched beneath a fallen tree. The forlorn creature had been on the lam for a cold, rainy two weeks after slipping her collar and bolting, and she could not have survived much longer before succumbing to the elements and the coyotes. Instead, she made a full recovery and found a life full of joy and love. The happy ending would not have been possible without my companion's intelligence and incredible nose, but above all, an instant of silent communication so compelling that I placed my complete trust in her. Trust is often beyond words, even between humans.

The role of trust in science communication has arisen throughout this book, but this chapter introduces a missing element: nonverbal messages – what I think of as the dark matter of communication. Just as the mysterious dark matter in the universe holds everything together and makes possible life as we know it, the dark matter of communication holds invisible power over our inner worlds and relations with others. This chapter explores the kinds of signals we send (usually inadvertently and often at odds with our words), delves into their psychological and physiological roots, and lays the groundwork to help us all become more self-aware, empathetic, effective communicators.

CHAPTER LEARNING OBJECTIVES: DARK MATTER OF COMMUNICATION

Knowledge: What mental and physical processes underpin emotion and empathy?

Skills: Practice active listening and perspective-taking to grasp what remains unspoken.

Habits of Mind: Cultivate awareness of breath, body, and cognitions during communication.

HOW COMMUNICATION DARK MATTER REVEALS OTHERS' EMOTIONS AND INTENTIONS

No one, whether scientist or nonscientist, can be well informed about everything. Often the best we can do is to rely on a credible expert. Scientists want to be viewed as credible, and they believe their expertise should give them credibility. It does, but that is only part of the trust equation, because it is insufficient for us to decide if someone will act in our best interests.[1] When a speaker walks out on stage or your new doctor enters the waiting room, chances are you make immediate judgments that influence how much you are willing to trust what they have to say based on how warm, kind, or benevolent they appear. Body language is a decisive factor in those judgments.

Nonverbal cues can be used deliberately in an act of communication, for example a wave to get someone's attention or a caring touch to comfort someone who has received bad news, but our bodies also communicate volumes without our conscious knowledge. Signals that inadvertently reveal something about our state of mind are known as **tells**.[2] The term "tell" comes from poker, where the ability to conceal one's feelings about one's cards – maintain a "poker face" – is an essential skill, as is the ability to read the tells of other players to figure out what kind of hand they are holding. Facial expressions, eye contact, gestures, stance and posture, muscle tone, and behavioral tics are examples of body-language tells. In anxiety-inducing situations, we may use self-comforting touch, such as stroking our own hair or neck. Feeling the need to restrain ourselves, we may bite our lips.

Tells can be expansive movements or small ones, involving just a single muscle group. They may be of an extended duration, such as a resolutely clenched jaw, or they may be fleeting, such as an eye flash – a quick widening of the eyelids without moving the eyebrows, often wide enough to reveal the sclera adjacent to the iris. Eye flashes last for an average of three-quarters of a second, and when used by a speaker, they accentuate the word being spoken.[3] Fleeting, miniature signals that appear for only a fraction of a second when we are trying to conceal our true feelings are known as **micro-tells**. In trying to put on a brave or nonchalant face, we may have our conflicting inner fear, grief, or disgust bubble to the surface as a micro-tell.[4] When we are being dishonest, our bodies tend to give us away even more than our facial expressions.[5]

Faking a tell to try to convince others that we are feeling something we are not feeling is known as a **counterfeit tell**.[6] For example, poker players may fake a fleeting smile to bluff their opponents into thinking they have a much better hand than they actually have. Politicians produce many counterfeit tells, such as turning down the corners of the mouth to project an image of compassion, striding out and exaggerating the backward swing of the arms with elbows moving laterally outward from the body to appear energetic and masculine, and waving to imaginary friends in the audience to come across as more likable. Counterfeit tells can succeed in conveying the image an individual wishes to convey, but the risk is coming across as disingenuous if the tells are identified as fake. Because our tells usually give us away regardless of our efforts to send a message at odds with our views, before engaging in a dialogue consider your consciously or unconsciously held views about the issue and your interlocutor(s).

THE ART OF CRUCIAL CONVERSATIONS AND THE ROLE OF COMMUNICATION DARK MATTER

High-Stakes Dialogues Call for Attention to the ABCs of Interactions

In dialogues about the personal and social implications of science, especially health and environmental issues, stakes are high, opinions vary, and emotions run strong. Dialogues with those three characteristics are dubbed "crucial conversations" in the book *Crucial Conversations: Tools for Talking When Stakes Are High.*[7] Although *Crucial Conversations* focuses on personal and workplace conversations and does not cover health or science communication, its practical recommendations are relevant across settings:

1. *Crucial conversations require a commitment by all parties to work together to seek mutual purpose.* Although the decision-making process and the dialogue to get the pertinent information on the table may be accomplished at different times with different stakeholders, conversations should never be held as a pretense when a decision has already been made. The relevant individuals should be involved early enough in the decision-making process that their input can be taken into consideration.

2. *During the conversation, individuals in the listening role should listen actively.* Listeners should avoid getting distracted by formulating the next thing they want to say when they transition to the speaking role. They can check their understanding by paraphrasing what the speaker is saying, for example, "So let me see if I am following you …" In addition to making the speaker feel heard, paraphrasing helps catch any misunderstandings.

3. *Individuals in the speaking role should speak with confidence, but also with humility.* Humility manifests itself as an openness to considering other perspectives, which involves distinguishing facts from the story we construct about those facts. In the context of science communication, this entails distinguishing evidence from our interpretation of the evidence and recognizing the influence of our values on our conclusions.

4. *The ABCs of crucial conversations are Agree, Build, Compare.* The parties having a crucial conversation may agree on much or even most aspects of what they are discussing, but when emotions run strong, it is easy to lose sight of the areas of agreement. For example, everyone may agree on the scope of the problem to be addressed. Acknowledge the agreement and build on it by adding relevant details that have not yet been discussed. When all the relevant information is on the table, compare positions and focus on uncovering the reasons for any areas of disagreement.

5. *For crucial conversations to succeed, all parties in the conversation must feel safe so that no one switches into fight-or-flight mode.* Verbally trying to shut someone down, either directly or more subtly through coercive language (as discussed in the context of the backfire effect in the previous chapter), violates safety, but so can the complex nonverbal tells that shape conversations.

Body Language Is Integral to Conversation Choreography

Like volleys in a well-played game of tennis, turn taking in a conversation can seem so natural as to not require an explanation, and yet the choreography of conversations is a complicated thing.[8] Listeners who are content to continue listening may signal so in several ways, such as with smiles, brief verbal reactions (yeah, oh, wow), repeating the speaker's words, asking questions, or remaining silent but orienting to the speaker.[9] Listeners often nod, slowly to show that they are following the speaker or more quickly to convey a sense of emphasis or urgency. Fast nodding can signal enthusiasm or agreement, or it can be a way for the listener to hurry the speaker along so that the listener can take over the speaking role. The direction of the listener's gaze distinguishes the two potential meanings of fast nodding: Supportive fast nodding is accompanied by a gaze directed at the speaker, while fast nodding to signal a wish to speak is accompanied by a gaze directed away from the speaker.[10] As with nodding, slow and rapid head shaking mean different things, with slow shaking indicating a shared reaction (incredulity, for instance) and fast shaking indicating a desire to interject. In contrast with attentive silent listening, in which the lips may be pressed together and the fingers or the hand may cover the mouth, a desire to transition to the speaking role may be signaled by opening the mouth and inhaling audibly, in an exaggeration of the normal preparatory movements for speech.[11] Alerting signals, such as raising a hand or finger, may be used as well.

A speaker's tells divulge a desire to hold the floor or a willingness to relinquish it. For example, a drop in vocal pitch can signal the end of a speaking turn. When a speaker's gaze comes to rest on a listener, this can be an indication that the baton is being passed to that individual. In a group setting, the next speaker is likely to be the listener on whom the speaker's gaze last came to rest.[12] Speakers maintain a claim on the speaking role by looking away from the listener, being emphatic, keeping the hands in motion, as well as freezing in mid-motion if interrupted and holding the frozen position.

Body language can leave us especially exposed in communication situations that make us uncomfortable or annoyed. Listeners bored or stressed by a conversation may avert their gaze from the speaker and steal glances around to find an exit. Because we are more conscious of our eye movements than we are of the rest of our bodies, when a listener is politely feigning continued interest, tells that give away the desire to escape may be the shifting of weight from foot to foot, the orientation of the body away from the speaker, and the feet pointing toward the planned escape.[13] A presenter bored with the audience's questions may inch away from the podium. A time-strapped doctor may try to maintain a compassionate expression while unconsciously turning toward the door from the waist down.

MIND, BODY, AND GENUINE EMPATHETIC CONNECTION

The book *Crucial Conversations* emphasizes the importance of distinguishing between a situation (the facts) and the story we tell ourselves about the situation (our interpretation of the facts). Intriguingly, not only is this distinction crucial in inferences we make about the external world, it is crucial when we are making sense of our own internal worlds. Conducive to the goal of becoming a more empathetic and effective communicator is an appreciation of how physiological responses and psychological responses interact with each other and with the external (physical and social) context.

Emotions Arise from an Interplay of Psychology and Physiology

Consider a now classic study that demonstrated the fascinating interplay between psychology, physiology, and context in emotion. Men who crossed the rocking, swaying Capilano suspension bridge, 200 feet above the Capilano River (near Vancouver, Canada) were more attracted to a female interviewer who met them on the other side than were men who were met by the same interviewer after they had crossed a low, sturdy bridge upstream.[14] Men who crossed the nerve-racking bridge introduced more sexual imagery into an ambiguous cognitive task conducted by the interviewer and were more likely to phone her afterward. To rule out the possibility of confounding effects in the real-world setting (namely differences in the adventurousness of the men crossing the two bridges), the researchers duplicated the findings in a controlled laboratory experiment, using the threat of an electric shock instead of a scary bridge crossing. This and many other studies demonstrate that bodily reactions elicited by one aspect of a situation can be reinterpreted and attributed to another.[15] In short, emotions arise from a combination of physiological responses and psychological inferences.

Although several regions of the brain are involved in the processing of emotion, from the evolutionarily ancient set of brain structures – the limbic system – that include the amygdala and hypothalamus to the higher cortical regions involved in cognitive control and decision-making, the body is central to the experience of emotion. Neuroscientist Antonio Damasio argues that an emotion begins when we are exposed to an external stimulus to which we respond physiologically, such as through changes in respiration, heart rate, and blood flow to the skin and muscles.[16] Feedback about the physiological response is sent to the brain, where it is mapped and interpreted, giving rise to the emotion felt. Figure 9.1 shows the interconnections among physiology, psychology, and the external content.

Assuming you are not reading this on the subway or in another public place where onlookers will think you are a bit odd, try on the following expressions and note how you feel after a few seconds of holding each:

- Raise your eyebrows, widen your eyes as much as you can, and draw your head back.

Figure 9.1. The Interplay of Psychology and Physiology

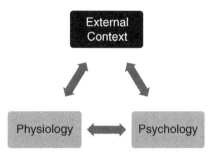

- Slightly raise your eyebrows without widening your eyes and cock your head to one side.
- Squint, lower your eyebrows, and clench your jaw.

The first expression is one of fear and surprise. Widened eyes allow more light to strike the retina to provide visual information about a potential danger.[17] The second expression is one of appeasement. Finally, the squint with lowered eyebrows may have been the same expression you made at the back of the person who was obliviously texting while blocking your way. It is an expression of anger. Without relevant context, these instructions would not trigger the corresponding emotions, but hopefully you did get an inkling of them. When people are given step-by-step instructions to make certain facial expressions (under a ruse to prevent them from knowing the true purpose of the experiment), the facial expressions influence their responses; for instance, with the corners of their lips upturned, they find cartoons funnier.[18] When individuals make facial expressions corresponding to emotions, they have measurable physiological responses that are distinct for each expression.[19]

As with facial expressions, body language regulates emotion. Putting people in a hunched, threatened position makes them more stressed about an upcoming test, and they are less likely to persist on a frustrating task after being in that posture.[20] Adopting open, expansive postures – power poses – has been shown to decrease levels of the stress hormone cortisol and increase testosterone; adopting threatened postures has the opposite effect.[21] These physiological changes only seem to occur when people are taking on the poses in the company of others – a relevant social context.[22] Interestingly, people often mirror one another's expressions and postures, and the mirroring appears to underlie empathy.

Effective Communication Is Rooted in Empathetic Connection

Effective communication requires emotional intelligence, which includes the ability to recognize and manage emotions in oneself, as well as the ability to recognize emotions in others and respond appropriately.[23] In short, emotional intelligence is a blend of self-awareness and empathy. The words "empathy" and "sympathy" are sometimes used interchangeably, but they do not have the same meaning. Carl Rogers, one of the founders of humanistic psychology, defined empathy as the ability to accurately perceive another person's frame of reference, including the emotional components and meanings.[24] Empathy is about perspective-taking, and as such it is a creative act of the imagination. With respect to the dark matter of communication, empathetic communicators do three things:

- Notice subtle verbal and nonverbal cues in an interlocutor.
- Correctly interpret these cues.
- Send back signals demonstrating that they understand.[25]

Empathy is a process, not a personality trait, and its essence is respectful, nonevaluative listening.[26] A lack of empathy causes devastating communication breakdowns across personal and professional settings.[27] Consider the complementary schismogenesis between cocktail party goers with different conversational styles discussed in Chapter 1. Such breakdowns could be avoided if the party goers used the three empathetic listening strategies instead of amping up their communication styles.

The impact of empathy is particularly profound in medicine. In a study involving hundreds of patients, in which both patients and independent observers rated physician empathy, physician empathy was shown to have direct, measurable effects on patient health outcomes.[28] Because all readers are patients (including those who are also doctors), you likely have personal experience consistent with this finding. The anecdote I shared in Chapter 1, of the orthopedic surgeon who was able to improve my compliance with medical advice by connecting with me through a shared identity, is a good example of the healing power of perspective-taking.

Empathy Involves Unconsciously Mirroring Others

Empathy is a multifaceted phenomenon, one aspect of which is the transmission of an emotional state from one individual to another without cognitive reflection. This is known as **affective empathy** and it involves mirroring another, especially the mirroring of facial expressions. The unconscious replication of another's nonverbal cues activates the same neural circuitry that would be involved in representing the corresponding emotion from a first-person perspective, allowing an observer to understand another through the mapping of that individual's actions onto the observer's own representation of that action.[29]

Individual "mirror neurons" have been discovered in the brains of nonhuman primates. Mirror neurons respond to specific actions but not others, and some of these cells respond to the same action when it is seen but not heard, and when it is heard but not seen.[30] Mirror neurons' activity is affected by the goal of an action and by social cues, such as gaze direction. Research supports the existence of a mirror neuron system in humans as well (although human studies are constrained by the dangers of doing invasive single cell recordings). Even before the discovery of mirror neurons, however, it was known that the accuracy with which an observer can rate another person's pain or anger is related to how closely the observer's own physiological responses match those of the distressed individual.[31]

Empathy Also Flows from Our Conscious Interpretations

Thus far, the discussion of emotions and empathy has glossed over their cognitive components. Consider an experimental study in which participants were injected with adrenaline, under the guise of testing a vitamin compound on vision.[32] Some participants were told about the side effects of the "vitamin shot" and some were not. When placed in the company of a stooge who acted either silly or angry, uninformed participants felt euphoric or angry in parallel with the behavior of the stooge; however, participants told exactly what symptoms they would feel did not respond emotionally to the stooge's behavior. They had an alternative rationale for their bodily sensations.

Empathy also has a cognitive component, **cognitive empathy**. While the cognitive component of emotion involves conscious appraisal of one's own bodily state in relation to the context, cognitive empathy is conscious appraisal of another's intentions and context. In a study in which subjects were treated rudely by an experimenter and later given the opportunity to retaliate, they were significantly less likely to retaliate if they were told that the experimenter was under a lot of stress from his preliminary doctoral examination.[33] Communication of the mitigating circumstances either before or after the rude behavior reduced the victims' physiological responses and retaliatory action; however, knowing about the mitigating circumstances beforehand had a much greater impact. In that scenario, the mitigating information could be considered during the conscious appraisal of the behavior as it occurred.

Use cognitive empathy to give others the benefit of the doubt: If you can change the story you tell yourself about the reasons for another person's behavior, you may be in a better position to develop an empathetic connection to succeed in crucial conversations. (Note that giving others the benefit of the doubt does not mean putting yourself at the mercy of someone who is cruel or disruptive or to put your energy into engaging when the outcome is unlikely to be fruitful. Conscious appraisal applies equally well to giving others grace as to giving oneself grace.)

It Is Not Always "Mind over Matter"

Cognitive empathy is powerful, and it is much easier to put it into practice when physiological responses are in check. If, as Louis Pasteur once said, "chance favors the prepared mind," then empathy favors the prepared body. For example, the sense of being endangered – whether by a real physical threat or a threat to self-esteem or dignity – is a universal trigger for anger, but how easy it is to trigger anger depends on your physiological state before being exposed to the threat. If the adrenal-cortical system is on high alert, even our cognitive assessment of a situation may fail to prevent a relatively small stressor from leading to fury – what Daniel Goleman refers to as an emotional hijacking.[34] Fortunately, exciting findings about the one vegetative life support function that is under both automatic and volitional control can help a communicator maintain composure.

THE SECRET TO COMMUNICATORS' COMPOSURE – NOT A LOT OF HOT AIR

Gasp of surprise, pants of laughter, sigh of contentment, yawn of boredom, snort of disgust, sobs of sadness, puffed-out chest of pride, rasps of rage, groan of annoyance, moan of resignation, uneven breathing of guilt … everyday experience tells us that our breathing patterns are influenced by our emotional state, and research demonstrates that the relationship between emotion and breathing is bidirectional.[35] Not only does our state of mind affect our breathing, our breathing affects our state of mind, a fact that has profound implications for anyone who suffers from stage fright or individuals trying to maintain their cool in the midst of a crucial conversation. Also of profound significance for communicators is the fact that breathing and voice are physiologically interconnected. Disturbances of breathing patterns contribute to the vocal tells that give us away. Illuminating these psychological aspects of breathing requires some fundamentals on the physiology of breathing.

It All Starts with an Intricately Beautiful Architecture

Lungs are not simple bellows; they contain a majestic fractal-like network of passageways, leading to the finest fabric through which our blood and the atmosphere engage in a life-sustaining caress. When we breathe in, the diaphragm descends and the intercostal muscles lift the chest up and out. The lungs expand, drawing in air. Entering through the nose or mouth, air passes the larynx (a valve that keeps food out of the airway and contains the delicate vocal cords) and enters the trachea. The trachea extends into the chest, where it bifurcates into two main bronchi, one to each lung. The bronchi each diverge into subbranches, which branch again and again into successively narrower passages called bronchioles. The final divisions of the bronchioles end in the air sacs where gas exchange occurs. The airway is structured like an inverted tree, with the trachea as the trunk and intricate branches fanning out into tiny twig-like bronchioles. At the end of the bronchioles the tiny sacs, called alveoli, are each approximately the size of a large water droplet. Human lungs have about 500 million alveoli with exceedingly fine membranes that collectively provide a vast surface area for gas exchange.[36]

Thin-walled capillaries, so narrow that red blood cells have to squeeze through, envelop the alveolar membranes. Because the concentration (or more accurately, the partial pressure) of atmospheric oxygen in the alveoli is much greater than in the blood returning from the body's tissues to the lung, oxygen passively diffuses through the alveolar membranes and the walls of the capillaries into the blood. A small amount of oxygen can dissolve in the blood, but hemoglobin in red blood cells is responsible for transporting most of the oxygen to the tissues. At the same time as oxygen is diffusing into the capillaries, carbon dioxide from the body's metabolic processes is diffusing in the other direction into the alveoli to be breathed into the atmosphere. This all happens in a heartbeat, literally, as a bolus of blood is passed through the capillaries with each pump of the heart.

Depleting Carbon Dioxide (Not Oxygen!) Makes You Lose Your Calm

Three regions of the brain control respiration: (1) A central pattern generator in the brainstem maintains unconscious control of the oscillatory inspiration-expiration rhythm; (2) the primary motor cortex takes command of the respiratory muscles when we consciously alter our breathing; and (3) the amygdala alters breathing in response to emotional stimuli, such as those that trigger a fight-or-flight response.[37] When we are scared or angry, an increase in breathing rate readies us for action. This response is adaptive when we are going to run or engage in combat, but in the case of stage fright and other stressful but sedentary communication situations it can generate a cascade of unpleasant and sometimes debilitating sensations. Although fear of public speaking is one of the most common phobias, the underlying respiratory mechanism tends to be misconceived by most people, including communication trainers.

The common advice "just take a deep breath" is based on the fallacy that we can fix the stress response by simply taking in more oxygen. Unless we are exercising intensely, standing on a mountaintop, or holding our breath, oxygen is not what regulates respiration. This is because, under normal rest conditions, hemoglobin is nearly fully saturated with oxygen. Contrary to popular belief, carbon dioxide is the culprit responsible for the symptoms experienced in a sedentary stress situation. To understand why, consider a normal (nonsedentary) fight-or-flight response. During physical exertion, the muscle cells produce extra carbon dioxide as a byproduct of metabolism. Carbon dioxide is readily converted to carbonic acid, which means that active tissues are more acidic (lower pH). In lower pH, hemoglobin has a reduced affinity for oxygen; thus, hemoglobin releases more oxygen into the active tissues where it is needed. Furthermore, as the carbon dioxide levels in the blood start to increase, the increase is detected by sensors called carotid bodies in the carotid arteries. The information is relayed to the central pattern generator in the brainstem. It increases ventilation rate or depth to remove the excess carbon dioxide.

Therefore, under conditions of physical exertion, this finely tuned system ensures that the muscles and brain get needed oxygen, while excess carbon dioxide is exhaled to maintain the pH of the blood. In stressful sedentary situations, the system gets destabilized, because respiration rate often increases above what is needed to meet metabolic demands – that is, people hyperventilate.[38] The body finds itself in the situation where carbon dioxide is being exhaled, but muscle activity has not changed, so the blood levels of carbon dioxide drop and blood pH rises. Under these conditions, hemoglobin binds oxygen more tightly, and this is where the horrible feeling of not being in full command of your faculties starts to arise. Although the blood is fully oxygenated, it cannot be released into the tissues where it is needed. The brain becomes starved of oxygen, leading to problems with attention and focus, light-headedness, the sensation of being out of your body and the feeling of being anxious or upset. These symptoms are familiar to those with stage fright, but individuals who do not usually experience public-speaking anxiety may be even more surprised and frustrated when they experience these symptoms for the first time in a high-stakes communication situation.

To synthesize, the symptoms of stage fright as well as the sense of losing control when a conversation turns contentious all come back to the breath, but not to a lack of breath. Although the blood is oxygenated, the conditions caused by the lack of carbon dioxide shift hemoglobin

Figure 9.2. Breath, Blood, and Stage Fright

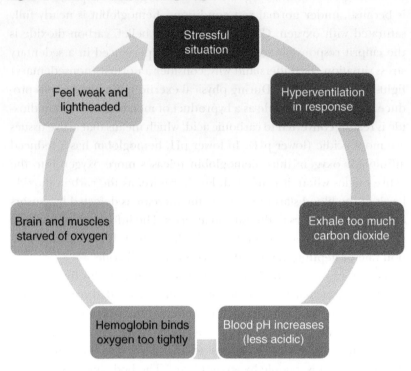

into its stingy shape, and it becomes like Gollum hanging onto his preciousss! Only by ending the loss of carbon dioxide will hemoglobin get back to doing its job properly. In the meantime, the hyperventilation-induced bodily sensations can fuel feelings of anxiety or exacerbate frustration, leading to more hyperventilation, setting up a vicious cycle (Figure 9.2). At its most severe, the vicious cycle can culminate in a panic attack, and even in less severe cases it can hamper your ability to fully engage in a communication situation. It makes it difficult to listen intently and alters our body language as well as our voices.

Vocal Confidence Is in the Breath

In its most narrow sense, nonverbal communication refers to actions that are distinct from speech.[39] Thus far, the nonverbal communication discussed – facial expressions, gestures, body postures, and positions of the legs and feet – fit this narrow definition. Discussions of nonverbal communication, however, have traditionally included a variety of subtle aspects of speech, making the term "nonverbal" somewhat of a misnomer.[40] "Dark matter of communication" feels more inclusive of these nonverbal acoustic properties of speech – also known as paralanguage or **paralinguistic cues**. These include volume, variation in volume, pitch, variation in pitch, inflection, speech rate, and use of pauses.[41] The voice is the intersection of verbal and nonverbal communication, and nonverbal vocal communication is both conscious and unconscious.

We can use paralinguistic cues deliberately (as discussed in Chapter 2), such as pausing or varying volume for emphasis, but we also unconsciously produce paralinguistic cues. This is why vocal coach Kristin Linklater asserts that the voice reveals our inner world to the outer world.[42] Indeed, even without the content of communication, for example when listening to nonsense syllables, people can judge anger, fear, happiness, sadness, and tenderness in voice audio with the same accuracy as these emotions can be detected from facial expressions.[43] Pitch is particularly revealing in stage fright and other stressful communication situations. Controlling for gender, higher pitch reduces perceptions of speaker confidence.[44] Encouragingly, in individuals successfully treated for speaking anxiety, mean and maximum voice pitch decreases, and listeners rate the post-treatment voices as sounding more confident.[45]

It all comes back to breathing, because it is within the stream of exhaled air moving through the larynx that contractions of the vocal fold muscles create patterns of vibrations. These sound waves are amplified by resonance within the throat and mouth, and the acoustics of speech are controlled by the up and down movement of the larynx, as well as movements of the jaw, tongue, and lips. Because anxiety increases the tautness of the laryngeal and vocal fold muscles, it results in faster vibrations and raises pitch.

For Stress and Stage Fright, Rethink What It Means to "Just Breathe"

When people are faced with an anxiety-inducing situation, they are often told to "just take a deep breath." If a communication situation is causing you to speak too quickly without taking time to breathe, this is sound advice. Unfortunately, when the feelings of light-headedness and disconnectedness are due to stress-induced hyperventilation, as is often the case, this advice can make things worse by further depleting carbon dioxide levels, particularly if the expiration is forced. Key to maintaining composure in a communication situation is aligning respiration rate with metabolic needs. Emotional stimuli activate the amygdala and increase respiration rate; consciously reducing your respiration rate may reduce amygdala activity and correspondingly reduce anxiety.[46] Stress-induced hyperventilation is reduced by various interventions, including mindfulness and meditation.[47]

MINDFULNESS AND MEDITATION CAN BUILD FUNDAMENTAL COMMUNICATION SKILLS

Mindfulness is the awareness of the present moment that results from paying attention purposefully with an attitude of openness and without judgment.[48] Mindfulness can be cultivated through meditation. A section on mindfulness and meditation may seem like a hippie interlude in a research-driven book on communication, but empathy and authentic connection to others is impossible without mindfulness. A wandering mind prevents you from connecting to another and truly listening to their words and attending to their body language. Learning to monitor and control shifts in your attention can help you be fully present in the moment and more attuned to others' spoken and unspoken communication. The growing body of research on the benefits of mindfulness and meditation is unequivocal. Mindfulness and meditation training measurably reduces biological markers of stress, both hormonal (adrenocorticotrophic hormone) and immunological (pro-inflammatory cytokines), as well the subjective experience of stress involved in the preparation and delivery of a speech.[49] A meta-analysis of studies on meditation techniques found that the benefits can be long lasting.[50]

Neuroimaging reveals that meditation activates areas of the brain involved in attention and motivation, and experienced meditators have structural changes in these brain regions.[51] Experienced meditators also have replicable patterns of brain activity that have never been observed in non-meditators.[52] Meditation and mindfulness practices also have benefits in the near term. In a study of individuals new to meditation, one 20-minute session of guided breath meditation per day for four days improved attention and working memory, and a single session reduced emotional volatility to a stressor that immediately followed the meditation.[53] Mindfulness and meditation has been shown to increase emotional intelligence, even among those new to meditation.[54]

Mindfulness-based stress reduction (MBSR) is often used as an umbrella term for a whole variety of secular mindfulness and meditation practices, with which many readers will be familiar. Most studies of mindfulness and meditation do not attempt to compare one MBSR technique to another, as techniques are often used in combination. In a rare study that compared two meditation practices, focus on the breath was shown to be more effective than focus on the emotions in the face of an immediate stressor, but both were equally beneficial in reducing emotional volatility to a stressor that followed the meditation.[55] With so many different practices and little research to distinguish their effects, the best advice is that the most effective practice is the one you will actually do. The following section introduces five practices relevant to communication. Because resources on MBSR techniques are widely available, this section is intended as a starting place. The five techniques are listed here and described in more detail below.

- *External awareness/five senses.* Turn your full conscious attention to experiencing the world through your senses. Notice details that the busy mind tends to miss.
- *Internal awareness/body scan.* Turn your full attention to your internal bodily state, noticing thermal and mechanical sensations (e.g., tightness, heaviness) throughout, as well as heart rate and respiration.
- *Mantra repetition.* Repeat a word or phrase with your attention focused on the sound or rhythm of the words. You may tie the repetitions to your breath.
- *Breath concentration.* Focus on your breath at the level of your nose, chest, or abdomen. If thoughts intrude, notice them with equanimity and return your focus to your breath.
- *Yogic breathing.* Gently slow your respiration rate. Slow the inspiration and expiration or lengthen the pauses between inspiration and expiration.

External Awareness / Five Senses

Method: This mindfulness practice involves turning your full attention to each of your senses, one at a time in gradual succession. Depending on where you are and how much there is to see, make a mental note of all the things you see, or look carefully at one thing and fastidiously note the details. As I look up from my laptop while writing this paragraph, I notice the tattered olive-green shag mat in the entryway. The shag is sticking up in sections and mashed down in others, giving it the appearance of a scaled-down model of a wild landscape. In all the times I have seen the mat, this is the first time I noticed its likeness to a landscape, attesting to how easy it is look without seeing as we rush about our business. Once you have focused your attention deeply to experience the world through one sense, move on to the next. What do you hear? What is the loudest thing that you hear? What is the softest thing that you hear? What do you smell? What do you taste? What tactile sensations are you experiencing?

Communication applications: This mindfulness exercise teaches you how to snap yourself back to actively engage in the moment. Vision and hearing are obviously most relevant to communication situations. Right before giving a talk, you can focus on noticing specific details in the room or out the window to settle the mind and reduce the psychological component of the stress response.

Internal Awareness / Body Scan

Method: This mindfulness exercise involves shifting your attention to sensations arising within the body. Because we tend to tune these out in our daily life, it is easiest to begin this practice in a quiet place with few distractions and your eyes closed. Once you are attuned to your physical sensations, it will be easier to use this practice as a check-in as you go about your business, including as you are anticipating an upcoming communication situation. Start with one area of your body and note any sensations arising from it before slowly moving to the next part of your body. Concentrate especially carefully when you get to the core (thorax and abdomen), because signs of stress manifest themselves there. What is the rate and depth of your breathing? How hard and fast is your heart beating? Do you have any constriction in your core? Shoulders, jaws, and foreheads also often hold much stress (and convey our stress to others). Gently ease any tensions you find.

Communication applications: By providing a window on the various physical sensations rising and falling within the body at any given moment, the internal awareness mindfulness teaches you to recognize when a situation is causing a shift from your normal homeostatic baseline. It also helps you learn to separate physical sensations from your cognitive assessment of them. For instance, since positive excitement and anxious excitement share some of the same physical sensations, the next time you feel butterflies before a big talk, try to imagine it as positive energy that you can channel into enthusiasm.

Mantra Repetition

Method: A mantra is a sound, a word, or a phrase that you repeat silently to yourself. Select a mantra that does not feel cumbersome to repeat. You may wish to choose something self-affirming. Repeat the mantra in a steady cadence, once on each exhalation if that feels comfortable. The idea is to focus your attention on the sound of the mantra and the rhythm of the repetitions. If it is difficult to focus, you may use beads or a meditation ring to mark each repetition. If your attention wanders, calmly turn it back to the repetitions.

Communication application: Over time, as you practice slipping into a tranquil state during the meditation, the mantra, through classical conditioning, becomes a signal for that physiological state. When it does, the mantra can be used as a conditioned stimulus to decrease nervousness in the face of a stressor, such as before a big presentation.

Breath Concentration

Method: Sit comfortably and focus on your breath, either the air flowing in and out of your nose or the expansion and contraction of your chest or abdomen with each inhalation and exhalation. If your attention wanders, notice your thoughts, but gently release them without judgment and return the mind to the breath. As you begin to meditate, you can envision the air flowing through the intricate branches of your air passages and the gas exchange across the alveoli. You may want to imagine stress leaving the body on the exhalation.

Communication applications: This meditation practice helps you become cognizant of when a tense situation has accelerated and shifted your breathing, because when people become stressed, hyperventilation is often accompanied by a shift in breathing from the abdomen to the chest.[56] Furthermore, the practice of learning to note when your attention has wandered develops a meta-awareness of your own mental fugues. This awareness helps us avoid the mental multitasking that, through body language, reveals that we are not fully committed to the conversation.

Yogic Breathing

Method: Yogic breathing is an umbrella term for a set of controlled breathing exercises, one of which is paced breathing. Navy SEALS use a paced breathing technique known as box breathing, which involves inhaling for four counts, pausing for four counts, exhaling for four counts, and pausing for four counts.[57] Another paced breathing technique is slowing the exhalation to twice the length of the inhalation (but keeping the amount of exhaled air the same, because you do not want to lose more carbon dioxide). A note of caution: Other yogic breathing techniques, particularly those involving rapid or forceful breathing, can trigger panic attacks in anxiety disorders.[58] To moderate stress and stage fright, subtle breathing changes can do the trick.

Communication applications: Yogic breathing can be used to stop the physiological and psychological stress cycle caused by hyperventilation.

Some Reflections on Getting Started and Sticking to It

Akin to Alan Alda,[59] who fortuitously realized that improvisation training was a route to improve science communicators' empathy, my initial interest in mindfulness and meditation had nothing to do with improving communication. I had turned to it seeking relief from a lifelong battle with (general) anxiety. Because anxiety is a state of hypervigilance, I found it challenging to begin with breath-concentration meditation. Meditation makes you feel less anxious in the long run, but only if you feel safe enough to let down your guard and meditate in the first place.

Figure 9.3. Check-Ins for Keeping Your Cool and Calming Your Nerves

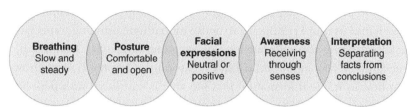

I was able to start (outdoors in nature) with the external-awareness five-senses mindfulness. Then I introduced the practice of body scan. I learned to sit and meditate with mantra repetition, and in stressful situations I combine yogic breathing and repetition of affirmations. Currently, my main practice (alone or guided) is breath meditation with body scan, but I use all five practices described here. During the pandemic, to feel closer to a larger community, I also began attending classes virtually, including a weekly loving-kindness meditation through the Dharma Bum Temple in San Diego. (Most of their classes are now both online and in person and are free and open to all.)

I have found the approach of the guides at the Dharma Bum Temple liberating. They emphasize starting small (even five minutes per day) and not judging your practice, especially when your mind wanders. They point out that if you notice your mind wandering, it is actually a win because it means you are learning to notice. I have been surprised by how much meditation helps me notice. For example, I did not notice how much tension I was holding in my forehead and jaw until I was following a guided meditation that focused attention on relaxing the muscles in the face and head. Obviously, crinkled stress-face is a tell, which draws us back to the dark matter of communication.

Dark matter underpins communication. No matter how well-honed your verbal delivery is, things will go awry if your nonverbal cues give away your disengagement, lack of empathy, or the anxiety that may make you seem disengaged, inauthentic, or untrustworthy. Figure 9.3 summarizes the check-ins that can help you remain poised and fully present. Becoming fully present as a communicator is an ongoing process of practice and self-reflection. Toward that goal, the lessons from the previous chapters complement this chapter in two ways. The first is by helping you develop the words, analogies, images, and stories to describe your work in audience-accessible terms (Chapters 1–5). Having these "in your back pocket" supplies the confidence to relax and be yourself. The previous chapters also help you develop the understandings and habits of mind conducive to active empathetic listening, especially acknowledging the complexities of weighing tradeoffs (Chapter 6), recognizing how emotion facilitates reasoning (Chapter 7), and knowing how to frame information in a way that is consistent with people's worldviews (Chapter 8). The concluding chapter of this book will help you polish and organize these tools to have them at the ready.

10

Collecting the Tools into the Toolbox

My canine companion has grown older and wiser in the years I have worked on this book. She can still root out feral tennis balls like nobody's business, but she has become less obstinate about her strategy for hunting human-made suburban prey. Instead of expecting success from revisiting the same old empty nesting sites over and over, she is always on the lookout for new hiding places, and instead of relying on intuition, she is receptive to guidance from her human companion. She even asks for it, with a slight tilt of her head and a furrow of the now-white eyebrows above her sparkling eyes. You *can* teach an old dog new tricks.

If the growth mindset of ability applies to my hunting dog's (mostly) genetically programmed skills, it most certainly applies to communication. Although the global pandemic has shone a spotlight on communication gone horribly awry, the problem is not new. Every day in our workplaces, homes, classrooms, doctors' offices, the media, the policy arena, and all the settings in which communication happens, communication failures occur even when all parties have the best of intentions. This book, and the substantial terrain it covers, was born from my frustration with the shallowness and narrowness of traditional communication guidance. Each chapter of this book is written to be self-contained and to dig deep into one set of knowledge, skills, and habits of mind, such that together the chapters build a toolkit applicable across a hierarchy of communication goals.

Achieving even the lowest goal on the hierarchy – conveying basic, uncontroversial information – calls for mastery of words and visuals. To move up the hierarchy and promote an understanding of concepts and processes, mastery must extend to development of apt comparisons and the construction of a logic story that meets learners where they are. If your audiences are to apply scientific findings and scientific thinking in their own lives, or to see themselves pursuing a career in science, you will need to convey the relevant aspects of the discovery story and humanize the discovery process. Supporting decision-making that involves analyzing costs, benefits, and unknowns means elucidating tradeoffs and clarifying uncertainty. Supporting evaluation of conflicting claims or information that conflicts with peoples' values requires the knowledge, skills, and habits of mind to navigate heuristics and the backfire effect. The goal, at the top of the hierarchy, of working collaboratively with others to develop shared solutions calls for embodied awareness and empathy.

The communication hierarchy was introduced in Chapter 1 in the shape of a pyramid, the way the general version of Bloom's Taxonomy is often illustrated to highlight the increasing challenge of reaching successively high-level goals. In Table 10.1, the hierarchy builds from bottom to top, with each row listing (respectively, across the columns) the communication goal as well as the foundational knowledge, communication skills, and habits of mind needed to achieve that goal. (The relevant chapters are indicated.)

The beauty of the hierarchy is that it draws attention to how the approach to communication must shift according to the communication goals. In doing so, it makes explicit the corresponding knowledge, skills, and habits of mind needed to meet those goals. By clearly articulating these competencies, this hierarchy can help you be strategic about your own professional journey. Instead of vague "communication skills" that most communication workshops reduce to "dejargonizing" and "distilling," the hierarchy makes clear that although reducing terminology and being concise are necessary skills, they are only sufficient for the most basic communication goals. Dissatisfaction with the deficit model of communication has led to calls for dialogue, sometimes to the extent that the pendulum swings far in the other

Table 10.1. Communication Toolkit Organized along Bloom's Taxonomy of Goals

Goal Taxonomy	Foundational Knowledge	Communication Skills	Habits of Mind
CREATE collaborative solutions	Know what factors underpin emotion and empathy.	Bridge divides through empathetic connection. (*Ch. 9*)	Work on awareness of physical state and inner dialogue, and re-center as needed.
EVALUATE conflicting claims	Determine situation-relevant heuristics and likely backfires.	Apply strategies to support deliberation and reduce backfires. (*Ch. 7 & 8*)	Attend to nuances of interpretation and the message behind the message.
ANALYZE pros, cons, unknowns	Understand how people assess risk and view tradeoffs.	Clarify the pros, cons, alternatives, and uncertainties. (*Ch. 6*)	Seek out the voices of constituencies that struggle to be heard.
APPLY to everyday situations	Recognize the flaws in portrayals of scientific discovery.	Bring the discovery journey and the discoverers to life. (*Ch. 5*)	Reflect with humility on your values, assumptions, and limits of expertise.
UNDERSTAND concepts, processes	Explore what misconceptions may arise and why.	Craft audience-appropriate stories and comparisons. (*Ch. 3 & 4*)	Critically examine the logic chain and predict potential confusions.
REMEMBER basic information	Identify audience expectations and entry points.	Optimize language and create clear, meaningful visuals. (*Ch. 1 & 2*)	Assess how communication is received and adapt accordingly.

direction, implying that dialogue is the only effective form of communication. This hierarchy provides nuance about what this means in practical terms, when not all communication contexts permit face-to-face interactions. Other than for those goals at the top of the hierarchy, which often require crucial conversations, the "dialogue" can take different forms, such as sleuthing to learn about the audience, getting survey feedback from a pilot group, and exploring the scholarship on how people learn certain concepts. Regardless of the form, however, effective communication always requires self-reflection and perspective-taking.

The hierarchy should not be taken to imply that these are the only possible communication goals. For example, not explicit here are aesthetic goals that might include savoring a beautiful scientific image, being moved by a visual metaphor, or learning to appreciate science as a cultural endeavor. These goals would draw (successively) on the knowledge, skills, and habits of mind listed under the first, second, and third levels of the hierarchy. The hierarchy is also not meant to imply that the knowledge, skills, and habits of mind listed at higher levels are never needed for goals lower in the hierarchy. After all, you may think you are presenting uncontroversial facts only to discover that the information is ideologically unwelcome for certain members of the audience. Furthermore, knowledge, skills, and habits of mind covered in later chapters, particularly those in the chapter on the dark matter of communication, are useful for giving better presentations and are necessary in any situation where trust is an issue. For example, a patient may tune out a physician whose body language suggests a lack of empathy, irrespective of what information the physician is providing. Therefore, think of the hierarchy as a map to a lifelong journey of personal and professional growth.

Even in the case of a face-to-face conversation, preparation is the most important aspect of communication, but that does not mean sticking rigidly to a script (not even when you have an actual script). Acting teacher Sanford Meisner emphasized the importance of being open and attentive to what is happening in the moment on stage and only responding after fully grasping the words or actions.[1] Responding in the moment, however, does not mean winging it. Before actors step on stage on opening night, they have analyzed, questioned, experimented, practiced, critiqued, rehearsed, and polished. Preparation does not inhibit spontaneity: Lack of preparation inhibits spontaneity. After all, you need to be comfortable in your role in order to listen to the audience. Then to respond, you need possible options from which to choose. To support your preparation by helping you collect the tools into the toolbox, the final sections of this chapter provide practice exercises and handy checklists. May you continue your communication journey with a healthy mix of optimism and wisdom, and the willingness to adapt your approach to the ever-evolving terrain.

EXERCISES

Chapter 1 Exercises: Planning for the Communication Dimensions

EXERCISE 1.1: TAKE STOCK OF YOUR AUDIENCE, CONTEXT, AND GOALS

a) Who are the audiences for your communication? If you have one main audience, such as patients or students, consider the heterogeneity within that audience. Do their expectations and needs differ by age, culture, science knowledge, lifestyle, or other factors? What opportunities do you have (or can you create) to learn more about them?

b) What are the existing and potential contexts for your communication? What are the affordances and constraints of these contexts and how will you optimize the context to reach and support your diverse potential audiences? Are any relevant modes of communication missing from your communication plan?

c) What are your communication goals? Where do your goals fall along Bloom's Taxonomy? What are the goals of your audience? If different, how will you reconcile your goals with those of the audience?

d) Use the brainstorming you did in a, b, and c to develop a communication plan that lists your planned activities, noting intended audiences and goals. Include a timeline of activities, which may be tied to pragmatic considerations, such as the length of a grant-funded project. Be realistic given the competing demands on your time and energy, but also specify one or more aspirational activities you could achieve with additional resources.

EXERCISE 1.2: ADVISOR OR ADVOCATE?

Communicators themselves may not be cognizant of when they cross the line between advising and advocating. For each of the following potential goals of a researcher working with a policymaker, where is the line between advising and advocating?

- Providing data that speak to the size of a public health or environmental problem

- Pointing out the need for more funds for a particular area of research
- Enumerating the possible solutions to a socio-scientific problem
- Explaining the outputs of a computational model that predicts the impact of different mitigation efforts
- Documenting the research on effectiveness of policy in lay-language terms

Chapter 2 Exercises: Optimizing Your Language and Visuals

EXERCISE 2.1: FIND THE RIGHT WORDS

List the terminology used in your work. Be sure to include terms applied in more familiar contexts with a different meaning. Also include phrases like "embryonic developmental program" or (from a business gobbledy-gook generator) "implement functional incremental options" in which the meaning of the individual words is familiar, but the meaning of the phrase is opaque. Once you have generated your list of specialist words and phrases, decide which can be eliminated when addressing an audience outside your field. For those that cannot, write clear definitions or identify synonyms. A thesaurus is a valuable tool for this, but if you are a non-native speaker (or if you are writing about a field in which you are not an expert), brainstorm with colleagues about the nuances of meaning.

EXERCISE 2.2: POLISH YOUR VISUALS AND MULTIMEDIA

Examine the images, diagrams, graphs, tables, and other visuals you use in your talks, papers, and grant proposals.

a) To what extent do they rely on your discipline's visual jargon? Would nonexperts seeing your figure for the first time know what they are looking at? What is the main message, and are you trying to show multiple things (e.g., structures, interactions, steps, variables, outcomes) at once? Are viewers expected to see differences between different parts of the graphic? How are they guided to see what you want them to see?

b) Consider the levels of abstraction, originality, redundancy, dimensionality, decoration, and density of your graphics. Which of these are mutable and what changes could be made to better support a nonexpert audience? For example, could a more familiar graphical form be used? If you are using decorative elements, do they draw attention to the graphic's essential information or away from it?

c) Review the principles of Gestalt psychology and color perception and use them to critique your own visuals. To improve your skills at critiquing your own work, look for common pitfalls in figures created by those in other fields. These may include inconsistent use of colors or symbols, inadequate use of white space, visually confusing layout, excessive use of borders or gridlines, limited cues (such as enclosures, connections, or highlights) to indicate relationships between elements, failure to ensure that colors differ in both brightness and hue, and the use of color gradients that have not been scientifically derived based on knowledge of human color perception.

d) Review the cognitive design principles for multimedia presentations and critique your slide presentations. What is the main message of each slide? Are the images and narration complementary? What extraneous details can be eliminated? What are the most conceptually challenging places where pausing or segmenting may be especially helpful?

Chapter 3 Exercises: Tapping into the Power of Comparisons

EXERCISE 3.1: WAR, INSURANCE, MECHANISM, OR MEDICINE?

Journalists use various themes of metaphors to discuss the application of geoengineering technologies to reverse global warming.[2] These include (1) metaphors of fighting and war, (2) metaphors about insurance, (3) mechanistic metaphors (such as thermostat, sunshade, and dimmer switch), and (4) medical metaphors (such as cure, treatment, and liposuction). Although all these themes of metaphors are used in stories that argue for or against the technology, as well as in neutral stories, the themes are not used evenly across positions.

a) If you were to write an editorial encouraging research on geoengineering technologies, what theme(s) of metaphors (if any) would you choose? Would you use different metaphors if you were to write a cautionary piece?

b) What is your rationale for your choices?

EXERCISE 3.2: CRAFT YOUR COMPARISONS

a) What metaphors or analogies are used in your field? (Be sure to consider any idiomatic metaphors that seem commonplace, such as the way "up" and "down" are used to describe mood. Note other metaphorical language that slips into your speech, like the fight/war metaphors discussed in Chapter 3.)

b) Do any of the comparisons present framings that inadvertently favor certain solutions or research approaches over others? Are the comparisons anachronistic or oversimplifying complexity?

c) What features from the source domain should audiences map to the target domain? What features should not be mapped? For what audiences and purposes are the comparisons suited?

d) If you were to use these comparisons, how would you use them and what context would you provide? Are any of the comparisons particularly visual metaphors? If so, consider working with an artist to create an image that you could use when communicating about your work.

e) Brainstorm other metaphors or analogies to communicate about the products or process of your work. Depending on your goals, the comparisons may be designed to add interest, or they may be designed to make accessible something that is complex or difficult to picture. If your work is highly theoretical or mathematical, a verbal or visual metaphor may be the most effective way to invite audiences in, so think about how you can use metaphorical imagery or other creative forms to foster an aesthetic or physical (embodied) appreciation of your work.

EXERCISE 3.3: MULL OVER YOUR METAPHORICAL MUSCLE

In the news media, the conceptual metaphor "monster" is often used to describe wildfires, and when "monster wildfire" is used instead of "major wildfire" people's perceptions of the risk are enhanced and they are more likely to opt to evacuate.[3] The mechanism by which the monster metaphor alters risk perception may be a direct effect on reasoning (because it highlights the erratic and destructive behavior of the fire) or an indirect effect by influencing emotions (creating more fear and anxiety).

a) In your opinion, is it ethical to use this metaphorical framing to increase compliance with evacuation orders? Why or why not? Does your response depend on whether the influence of the metaphor is on reasoning or on emotion?
b) How do you respond to "major," "monster," and other words used to grab your attention. When do these words become hype?
c) Does your field have any metaphors that may influence people's decision-making? How are these metaphors used, and what are the ethical considerations?

Chapter 4 Exercises: Connecting the Dots to Facilitate Understanding

EXERCISE 4.1: IDENTIFY AND BUILD ON PRIOR KNOWLEDGE

a) What prior knowledge do people have about your field or the topic about which you are communicating? Consider both knowledge assets they may bring and potential misconceptions they may have or could develop during learning.
b) How will you acknowledge and build on the knowledge they have? How will you take possible misconceptions into account?

EXERCISE 4.2: PLAN YOUR PREVIEW, PITCH, AND PLOT

a) Craft one or more encapsulate one-liners that can be a preview of your work (or the topic you are working on) or a stand-alone summary.
b) Prepare at least one clear, concise essence synopsis.
c) For a longer story (choose a format relevant to you), identify your tantalize one-liner, take-home one-liner, last line, and the plot logic outline.

Chapter 5 Exercises: Telling Stories of Inspiration and Discovery

EXERCISE 5.1: RECONNECT WITH YOUR PASSION

a) Who or what initially motivated you or sparked your interest? What keeps you going when the going gets tough?

b) Recall a moment of wonderment, awe, or fascination that you have had in your work. Do your best to rekindle the emotions you experienced in that moment. Think about how you might convey (through words, visuals, movement, or gestures) that experience to others.

EXERCISE 5.2: UNCOVER "HIDDEN FIGURES"

a) Within the history of your field, has anyone identified individuals who did not get credit for their intellectual or technical contributions? Can you introduce some of their stories into your teaching, writing, or other communication?

b) Within your field today, can you think of any practices or conventions that continue to marginalize some (such as what contributions do and do not merit authorship credit)? How can your communication draw attention to their contributions and emphasize the many kinds of opportunities for budding scientists to contribute to the discovery process?

EXERCISE 5.3: CONSIDER DIVERSE EXPERTISE

What kinds of expertise or cultural or institutional knowledge might give you a fresh perspective on your work or its application, and how can you seek it out?

EXERCISE 5.4: MAP THE HIDDEN SCIENTIFIC CLIMB

If you are a researcher, map the hidden scientific climb for one of your published or forthcoming studies (noting the timeline, ordering of steps in the paper versus in reality, paths taken and abandoned, foundational tools and techniques, and serendipitous intellectual contributions). As you do so, consider the big-picture lessons about the process of science and how you can do more to convey them to students, teachers, and publics.

Chapter 6 Exercises: Discussing Tradeoffs and Uncertainty

EXERCISE 6.1: IDENTIFY TRADEOFFS

a) For the topic you are communicating about, what are the tradeoffs of i) funding the work, ii) conducting the work, and iii) applying the work?
b) How does the prioritization, completion, and application of the work reduce or exacerbate inequities?
c) Who are the voices missing from discussions about the work or field of research? How might you seek their input?

EXERCISE 6.2: CLARIFY UNCERTAINTY

a) What uncertainties arise in the work or its application? (Use the documenting uncertainty framework in Chapter 6 to systematically document them.)
b) Of these uncertainties, which are currently communicated (to those in or out of field) and which are not?
c) Write a clear, concise paragraph to summarize the uncertainty you have documented using the framework. Also craft a one-line summary (take-home message) of the paragraph.

EXERCISE 6.3: ROGUE CERTAINTY

Uncertainty is often glossed over in health reporting – for example, by giving spuriously precise numbers instead of range estimates, by not disclosing potential individual differences in benefits, by making overly certain causal links between behaviors and outcomes, or by failing to specify whether the statement "there is no evidence to suggest" means there has not been a study done or a study that has been done has disconfirmed the link.[4] Consider any current health fad. How is rogue certainty being used in communication about it?

Chapter 7 Exercises: Making Information Intuitive and Presenting Data

EXERCISE 7.1: DESIGNED DATA AND EXEMPLARY EXAMPLES

a) What kind of data or evidence do you need to communicate? If you have numerical or statistical data, what format(s) can you use? If you have qualitative data, what examples will you use and how much depth will you provide? Think about helping audiences understand the scope of the problem and the reality of an individual case.

b) What context do you need to provide to help audiences make sense of the evidence? What challenges may people encounter as they try to make sense of the numerical data? What confounds are hidden in the data and how will you communicate them?

c) Consider (and discuss with a colleague if possible) your different options for presenting data and examples. Which are most accessible? Which are most informative? Which best convey what you want to convey? Which are most transparent?

EXERCISE 7.2: DATA IN THE WILD

a) Choose a science or health topic that has received media coverage positing recommendations for individual or policy actions. Read articles about it published by a variety of sources.

b) How do the articles treat causation? Are the potential causal mechanisms clearly explained? What confounds may be lurking in the evidence being used to infer causation? Are the potential confounds discussed?

c) How do the articles treat context? Do they describe the study population, conditions, or location? Do they provide caveats about generalizing the results to new contexts?

d) How do the articles treat potential harms? Are the economic costs and the health or environmental risks of the intervention discussed? Is coverage of the pros and cons balanced, or are the cons presented less prominently than the pros, or presented in absolute terms while the pros are presented in relative terms?

e) Are any of the articles treating causation, context, effect size, or potential harms in a way that deliberately or inadvertently misrepresents the data? What is the original source of the misrepresentation (e.g., the media outlet, the original press release, the researcher, a public official)?

EXERCISE 7.3: CORRECTING MISCONCEPTIONS

Identify at least one factual misconception that people hold about your research or something important to you.

a) State the *misconception.*
b) Identify the *thinking* behind it.
c) Affirm the *fact* without repeating the misconception.
d) Provide a causal story or *mechanism* that supports the correct idea.
e) Identify any *heuristics* contributing to the misconception.
f) Describe any *data or examples* that may reduce reliance on heuristics.

Table 10.2 presents an example for a topic near and dear to my heart.

Table 10.2. Example of Correcting Misconceptions

Misconception	Running causes arthritis.
Thinking	Moving parts in machines and vehicles wear with use.
Fact	Running protects against arthritis.
Mechanism	Exercise supports joint health by strengthening the muscles, increasing blood flow, and stimulating the production of lubricating synovial fluid.
Heuristics	Availability – "I know runners who have arthritis."
Data/Examples	Statistical data showing lower rates of arthritis in runners. Examples of marathon runners continuing into their 60s, 70s, 80s, and beyond.

Chapter 8 Exercises: Reducing Polarization, Myths, and Backfires

EXERCISE 8.1: BEYOND BACKFIRES

a) What language used to describe your work, or a societal problem related to it, reflects individual or group ideologies? This may be slogans or virtue signaling, but it could also be more subtle terms.

b) What kinds of backfires may arise (clashes with cultural affiliations, threats to autonomy, incompatibility with self-concept, normalizing the problem, mismatched argument strength, hidden unintended messages, or superficial myth debunking)?

c) For each of the potential backfires you have identified, determine how you can apply one or more of the strategies for avoiding backfires discussed in Chapter 8.

EXERCISE 8.2: GIVING MYTHS THE SILENT TREATMENT

Chapter 8 explored how superficial myth debunking can backfire. Another risk of repeating falsehoods to debunk them is that you can be quoted out of context to make it seem like you are endorsing the falsehood. If your work involves debunking falsehoods, what debunking strategies from Chapter 8 will you apply to avoid advertising the falsehoods?

EXERCISE 8.3: SCHISMOGENESIS IN ACTION

What starts out as a small divide can grow into a yawning chasm when, instead of working toward common ground, both parties step up the ante in response to one another. Can you identify an example of this occurring in a historical or contemporary issue? How did the creation of division play out? Were there missed opportunities to bridge the divide before it escalated (e.g., using neutral language, affirming another's good intentions, connecting through a shared identity)?

Chapter 9 Exercises: Presenting with Poise and Cultivating Empathy

EXERCISE 9.1: KEEPING IT REAL

a) What emotional responses may audiences have in learning about your work? Might they experience joy or a feeling of awe? Could they experience anger because your conclusions seem contrary to an important belief? Is it possible that learning about your work could bring up deep trauma associated with the loss of a loved one or first-hand experience of a natural disaster?

b) As you imagine these possible audience reactions, think about how you feel about your work. Can you create a bond with the audience through shared feelings? Can you empathetically connect with someone who does not share your feelings by making the sincere effort to understand theirs?

c) Role-play with a colleague to practice a realistic emotional scenario that could arise about your work, such as communicating unwelcome information or discussing research findings with individuals who have first-hand traumatic experience with the problems your research is aimed at (ultimately) solving.

EXERCISE 9.2: TICS AND NERVES

When you are giving a presentation or interview, the most important thing is to be yourself because there is no single "correct" communication style. For example, you can be effective whether you are a highly animated speaker or a serenely still one, and you will find successful historical figures or celebrities who share your style. By being yourself, you can be authentically present in the moment with your audience. In our workshops, when participants observe themselves on camera, they often become overly critical about mannerisms that none of the trainers or fellow participants found troublesome. That said, you may have something you want to change about the way you communicate. The trick is not to focus on the thing you want to change, but to focus on what you can do to change it by altering the context or by substituting one behavior for another. Do you have any behaviors that you would like to change? If so, consider what you could do instead. Table 10.3 provides some ideas.

Table 10.3. Presentation Difficulties and Alternatives

Difficulty	Alternatives
Shaking laser pointer	If you must use a pointer, use it sparingly. It is normal for your arm to shake if you hold it at right angles to your body for too long. Instead, in one gradual motion, lift your arm up, circle the important feature twice and then lower your arm. Alternatively, do away with the laser pointer entirely. Simplify your slides so people know where to look. Use the affordances of the presentation software (e.g., bring in an arrow or use an opaque shape to mask a feature and then remove it to reveal it in sync with your narration).
Getting out of breath	Pausing for emphasis supports learning, so as you are planning your presentation, note the places where you want to give the audience a moment to take in what you have just said. That way, you can relax and take a breath, knowing that you are helping the audience. While you are waiting to give your presentation, practice paced breathing to keep from hyperventilating.
Overly quiet voice	Even if you think you do not need a microphone, it is best to use one if available because this helps audience members who are hard of hearing. Looking at your audience or toward the back of the auditorium can help you better project. Imagine that your words have momentum and travel in the direction you send them and with the energy you give them.
Sentences trailing off	It is easier to treat sentences as a distinct unit of thought (instead of mushing them together like overcooked linguini noodles) if you have come up with meaningful sentences ahead of time. Practice your one-liners and essence synopsis by saying them in different ways. Think about how you deliver the punchline of a joke. Take us all the way to the last word.
Habitually nodding or saying yes when listening to questions	This is not necessarily a problem, but it can be a problem in a "gotcha" interview situation. (The interviewer asks you a controversial question and they cut to you nodding what seems to be "yes" but that was not what you intended.) Other signals can be used to signal attention; for example, think about the contemplative expression on Auguste Rodin's "The Thinker" statues.
Fidgeting, quirks, appearing stiff or using excessive body language	If you tend to be an animated speaker who uses a lot of nonspecific gestures, coming up with specific gestures can help you rein it in without becoming overly self-conscious about your style. Likewise, if you tend to feel a bit stiff when you are speaking, adding a few meaningful gestures can gently animate you. Instead of placing your focus on the thing to avoid, like fiddling with clothing, try to shift your focus to ways you can use your hands and body to support audience engagement and comprehension.

CHECKLISTS

Planning for the Audience, Context, and Goals

- Identify the audience(s) to be reached.
- Consider the audience's audience, if relevant.
- Consider the audience's interests, knowledge, and goals.
- Identify your communication goals.
- Examine any discrepancies between the goals.
- Revise your goals as appropriate.
- Use backward design to plan communication.
- Select or optimize the context or medium:
    - Directionality
    - Modes
    - Time
    - Story
    - Style and tone
- Support accessibility for neurodiversity.
- Consider how you will assess communication outcomes.

Selecting, Creating, and Combining Words and Visuals

- Identify jargon and hidden jargon.
- Tailor language to the audience.
- Support learning of new terms with pacing, articulation, and explaining concepts first.
- Analyze your discipline's visual vocabulary.
- Balance complexity and depth of graphics:
    - Concreteness
    - Familiarity
    - Redundancy
    - Dimensionality
    - Density
    - Adornment
- Apply the principles of Gestalt psychology and color perception.
- Synchronize words and visuals.
- Eliminate interference in visual and verbal channels.

- Signal important information visibly or audibly.
- Segment information strategically.
- Weed out extraneous details.

Crafting Comparisons and Clarifying Concepts through Logic Stories

- Choose apt comparisons and treat less apt ones as teachable moments.
- Be alert to anachronism, oversimplification, and unfamiliar comparisons.
- Align framing of problems and solutions when selecting comparisons.
- Research common confusions and misconceptions about your field.
- Start with the learner's prior knowledge and build logic stories.
- Examine your logic chain for missing links from the learner's perspective.
- Develop an essence synopsis that helps the audience connect to your work.
- Develop one-liners to encapsulate, tantalize, and scaffold.
- Streamline the plot but tier your story depth as learning progresses.
- Promote a growth mindset, metacognition, and knowledge integration.

Telling the Story of Discovery and Discoverers

- Reconnect with and share your own sense of awe and wonder.
- Establish the setting with vivid details.
- Share stories about overcoming personal or professional challenges.
- Highlight diversity in the broadest sense of the word.
- Portray community aspects, including collegial contributions and critique.
- Provide the big picture of the real discovery journey with relevant insights.

- Showcase the craft of the process and the satisfaction of figuring things out.
- Allow students and teachers to learn "with" and "about" scientific inquiry.
- Communicate inherent motivations to humanize the discovery journey.

Informing Complex Decisions in the Face of Uncertainty

- Elucidate the complete range of tradeoffs:
  - Health
  - Well-being
  - Environment
  - Economic
- Examine the boundedness of assessments:
  - Long term/short term
  - Geographical reach
  - Population separation
- Communicate both individual and societal tradeoffs.
- Articulate inherent value assumptions and explore problem framings.
- Broaden risk assessments to considerations beyond severity and likelihood:
  - Familiarity
  - Control
  - Understanding
  - Equitability
- Explain the purpose and limitations of models used in the work.
- Provide insight into (and mental models for considering) causal mechanisms.
- Portray uncertainty understandably and realistically:
  - Source(s)
  - Magnitude
  - Resolvability
  - Disagreements
- Cultivate conversations with clarity, humility, humanity, and perspective-taking.

Presenting Numerical Data and Statistics

- Beware of confounds, such as base rates, lead-time bias, and amalgamation.
- Define the object of probability statements.
- Provide absolute risk, not just relative risk.
- Present numbers with the same format and denominators.
- Suggest comparisons that provide a sense of scale.
- Consider the familiarity of data displays and provide time for sensemaking.
- Explain the meaningfulness, not just the significance.
- Show or describe the shape of data distributions.
- Express data in understandable units or explain what the units measure.
- Use apt formulations for small numbers and expressing losses/gains.
- Share appropriate contextual information to support meaning-making:
  - Compare options
  - Trends
  - Regions
  - Populations
  - Threshold
- Consider juxtaposing quantitative and qualitative information.

Avoiding Ideological Clashes and Backfires

- Foster authentic connection across potential divides:
  - Neutrality
  - Solution focused
  - Alliances
  - Shared identity
  - Safety
- Understand that autonomy is a valued commodity:
  - Noncoercive language
  - Emphasize options

- Demonstrate consistency with self-concept:
  - Show alignment
  - Be affirming
- Focus on positive examples instead of emphasizing the undesired norm.
- Put forth arguments optimized for the audience and relevant to the goals.
- Beware of hidden messages when selecting characters or examples.
- Be strategic when addressing myths and false information:
  - Information inoculation
  - NO state-and-negate
  - Scaffold sensemaking

Establishing Trust through Pertinent Expertise, Integrity, and Benevolence

- Provide clear conceptual explanations.
- Explain how the results were obtained and vetted.
- Endeavor to collect all relevant expertise.
- Reveal the magnitude and source(s) of uncertainties.
- Avoid incredible certitude and false assurances.
- Share your own motivating values.
- Accept that trust is a leap of faith.
- Build relationships with relevant communities.
- Empathize with others' perspectives, values, and feelings.
- Monitor your own inner dialogue and physiological responses.

Summary of Learning Objectives

CHAPTER 1 LEARNING OBJECTIVES: MAPPING THE LANDSCAPE

Knowledge: What are the affordances and constraints of potential communication contexts?

Skills: Begin to optimize communication for the audience and to design for diversity.

Habits of Mind: Compare goals of all involved in the communication and assess outcomes.

CHAPTER 2 LEARNING OBJECTIVES: WORDS AND VISUALS

Knowledge: What cognitive and perceptual principles are relevant to multimedia learning?

Skills: Optimize your verbal and visual language to reach the audience and meet the goals.

Habits of Mind: Distinguish clarification from simplification to maximize comprehensibility.

CHAPTER 3 LEARNING OBJECTIVES: METAPHORS AND ANALOGIES

Knowledge: How do metaphors and analogies shape thought and when do they go awry?

Skills: Craft comparisons that offer productive frames and make the intangible tangible.

Habits of Mind: Beware of anachronism and other potential metaphor and analogy pitfalls.

CHAPTER 4 LEARNING OBJECTIVES: MISCONCEPTIONS AND STORY

Knowledge: How is conceptual understanding constructed and what misconceptions arise?

Skills: Develop preview, pitch, and plot stories with logical progression, without logic gaps.

Habits of Mind: Recognize, respect, and build on knowledge assets that others bring.

CHAPTER 5 LEARNING OBJECTIVES: HIDDEN CLIMB

Knowledge: How do popular portrayals of discovery and discoverers mislead, and why should you care?

Skills: Reveal the humanity and the untold stories in the retelling of the research journey.

Habits of Mind: Reflect on your (or the field's) implicit motivations and assumptions.

CHAPTER 6 LEARNING OBJECTIVES: TRADEOFFS AND UNCERTAINTIES

Knowledge: How should potential costs, benefits, and uncertainties be identified and discussed?

Skills: Clarify complexity with humility, humanity, and room for multiple perspectives.

Habits of Mind: Cultivate awareness of value judgments made in assessments of tradeoffs.

CHAPTER 7 LEARNING OBJECTIVES: HEURISTICS

Knowledge: What kinds of shortcuts in reasoning do people use and under what conditions?

Skills: Provide relevant context and intelligible statistical information to support reasoning.

Habits of Mind: Recognize the adaptive benefits of intuition and emotion in decision-making.

CHAPTER 8 LEARNING OBJECTIVES: BACKFIRE EFFECT

Knowledge: What is the backfire effect and what are the many possible causes of backfires?

Skills: Be proactive to avoid or reduce the cognitive and ideological triggers of backfires.

Habits of Mind: Avoid broad conclusions about group affiliation and seek shared identities.

CHAPTER 9 LEARNING OBJECTIVES: DARK MATTER OF COMMUNICATION

Knowledge: What mental and physical processes underpin emotion and empathy?

Skills: Practice active listening and perspective-taking to grasp what remains unspoken.

Habits of Mind: Cultivate awareness of breath, body, and cognitions during communication.

Notes

Introduction

1 Dweck, 2015.
2 Lönngren & Van Poeck, 2021.
3 United Nations, 1948, Article 27.
4 Canfield & Menezes, 2020.

1. Mapping the Landscape of Audiences, Contexts, and Goals

1 Mandelbrot, 1983.
2 Chirico, Glaveanu, Cipresso, Riva, & Gaggiloi, 2018.
3 Lippman, 1922, p. 400.
4 Rabin et al., 2021.
5 Besley & Nisbet, 2013.
6 Tannen, 2005.
7 Tannen, 1981a.
8 Tannen, 1981b.
9 Tannen, 1981a.
10 Bateson, 1935.
11 Bennett, 2017.
12 Bennett, 1979.
13 Greeno, 1994.
14 National Academies of Sciences, Engineering, and Medicine, 2017.
15 Núñez, 2008.
16 Weisberg & Newcombe, 2017.

17 Moreno, 2006.
18 Key & Hendry, 2016.
19 Wall, 2016.
20 Walters, 2016.
21 Achenbach & Feltman, 2016.
22 Bennett, 2016.
23 Key & Hendry, 2016.
24 Inzunza, 2020.
25 Greene, 2012; Kamizasa, Terashima, & Awaki, 2012.
26 Méndez & Alcaraz, 2015.
27 Tufte, 2006.
28 Center for Universal Design, 1997.
29 Story, 2001.
30 Smith & Harvey, 2014.
31 Sucharov, 2019.
32 Canfield et al., 2020.
33 Phillips, Kanter, Bednarczyk, & Tastad, 1991.
34 Martínez & Mammola, 2021.
35 Davies, McCallie, Simonsson, Lehr, & Suensing, 2009.
36 Molek-Kozakowska, 2017.
37 Stuckey, Hofstein, Mamlok-Naaman, & Eilks, 2013.
38 Priest, Goodwin, & Dahlstrom, 2018.
39 Kearns, 2021.
40 Wailoo, 2021.
41 Krathwohl, 2002.
42 Wiggins & McTighe, 2005.

2. Masterful Use of Words and Images, the Fundamental Tools of the Communication Artisan

1   Groves, 1995.
2   Wilkinson, 1992.
3   Miller, 1956.
4   Gowaty, 1982.
5   Ryan, 1985.
6   Gowaty, 1982.
7   Feasey, 2021.
8   Mattys & Melhorne, 2007.
9   Sanders & Neville, 2000.
10 Umeda & Coker, 1974.
11 Brown & Ryoo, 2008; McDonnell, Barker, & Wieman, 2016.
12 Ziman, 2000.
13 Edelstein, 2018.
14 Shakespeare, 1603, *Hamlet*, 1.4.1, as cited in Edelstein, 2018.
15 Boerner, 2021.

16   Eick & King, 2012; Tversky, Morrison, & Betrancourt, 2002.
17   Thompson, 2016.
18   Ericsson, 2018.
19   Cook, 2006; Tasker, 2016.
20   Johnstone, 1991; Johnstone, 1993.
21   Cairo, 2012.
22   Tufte, 1983.
23   Mayer & Estrella, 2014; Plass, Heidig, Hayward, Homer, & Um, 2014.
24   Heidig, Müller, & Reichelt, 2015.
25   Mayer, 2014.
26   Rock & Palmer, 1990.
27   Frankel & DePace, 2012.
28   Crameri, Shephard, & Heron, 2020.
29   Crameri, Shephard, & Heron, 2020.
30   Crameri, Shephard, & Heron, 2020.
31   Chandler & Sweller, 1991.
32   Moreno, 2006.
33   Núñez, 2008.
34   Mayer & Moreno, 2003.
35   Chen & Wu, 2015.
36   Hegarty, 2005.
37   Mayer & Moreno, 2003; Moreno & Mayer, 1999.
38   Moreno, 2006; Mayer, Bove, Bryman, Mars, & Tapangco, 1996.
39   Mayer & Moreno, 2003.
40   Wright, Cardenas, Liang, & Newman, 2017.
41   Bussey & Orgill, 2015.
42   Edelstein, 2018.
43   Guo, Kim & Rubin, 2014; Newman & Schwarz, 2018.
44   Lieberman, Schroeder, & Amir, 2022.
45   Mayer & Moreno, 2003.
46   Mayer & Moreno, 2003.
47   Moreno & Mayer, 2000.

3.   Metaphors and Analogies: Uncovering How They Frame Thought

1   Jarvis, 2017, p. 43.
2   Bush, 1945; Flusberg, Matlock, & Thibodeau, 2018.
3   Nerlich & James, 2009.
4   Thibodeau, Hendricks, & Boroditsky, 2017.
5   Sopory & Dillard, 2002.
6   Eddington, 1931, p. 316.
7   Lightman, 1989.
8   Lakoff & Johnson, 1980.
9   Thibodeau & Boroditsky, 2011.
10   Kandel, Schwartz, & Jessell, 1991.

11 Fresnel & Arago, 1900.
12 Brown, 2003.
13 Brown, 2003.
14 Arrhenius, 1908, pp. 51–52.
15 Vollmer, 1984.
16 Niebert & Gropengießer, 2015.
17 Brown, 2003.
18 Kuhn, 1993.
19 Clement, 1993.
20 Gick & Holyoak, 1983.
21 Thibodeau, Hendricks, & Boroditsky, 2017.
22 Citron & Goldberg, 2014.
23 Desai, Conant, Binder, Park, & Seidenberg, 2013.
24 Sopory & Dillard, 2002.
25 Aziz-Zadeh & Damasio, 2008.
26 Desai, Conant, Binder, Park, & Seidenberg, 2013.
27 Lightman, 1989.
28 Taber, 2001.
29 Gericke & Smith, 2014.
30 Watson & Crick, 1953.
31 Gericke & Smith, 2014; Keller, 2000.
32 Strauss, 2009.
33 Hoh, 2017.
34 Reynolds, 2018.
35 Pigliucci & Boudry, 2011.
36 Balmer & Herreman, 2009.
37 Ancillotti, Holmberg, Lindfelt, & Eriksson, 2017.
38 Pigliucci & Boudry, 2011.
39 Ancillotti, Holmberg, Lindfelt, & Eriksson, 2017.
40 Hebert, Cywinska, Ball, & DeWaard, 2003.
41 Strauss, 2009; Larson, 2009.
42 Keefer, Landau, Sullivan, & Rothschild, 2014.
43 Landau, Arndt, & Cameron, 2017.
44 Flusberg, Matlock, & Thibodeau, 2017.
45 Flusberg, Matlock, & Thibodeau, 2018.
46 Degner, Hack, O'Neil, & Krisjanson, 2003.
47 Hauser & Schwarz, 2015.
48 Larson, 2005.

4. So We Live in a Snow Globe? Misconception Mishaps and Designing Stories for Learning

1 Bourke, 1997.
2 Schneps, & Sadler, 2010.

3 Vosniadou & Brewer, 1992.
4 Bailey & Kandel, 2008.
5 Sfard, 1998.
6 Francek, 2013.
7 Minstrell, 1982.
8 DiSessa, 2014.
9 Stern & Kampourakis, 2017.
10 Leach, Driver, Scott, & Wood-Robinson, 1996.
11 Nakhleh, 1992.
12 Schneps, & Sadler, 2010.
13 Francek, 2013.
14 Rickinson, 2001; Seethaler, Czworkowski, & Wynn, 2018.
15 Stern & Kampourakis, 2017.
16 Nakhleh, 1992.
17 Meadows & Wiesenmayer, 1999; Boyes & Stanisstreet, 1997.
18 Gruber & Vonèche, 1977; Bransford, Brown, & Cocking, 2000.
19 Kuhn, 1996.
20 Posner, Strike, Hewson, & Gertzog, 1982.
21 DiSessa, 2014; Toulmin, 1972.
22 Chinn & Brewer, 1993.
23 Hammer, 2000.
24 Minstrell, 1992.
25 DiSessa, 2014.
26 Brown, 2014.
27 Pintrich, Marx, & Boyle, 1993.
28 Vygotsky, 1978.
29 Linn, Eylon & Davis, 2013; Seethaler & Linn, 2004.
30 Shulman, 1986.
31 Carpenter, Franke, Jacobs, Fennema, & Empson, 1998.
32 Shindell, Rind, & Lonergan, 1998; Seethaler, 2016a.
33 White & Frederiksen, 1998.
34 Hershey, 2003.
35 Burton, 1991.
36 Katsumoto et al., 2007.
37 Llopart & Esteban-Guitart, 2018.
38 Calabrese Barton & Tan, 2019.
39 Ojalehto, Medin, & García, 2017; Biedrzycki & Bais, 2010.
40 Crouch, Fagen, Callan, & Mazur, 2004.
41 Zee & Minstrell, 1997.
42 Aguilar, Walton, & Wieman, 2014.
43 Brown, 1987.
44 White & Frederiksen, 1998.
45 Cook, Kennedy, & McGuire, 2013.
46 Kemper, 1984; Bruner, 1987.

47 Dahlstrom, 2014.
48 Bower & Clark, 1969.
49 Olson, 2015; Angler, 2020.
50 Cohen, 2011.
51 Birkenstein & Graff, 2018.
52 Olson, 2015.
53 Bruner, 1960.
54 American Association for the Advancement of Science, 2013.

5. The Hidden Climb Revealed: Giving Voice to People and Process

1 Koenigsberger, 1906, pp. 181–182.
2 Turner & Sullenger, 1999; Osborne, 2014.
3 Barrow, 2006; Dewey, 1910.
4 Mead & Métraux, 1957; Beardslee & O'Dowd, 1961.
5 Abd-El-Khalic, Waters, & Le, 2008; Binns & Bell, 2015.
6 Nelkin, 1995.
7 Tudor, 1989.
8 Haynes, 2003.
9 Weingart, Muhl, & Pansegrau, 2003.
10 Dudo et al., 2011.
11 Haynes, 2016; Kirby, 2017.
12 Weingart, Muhl, & Pansegrau, 2003.
13 Dudo, Cicchirillo, Atkinson, & Marx, 2014.
14 Lederman, 1992; National Science Board, 2016.
15 Osborne, Simon, & Collins, 2003.
16 Weisberg, Landrum, Hamilton, & Weisberg, 2021.
17 Reichenbach, 1938.
18 Oreskes, 2004.
19 Lin-Siegler, Ahn, Chen, Fang, & Luna-Lucero 2016.
20 Stefan, 2010.
21 Longino, 1990.
22 Ryder, Leach, & Driver, 1999.
23 Nersessian, 2008.
24 Lave & Wenger, 1991.
25 Simpson, Beatty, & Ballen, 2020.
26 Chambers, 1983; Finson, 2002.
27 Yong, 2018.
28 Ong, Wright, Espinosa, & Orfield, 2011.
29 Cobern & Loving, 2001.
30 Johnson et al., 2014.
31 Daston & Galison, 2007.
32 Latour & Woolgar, 1979.
33 Medawar, 1999 (1963).

34 Kuhn, 1996.
35 Knorr-Cetina, 1981.
36 Osborne, Collins, Ratcliffe, Millar, & Duschl, 2003.
37 Yaqub, 2018.
38 Pearce, 1912.
39 Watson, 1968.
40 Latour, 1987.
41 Lederman, 1992.
42 Schwartz, Lederman, & Crawford, 2004.
43 Abd-El-Khalick, 2013.
44 National Research Council, 2012.
45 Schooler, 2014.
46 *Chemical and Engineering News*, 2007.
47 Wheeler, Mulvey, Maeng, Librea-Carden, & Bell, 2019.
48 Sverdlik, Hall, McAlpine, & Hubbard, 2018.
49 Devos et al., 2017; Litalien & Guay, 2015.
50 Ross, 1962.
51 Popper, 1959.
52 Kuhn, 1996.
53 Laudan, 1983.
54 Merton, 1973.
55 Resnik & Elliott, 2016.
56 Seymour & Hewitt, 1997.
57 Carlone & Johnson, 2007.
58 Rothman, 2020.
59 Tudor, 1989.
60 Nelkin, 2001.
61 Bang, Marin, & Medin, 2018.
62 Longino, 2013.
63 Ivlev, Hickman, McDonagh, & Eden, 2017.
64 Kotcher, Myers, Vraga, Stenhouse, & Maibach, 2017.
65 Hutchings & Stenseth, 2016.
66 Weber & Schell Word, 2001.
67 Wynne, 1989.
68 De Laet & Mol, 2000; Haywood & Besley, 2014.
69 Collins & Evans, 2007.
70 Collins & Evans, 2007.
71 Snow, 1959.
72 Franklin, 2007.
73 Sarewitz, 2011.
74 Priest, Bonfadelli, & Rusanen, 2003.
75 Jasanoff, 2005.
76 Oreskes, 2003.
77 Jones & Radaelli, 2015.

78 Cairney, 2016.
79 Cairney, 2016.
80 Wagner, Fisher, & Pascual, 2018.
81 Elliott & Resnik, 2014.
82 Scharrer, Rupieper, Stadtler, & Bromme, 2017.
83 Dunning, 2011.

6. Negotiating Uncertainty and the Intricacies of Tradeoffs

1   Fischhoff, 2015.
2   Hardin, 1968.
3   Fine & Clarkson, 1986.
4   Poland, Jacobson, Opel, Marcuse, & Poland, 2015.
5   Hansson, 2017.
6   Clarke & Short, 1993.
7   National Research Council, 1996.
8   Slovic, 2000.
9   Kasperson, Slovic, Pidgeon, & Renn, 2017.
10 Fischhoff, Slovic, Lichtenstein, Reid, & Combs, 1978.
11 Zehr, 2000.
12 Starr, 1969.
13 Fischhoff, Slovic, Lichtenstein, Reid, & Combs, 1978.
14 Kasperson, Slovic, Pidgeon, & Renn, 2017.
15 Fischhoff, Slovic, Lichtenstein, Reid, & Combs, 1978; Fox-Glassman & Weber, 2016.
16 Kasperson, Slovic, Pidgeon, & Renn, 2017.
17 Sjöberg, 2000.
18 Fischhoff & Davis, 2014.
19 Slovic, 2000.
20 Alvarez & Evans, 2021.
21 Fischhoff, 1995.
22 D'Olimpio, 2016.
23 Wiens et al., 2021.
24 Hofstede, 2011.
25 Kahan, Jenkins-Smith, Tarantola, Silva, & Braman, 2015.
26 Signorini, Wiesemes, & Murphy, 2009.
27 Keohane, Lane, & Oppenheimer, 2014.
28 Manski, 2020.
29 Cairns, deAndrade, & MacDonald, 2013.
30 Jensen, 2004.
31 Han, 2016.
32 Zehr, 2000.
33 Pinto, 2015; Zehr, 2017.
34 Oreskes & Conway, 2010.

35 Pearce, Brown, Nerlich, & Koteyko, 2015.
36 Jensen & Hurley, 2010.
37 Dunwoody & Peters, 1992.
38 Dearing, 1995.
39 Dixon & Clarke, 2013.
40 Chang, 2015.
41 Clarke, Weberling McKeever, Holton, & Dixon, 2015; Kohl et al., 2016.
42 Boykoff, 2007.
43 Ioannidis, 2005.
44 Kimmerle, Flemming, Feinkohl, & Cress, 2015.
45 Gustafson & Rice, 2019.
46 Winter, Krämer, Rösner, & Neubaum, 2015.
47 Binder, Hillback, & Brossard, 2016; Jensen et al., 2017.
48 Smithson, 1989.
49 Van der Bles et al., 2019.
50 Saltelli & Funtowicz, 2014.
51 Van Asselt & Rotmans, 2002.
52 Walker et al., 2003.
53 Pinker, 2021.
54 Van der Bles et al., 2019.
55 Walker et al., 2003.
56 Walker et al., 2003; Miles & Frewer, 2003; Han, Klein, & Arora, 2011.
57 Van der Bles et al., 2019.
58 Rocha Souza, Dorn, Pringer, & Wandl-Vogt, 2019.
59 Schwartz, Fischhoff, Krishnamurti, & Sowell, 2013.
60 Van Asselt & Rotmans, 2002.
61 Van der Bles et al., 2019.
62 Van der Bles et al., 2019.
63 Fischhoff & Davis, 2014.
64 Slovic, 1993.
65 Pielke & Conant, 2003.
66 Jasanoff, 2009.
67 Beck & Krueger, 2016.
68 Patterson, Grenny, McMillan, & Switler, 2002.
69 National Commission for the Protection of Human Subjects of Biomedical and Behavioral Research, 1979.
70 Gere, 2017.
71 Kahlor et al., 2015.
72 Wong-Parodi, Krishnamurti, Davis, Schwartz, & Fischhoff, 2016.

7. How (Not) to Trigger Audiences' Decision-Making Survival Tactics

1 Brissiaud, 1988.
2 Schoenfeld, 1988.

3 Brissiaud, 1988.
4 Tversky & Kahneman, 1974.
5 Kahneman, 2011.
6 Shah & Oppenheimer, 2008.
7 Chen, 2015.
8 Chaiken & Maheswaran, 1994.
9 Chaiken, Liberman, & Eagly, 1989.
10 Damasio, 1994.
11 Duncan & Barrett, 2007.
12 Chen & Chaiken, 1999.
13 Gigerenzer, 2007.
14 Gigerenzer, 2015a.
15 McKenzie & Nelson, 2003.
16 Potter, 2011.
17 Schwarz, 2011.
18 Slovic, 1999.
19 Gilovich, Griffin, & Kahneman, 2002.
20 Tversky & Kahneman, 1971.
21 Gilovich, Griffin, & Kahneman, 2002.
22 Hoffrage, Lindsey, Hertwig, & Gigerenzer, 2000.
23 Gigerenzer, Hoffrage, & Ebert, 1998.
24 Gigerenzer, Gaissmaier, Kurz-Milcke, Schwartz, & Woloshin, 2007.
25 Seethaler, 2016b.
26 Ritov & Baron, 1990.
27 Bond & Nolan, 2011.
28 Poland & Jacobson, 1994.
29 Tversky & Kahneman, 1974.
30 Betsch, Ulshöfer, Renkewitz, & Betsch, 2011.
31 Nickerson, 1998.
32 Ruiz & Bell, 2014.
33 Leask, Chapman, & Robbins, 2010.
34 Kata, 2012.
35 Brown et al., 2010.
36 Weinstein, 1989.
37 Krawczyk, Knäuper et al., 2015; Krawczyk, Perez et al., 2015.
38 Kata, 2012; Dickstein, 1980.
39 Tversky & Kahneman, 1981.
40 Seethaler, 2016b.
41 DiSessa, 1993.
42 Taber & García-Franco, 2010; Southerland, Abrams, Cummins, &
    Anzelmo, 2001.
43 Polya, 1957.
44 Pronin, 2009.
45 Johnson & Tversky, 1983.

46 Pronin & Kugler, 2007.
47 Gigerenzer, 2015b.
48 Sherman, Cialdini, Schwartzman, & Reynolds, 1985.
49 Reber & Schwarz, 1999.
50 Davis et al., 2017.
51 Linquist & Bartol, 2013.
52 Hart, 2011.
53 Knobloch-Westerwick, Johnson, Silver, & Westerwick, 2015.
54 Crow & Jones, 2018.
55 Dunwoody & Peters, 1992.
56 Lipkus, 2007.
57 Cialdini, 2016.
58 Karlsson, Loewenstein, & Seppi, 2009.
59 Sumner et al., 2014.
60 Meadows, Sweeney, & Mahers, 2016.
61 Hoffrage & Gigerenzer, 1998.
62 Gigerenzer, 2015b.
63 Welch, Schwartz, & Woloshin, 2000.
64 Simpson, 1951; Wagner, 1982.
65 Hernán, Clayton, & Keiding, 2011.
66 Murphy, Lichtenstein, Fischhoff, & Winkler, 1980.
67 Juanchich & Sirota, 2019.
68 Gigerenzer & Galesic, 2012.
69 Cassels et al., 2003; Moynihan et al., 2000.
70 Furedi, 1999.
71 Dieckmann, Gregory, Peters, & Harrtman, 2017.
72 Tversky & Kahneman, 1974.
73 Keohane, Lane, & Oppenheimer, 2014.
74 Thaler & Sunstein, 2008.
75 Gigerenzer, 2015a.
76 Thaler & Sunstein, 2008.
77 Johnson & Goldstein, 2003.
78 Gigerenzer, 2015a.
79 Wood & Rünger, 2016.
80 Priest, Goodwin, & Dahlstrom, 2018.
81 Stucki & Sager, 2018.
82 Baier, 1986.
83 Engdahl & Lidskog, 2014.
84 Hendriks, Kienhues, & Bromme, 2016.
85 Evans & Hargittai, 2020.
86 Peterson, Chou, Kelley, & Hesse, 2020.
87 Casiday, 2006.
88 Chaiken, 1980.
89 Durlak & DuPre, 2008.

90 Goldsteen, Goldsteen, & Schorr, 1992.
91 Cairns, deAndrade, & Macdonald, 2013.
92 Gigerenzer, 2015b.
93 Kunda, 1990.
94 Botterill, Lake, & Walsh, 2021.
95 Montibeller & Von Winterfeldt, 2015.

8. Obvious but Wrong: The Perils of the Backfire Effect and Tips to Prevent It

1 Van Bavel & Pereira, 2018.
2 Pew Research Center, 2017.
3 Jost & Amodio, 2012; Carney, Jost, Gosling, & Potter, 2008.
4 Kahan, 2013.
5 Nisbet, Cooper, & Garrett, 2015.
6 Nisbet & Markowitz, 2014.
7 Kahan, 2010.
8 Cohen, 2003.
9 Campbell, Converse, Miller, & Stokes, 1960.
10 Sniderman & Bullock, 2004.
11 Leeper & Slothuus, 2014.
12 Menon, 2019.
13 Kunda, 1990.
14 Ruiz & Bell, 2014.
15 Lord, Ross, & Lepper, 1979.
16 Taber & Lodge, 2006.
17 Kahan et al., 2012.
18 Pew Research Center, 2018.
19 Pew Research Center, 2014.
20 Pew Research Center, 2015.
21 National Science Board, 2016.
22 Evans, 2018.
23 Gere, 2017.
24 Nyhan & Reifler, 2010.
25 Hart et al., 2009.
26 Zuwerink Jacks & Cameron, 2003.
27 Bensley & Wu, 1991.
28 Goldfarb & Kriner, 2017.
29 Wood & Porter, 2019.
30 Dillard & Shen, 2005.
31 Witte & Allen, 2000.
32 Trevors, Muis, Pekrun, Sinatra, & Winne, 2016.
33 Roser & Gazzaniga, 2006.

34 Reich & Robertson, 1979; Schultz, Nolan, Cialdini, Goldstein, & Griskevicius, 2007; Stibe & Cugelman, 2016.
35 Sniderman & Theriault, 2004.
36 Chong & Druckman, 2007.
37 Byrne & Hart, 2009.
38 Stibe & Cugelman, 2016.
39 Schwarz, Sanna, Skurnik, & Yoon, 2007.
40 Schwarz, Sanna, Skurnik, & Yoon, 2007.
41 Fragale & Heath, 2004.
42 Ehret, Van Boven, & Sherman, 2018.
43 Van Boven, Ehret, & Sherman, 2018.
44 Hart et al., 2009.
45 Shepherd & Kay, 2012.
46 Jones, 2014.
47 Kahan, Jenkins-Smith, Tarantola, Silva, & Braman, 2015.
48 Kahan, 2010.
49 Nisbet, 2018.
50 Danielsen, 2013.
51 Nisbet, 2018.
52 Klar, 2013.
53 Nisbet, 2009.
54 Klar, 2014.
55 Jones, 2019.
56 Fowler & Kam, 2007.
57 Estrada, Schultz, Silva-Send, & Boudrias, 2017.
58 Lee, 2021.
59 Bensley & Wu, 1991.
60 Miller, Lane, Deatrick, Young, & Potts, 2007.
61 Witte & Allen, 2000.
62 National Academy of Sciences and Institute of Medicine, 2008.
63 Zimmerman, n.d.
64 Schüz, Schüz, & Eid, 2013.
65 Kogut & Beyth-Maron, 2008.
66 Wolske, Gillingham, & Schultz, 2020.
67 Druckman & Bolsen, 2011.
68 Nisbet, 2009.
69 Myers, Nisbet, Maibach, & Leiserowitz, 2012.
70 Mossler, Bostrom, Kelly, Crossman, & Moy, 2017.
71 Hart & Nisbet, 2012.
72 Kelly, Cooley, & Klinger, 2013.
73 Hart, 2011.
74 Manning, 2013.
75 Byrne & Hart, 2009.

76 Wakefield et al., 2006.
77 Moyer-Gusé & Nabi, 2010.
78 Lewandowsky, Ecker, Seifert, Schwartz, & Cook, 2012.
79 Schwarz, Sanna, Skurnik, & Yoon, 2007.
80 Tippett, 2010.
81 Peter & Koch, 2015.
82 Bolsen & Druckman, 2015.
83 McGuire & Papageorgis, 1961.
84 Barthel, Mitchell, & Holcomb, 2016.
85 Van der Linden, Leiserowitz, Rosenthal, & Maibach, 2017.
86 Lewandowsky & Van Der Linden, 2021.
87 Roozenbeek & Van der Linden, 2019.
88 Dudo & Besley, 2016.

9. Crucial Conversations, Trust, and the Dark Matter of Communication

1 Fiske & Dupree, 2014.
2 Collett, 2003.
3 Walker & Trimboli, 1983.
4 Ekman & Friesen, 1969.
5 Ekman & Friesen, 1974.
6 Collett, 2003.
7 Patterson, Grenny, McMillan, & Switzler, 2002.
8 Sacks, Schlegoff, & Jefferson, 1974; Walker, 1982.
9 Duncan, 1972.
10 Kendon, 1967.
11 Collett, 2003.
12 Harrigan & Steffen, 1983; Kalma, 1992.
13 Lockard, Allen, Schiele, & Wiemer, 1978.
14 Dutton & Aron, 1974.
15 Foster, Witcher, Campbell, & Green, 1998.
16 Damasio, 2003.
17 Collett, 2003.
18 Laird, 1974.
19 Levenson, Ekman, & Friesen, 1990.
20 Riskind & Gotay, 1982.
21 Carney, Cuddy, & Yap, 2010.
22 Carney, Cuddy, & Yap, 2015.
23 Salovey & Mayer, 1990.
24 Rogers, 1959.
25 Comer & Drollinger, 1999.
26 Yaseen & Foster, 2019.
27 Alda, 2018.

28 Mercer et al., 2016.
29 Ferrari & Coudé, 2018.
30 Ferrari & Coudé, 2018.
31 Levenson & Ruef, 1992.
32 Schachter & Singer, 1962.
33 Zillmann, 1993.
34 Goleman, 1995.
35 Timmons & Ley, 1994.
36 Del Negro, Funk, & Feldman, 2018.
37 Masaoka, Izumizaki, & Homma, 2014.
38 Boiten, Frijda, & Wientjes, 1994.
39 Mehrabian, 1972.
40 Mehrabian, 1972.
41 Van Zant & Berger, 2019.
42 Linklater, 2006.
43 Juslin & Laukka, 2003.
44 Guyer, Fabrigar, & Vaughan-Johnston, 2019.
45 Laukka et al., 2008.
46 Masaoka, Izumizaki, & Homma, 2014.
47 Timmons & Ley, 1994.
48 Kabat-Zinn, 2003.
49 Hoge et al., 2018.
50 Montero-Marin, Garcia-Campayo, Pérez-Yus, Zabaleta-del-Olmo, & Cuijpers, 2019.
51 Grecucci, Pappaianni, Siugzdaite, Theuninck, & Job, 2015.
52 Kabat-Zinn, 2003.
53 Zeidan, Johnson, Diamond, David, & Goolkasian, 2010; Arch & Craske, 2006.
54 Chu, 2010.
55 Beblo et al., 2018.
56 Boiten, Frijda, & Wientjes, 1994.
57 Nazish, 2019.
58 Brown, Gerbarg, & Muench, 2013.
59 Alda, 2018.

10. Collecting the Tools into the Toolbox

1 Edelstein, 2018.
2 Luokkanen, Huttunen, & Hildén, 2014.
3 Matlock, Coe, & Westerling, 2017.
4 Brown & de Barra, 2023.

References

Abd-El-Khalick, F. (2013). Teaching with and about nature of science, and science teacher knowledge domains. *Science & Education, 22*, 2087–2107. https://doi.org/10.1007/s11191-012-9520-2

Abd-El-Khalick, F., Waters, M., & Le, A.P. (2008). Representations of nature of science in high school chemistry textbooks over the past four decades. *Journal of Research in Science Teaching, 45*(7), 835–855. https://doi.org/10.1002/tea.20226

Achenbach, J., & Feltman, R. (2016, February 11). Cosmic breakthrough: Physicists detect gravitational waves from violent black-hole merger. *The Washington Post.* Retrieved from www.washingtonpost.com/news/speaking-of-science/wp/2016/02/11/cosmic-breakthrough-physicists-detect-gravitational-waves-from-violent-black-hole-merger

Aguilar, L., Walton, G., & Wieman, C. (2014). Psychological insights for improved physics teaching. *Physics Today, 67*(5), 43–49. https://doi.org/10.1063/pt.3.2383

Alda, A. (2018). *If I understood you, would I have this look on my face? My adventures in the art and science of relating and communicating.* Random House Trade Paperbacks.

Alvarez, C.H., & Evans, C.R. (2021). Intersectional environmental justice and population health inequalities: A novel approach. *Social Science & Medicine, 269*, 113559. https://doi.org/10.1016/j.socscimed.2020.113559. Medline:33309156

American Association for the Advancement of Science. (2013). *Atlas of science,* Volumes 1 and 2. Mapping K-12 science learning. Retrieved from www.project2061.org/publications/atlas/default.htm

Ancillotti, M., Holmberg, N., Lindfelt, M., & Eriksson, S. (2017). Uncritical and unbalanced coverage of synthetic biology in the Nordic press. *Public Understanding of Science, 26*(2), 235–250. https://doi.org/10.1177 /0963662515609834. Medline:26481730

Angler, M.W. (2020). *Telling science stories: Reporting, crafting and editing for journalists and scientists.* Routledge.

Arch, J.J., & Craske, M.G. (2006). Mechanisms of mindfulness: Emotion regulation following a focused breathing induction. *Behaviour Research and Therapy, 44*(12), 1849–1858. https://doi.org/10.1016/j.brat.2005.12.007. Medline:16460668

Arrhenius, S. (1908). *Worlds in the making: The evolution of the universe.* H. Borns (Trans.). Harper & Brothers.

Aziz-Zadeh, L., & Damasio, A. (2008). Embodied semantics for actions: Findings from functional brain imaging. *Journal of Physiology-Paris, 102*(1–3), 35–39. https://doi.org/10.1016/j.jphysparis.2008.03.012. Medline:18472250

Baier, A. (1986). Trust and antitrust. *Ethics, 96*(2), 231–260. https://doi.org /10.1086/292745

Bailey, C.H., & Kandel, E.R. (2008). Synaptic remodeling, synaptic growth and the storage of long-term memory in aplysia. *Progress in Brain Research, 169*, 179–198. https://doi.org/10.1016/s0079-6123(07)00010-6. Medline: 18394474

Balmer, A., & Herreman, C. (2009). Craig Venter and the re-programming of life: How metaphors shape and perform ethical discourses in the media presentation of synthetic biology. In B. Nerlich, R. Elliott, & B. Larson (Eds.), *Communicating biological sciences: Ethical and metaphorical dimensions* (pp. 219–234). Ashgate Publishing.

Bang, M., Marin, A., & Medin, D. (2018). If Indigenous peoples stand with the sciences, will scientists stand with us? *Daedalus, 147*(2), 148–159. https:// doi.org/10.1162/daed_a_00498

Barrow, L.H. (2006). A brief history of inquiry: From Dewey to standards. *Journal of Science Teacher Education, 17*(3), 265–278. https://doi.org/10.1007 /s10972-006-9008-5

Barthel, M., Mitchell, A., & Holcomb, J. (2016). Many Americans believe fake news is sowing confusion. Pew Research Center, *15*, 12.

Bateson, G. (1935). Culture contact and schismogenesis. *Man*, 178–183.

Beardslee, D.C., & O'Dowd, D.D. (1961). The college-student image of the scientist. *Science, 133*(3457), 997–1001. https://doi.org/10.1126/science .133.3457.997. Medline:17743790

Beblo, T., Pelster, S., Schilling, C., Kleinke, K., Iffland, B., Driessen, M., & Fernando, S. (2018). Breath versus emotions: The impact of different foci of attention during mindfulness meditation on the experience of negative and positive emotions. *Behavior Therapy, 49*(5), 702–714. https://doi.org /10.1016/j.beth.2017.12.006. Medline:30146138

Beck, M., & Krueger, T. (2016). The epistemic, ethical, and political dimensions of uncertainty in integrated assessment modeling. *Wiley*

Interdisciplinary Reviews: Climate Change, 7(5), 627–645. https://doi.org/10.1002/wcc.415

Bennett, J. (2016, February 18). What are gravitational waves and why should you care? *The Huffington Post.* www.huffpost.com/entry/what-are-gravitational-waves_b_9253680

Bennett, M.J. (1979). Overcoming the golden rule: Sympathy and empathy. *Annals of the International Communication Association, 3*(1), 407–422. https://doi.org/10.1080/23808985.1979.11923774

Bennett, M.J. (2017). Developmental model of intercultural sensitivity. *The International Encyclopedia of Intercultural Communication,* 1–10.

Bensley, L.S., & Wu, R. (1991). The role of psychological reactance in drinking following alcohol prevention messages. *Journal of Applied Social Psychology, 21*(13), 1111–1124. https://doi.org/10.1111/j.1559-1816.1991.tb00461.x

Besley, J.C., & Nisbet, M. (2013). How scientists view the public, the media and the political process. *Public Understanding of Science, 22*(6), 644–659. https://doi.org/10.1177/0963662511418743. Medline:23885050

Betsch, C., Ulshöfer, C., Renkewitz, F., & Betsch, T. (2011). The influence of narrative v. statistical information on perceiving vaccination risks. *Medical Decision Making, 31*(5), 742–753. https://doi.org/10.1177/0272989x11400419. Medline:21447730

Biedrzycki, M.L., & Bais, H.P. (2010). Kin recognition in plants: a mysterious behaviour unsolved. *Journal of Experimental Botany, 61*(15), 4123–4128. https://doi.org/10.1093/jxb/erq250. Medline:20696656

Binder, A.R., Hillback, E.D., & Brossard, D. (2016). Conflict or caveats? Effects of media portrayals of scientific uncertainty on audience perceptions of new technologies. *Risk Analysis, 36*(4), 831–846. https://doi.org/10.1111/risa.12462. Medline:26268067

Binns, I.C., & Bell, R.L. (2015). Representation of scientific methodology in secondary science textbooks. *Science & Education, 24*(7), 913–936. https://doi.org/10.1007/s11191-015-9765-7

Birkenstein, C., & Graff, G. (2018). *They say/I say: The moves that matter in academic writing.* W.W. Norton & Company.

Boerner, L.K. (2021, July 5). Expanding American Sign Language's scientific vocabulary. *Chemical and Engineering News.* Retrieved from https://cendigitalmagazine.acs.org/2021/07/11/expanding-american-sign-languages-scientific-vocabulary-2/content.html?utm_email+=45939593A495C49555D42438D2

Boiten, F.A., Frijda, N.H., & Wientjes, C.J. (1994). Emotions and respiratory patterns: Review and critical analysis. *International Journal of Psychophysiology, 17*(2), 103–128. https://doi.org/10.1016/0167-8760(94)90027-2. Medline:7995774

Bolsen, T., & Druckman, J.N. (2015). Counteracting the politicization of science. *Journal of Communication, 65*(5), 745–769. https://doi.org/10.1111/jcom.12171

Bond, L., & Nolan, T. (2011). Making sense of perceptions of risk of diseases and vaccinations: A qualitative study combining models of health beliefs, decision-making and risk perception. *BMC Public Health*, *11*(1), 1–14. https://doi.org/10.1186/1471-2458-11-943. Medline:22182354

Botterill, L.C., Lake, J., & Walsh, M.J. (2021). Factors affecting public responses to health messages during the COVID-19 pandemic in Australia: Partisanship, values, and source credibility. *Australian Journal of Political Science*, *56*(4), 358–375. https://doi.org/10.1080/10361146.2021.1978389

Bourke, A.F. (1997). Sex ratios in bumble bees. *Philosophical Transactions of the Royal Society of London. Series B: Biological Sciences*, *352*(1364), 1921–1933. https://doi.org/10.1098/rstb.1997.0179

Bower, G.H., & Clark, M.C. (1969). Narrative stories as mediators for serial learning. *Psychonomic Science*, *14*(4), 181–182. https://doi.org/10.3758/bf03332778

Boyes, E., & Stanisstreet, M. (1997). Children's models of understanding of two major global environmental issues (ozone layer and greenhouse effect). *Research in Science & Technological Education*, *15*(1), 19–28. https://doi.org/10.1080/0263514970150102

Boykoff, M.T. (2007). Flogging a dead norm? Newspaper coverage of anthropogenic climate change in the United States and United Kingdom from 2003 to 2006. *Area*, *39*(4), 470–481. https://doi.org/10.1111/j.1475-4762.2007.00769.x

Bransford, J.D., Brown, A.L., & Cocking, R.R. (2000). *How people learn*. National Academy Press.

Brissiaud, R. (1988). De l'âge du capitaine à l'âge du berger [Quel contrôle de la validité d'un énoncé de problème au CE2?]. *Revue Française de Pédagogie*, *82*, 23–31. https://doi.org/10.3406/rfp.1988.1457

Brown, A. (1987). Metacognition, executive control, self-regulation, and other more mysterious mechanisms. In F. Reiner & R. Kluwe (Eds.), *Metacognition, motivation, and understanding* (pp. 65–116). Erlbaum.

Brown, B.A., & Ryoo, K. (2008). Teaching science as a language: A "content-first" approach to science teaching. *Journal of Research in Science Teaching*, *45*(5), 529–553. https://doi.org/10.1002/tea.20255

Brown, D.E. (2014). Students' conceptions as dynamically emergent structures. *Science & Education*, *23*(7), 1463–1483. https://doi.org/10.1007/s11191-013-9655-9

Brown, K.F., Kroll, J.S., Hudson, M.J., Ramsay, M., Green, J., Vincent, C.A., … & Sevdalis, N. (2010). Omission bias and vaccine rejection by parents of healthy children: Implications for the influenza A/H1N1 vaccination programme. *Vaccine*, *28*(25), 4181–4185. https://doi.org/10.1016/j.vaccine.2010.04.012. Medline:20412878

Brown, R.C., & de Barra, M. (2023). A taxonomy of non-honesty in public health communication. *Public Health Ethics*, *16*(1), 86–101. https://doi.org/10.1093/phe/phad003

Brown, R.P., Gerbarg, P.L., & Muench, F. (2013). Breathing practices for treatment of psychiatric and stress-related medical conditions. *Psychiatric Clinics, 36*(1), 121–140. https://doi.org/10.1016/j.psc.2013.01.001. Medline:23538082

Brown, T.L. (2003). *Making truth: Metaphor in science.* University of Illinois Press.

Bruner, J.S. (1960). *The process of education.* Harvard University Press.

Bruner, J.S. (1987). Life as narrative. *Social Research, 54*(1), 11. https://doi.org/10.1353/sor.2004.0045

Burton, R.J. (1991). *Inventing the flat earth: Columbus and modern historians.* Praeger.

Bush, V. (1945). Science – The endless frontier: A report to the president on a program for postwar scientific research. United States Government Printing Office. Retrieved from www.nsf.gov/od/lpa/nsf50/vbush1945.htm

Bussey, T.J., & Orgill, M. (2015). What do biochemistry students pay attention to in external representations of protein translation? The case of the Shine–Dalgarno sequence. *Chemistry Education Research and Practice, 16*(4), 714–730. https://doi.org/10.1039/c5rp00001g

Byrne, S., & Hart, P.S. (2009). The boomerang effect: A synthesis of findings and a preliminary theoretical framework. *Annals of the International Communication Association, 33*(1), 3–37. https://doi.org/10.1080/23808985.2009.11679083

Cairney, P. (2016). *The politics of evidence-based policy making.* Springer.

Cairns, G., De Andrade, M., & MacDonald, L. (2013). Reputation, relationships, risk communication, and the role of trust in the prevention and control of communicable disease: a review. *Journal of Health Communication, 18*(12), 1550–1565. https://doi.org/10.1080/10810730.2013.840696. Medline:24298887

Cairo, A. (2012). *The functional art: An introduction to information graphics and visualization.* New Riders.

Calabrese Barton, A., & Tan, E. (2019). Designing for rightful presence in STEM: The role of making present practices. *Journal of the Learning Sciences, 28*(4–5), 616–658. https://doi.org/10.1080/10508406.2019.1591411

Campbell, A., Converse, P., Miller, W.E., & Stokes, D. (1960). *The American voter.* John Wiley & Sons.

Canfield, K., & Menezes, S. (2020). *The state of inclusive science communication: A landscape study.* Metcalf Institute, University of Rhode Island.

Canfield, K.N., Menezes, S., Matsuda, S.B., Moore, A., Mosley Austin, A.N., Dewsbury, B.M., … & Taylor, C. (2020). Science communication demands a critical approach that centers inclusion, equity, and intersectionality. *Frontiers in Communication, 5*, 2. https://doi.org/10.3389/fcomm.2020.00002

Carlone, H.B., & Johnson, A. (2007). Understanding the science experiences of successful women of color: Science identity as an analytic lens. *Journal of Research in Science Teaching, 44*(8), 1187–1218. https://doi.org/10.1002/tea.20237

Carney, D.R., Cuddy, A.J., & Yap, A.J. (2010). Power posing: Brief nonverbal displays affect neuroendocrine levels and risk tolerance. *Psychological Science, 21*(10), 1363–1368. https://doi.org/10.1177/0956797610383437. Medline:20855902

Carney, D.R., Cuddy, A.J., & Yap, A.J. (2015). Review and summary of research on the embodied effects of expansive (vs. contractive) nonverbal displays. *Psychological Science, 26*(5), 657–663. https://doi.org/10.1177/0956797614566855. Medline:25841000

Carney, D.R., Jost, J.T., Gosling, S.D., & Potter, J. (2008). The secret lives of liberals and conservatives: Personality profiles, interaction styles, and the things they leave behind. *Political Psychology, 29*(6), 807–840. https://doi.org/10.1111/j.1467-9221.2008.00668.x

Carpenter, T.P., Franke, M.L., Jacobs, V.R., Fennema, E., & Empson, S.B. (1998). A longitudinal study of invention and understanding in children's multidigit addition and subtraction. *Journal for Research in Mathematics Education, 29*(1), 3–20. https://doi.org/10.5951/jresematheduc.29.1.0003

Casiday, R. (2006). Uncertainty, decision-making and trust: Lessons from the MMR controversy. *Community Practitioner, 79*(11), 354–357.

Cassels, A., Hughes, M.A., Cole, C., Mintzes, B., Lexchin, J., & McCormack, J.P. (2003). Drugs in the news: An analysis of Canadian newspaper coverage of new prescription drugs. *Canadian Medical Association Journal, 168*(9), 1133–1137.

Center for Universal Design. (1997). The principles of universal design. Retrieved from https://projects.ncsu.edu/ncsu/design/cud/pubs_p/docs/poster.pdf

Chaiken, S. (1980). Heuristic versus systematic information processing and the use of source versus message cues in persuasion. *Journal of Personality and Social Psychology, 39*(5), 752–766. https://doi.org/10.1037/0022-3514.39.5.752

Chaiken, S., Liberman, A., & Eagly, A.H. (1989). Heuristic and systematic processing within and beyond the persuasion context. In J.S. Uleman & J.A. Bargh (Eds.) *Unintended thought* (pp. 212–252). Guilford Press.

Chaiken, S., & Maheswaran, D. (1994). Heuristic processing can bias systematic processing: Effects of source credibility, argument ambiguity, and task importance on attitude judgment. *Journal of Personality and Social Psychology, 66*(3), 460. https://doi.org/10.1037/0022-3514.66.3.460. Medline:8169760

Chambers, D.W. (1983). Stereotypic images of the scientist: The draw-a-scientist test. *Science Education, 67*(2), 255–265 https://doi.org/10.1002/sce.3730670213

Chandler, P., & Sweller, J. (1991). Cognitive load theory and the format of instruction. *Cognition and Instruction, 8*(4), 293–332. https://doi.org/10.1207/s1532690xci0804_2

Chang, C. (2015). Motivated processing: How people perceive news covering novel or contradictory health research findings. *Science Communication, 37*(5), 602–634. https://doi.org/10.1177/1075547015597914

Chemical and Engineering News (2007). A cautionary tale on reproducibility. Retrieved from https://cen.acs.org/articles/85/i4/cautionary-tale-reproducibility.html

Chen, C.M., & Wu, C.H. (2015). Effects of different video lecture types on sustained attention, emotion, cognitive load, and learning performance. *Computers & Education, 80*, 108–121. https://doi.org/10.1016/j.compedu.2014.08.015

Chen, N.T. (2015). Predicting vaccination intention and benefit and risk perceptions: The incorporation of affect, trust, and television influence in a dual-mode model. *Risk Analysis, 35*(7), 1268–1280. https://doi.org/10.1111/risa.12348. Medline:25808562

Chen, S., & Chaiken, S. (1999). The heuristic-systematic model in its broader context. In D. Chaiken & Y. Trope (Eds.), *Dual process theories in social psychology* (pp. 73–96). Guilford Press.

Chinn, C.A., & Brewer, W.F. (1993). The role of anomalous data in knowledge acquisition: A theoretical framework and implications for science instruction. *Review of Educational Research, 63*(1), 1–49. https://doi.org/10.3102/00346543063001001

Chirico, A., Glaveanu, V.P., Cipresso, P., Riva, G., & Gaggioli, A. (2018). Awe enhances creative thinking: an experimental study. *Creativity Research Journal, 30*(2), 123–131. https://doi.org/10.1080/10400419.2018.1446491

Chong, D., & Druckman, J.N. (2007). Framing public opinion in competitive democracies. *American Political Science Review, 101*(4), 637–655. https://doi.org/10.1017/s0003055407070554

Chu, L.C. (2010). The benefits of meditation vis-à-vis emotional intelligence, perceived stress and negative mental health. *Stress and Health: Journal of the International Society for the Investigation of Stress, 26*(2), 169–180. https://doi.org/10.1002/smi.1289

Cialdini, R. (2016). *Pre-suasion: A revolutionary way to influence and persuade.* Simon and Schuster.

Citron, F.M., & Goldberg, A.E. (2014). Metaphorical sentences are more emotionally engaging than their literal counterparts. *Journal of Cognitive Neuroscience, 26*(11), 2585–2595. https://doi.org/10.1162/jocn_a_00654. Medline:24800628

Clarke, C.E., Weberling McKeever, B., Holton, A., & Dixon, G.N. (2015). The influence of weight-of-evidence messages on (vaccine) attitudes: A sequential mediation model. *Journal of Health Communication,*

20(11), 1302–1309. https://doi.org/10.1080/10810730.2015.1023959.
Medline:26214547

Clarke, L., & Short Jr, J.F. (1993). Social organization and risk: Some current controversies. *Annual Review of Sociology, 19*(1), 375–399. https://doi .org/10.1146/annurev.so.19.080193.002111

Clement, J. (1993). Using bridging analogies and anchoring intuitions to deal with students' preconceptions in physics. *Journal of Research in Science Teaching, 30*(10), 1241–1257. https://doi.org/10.1002/tea.3660301007

Cobern, W.W., & Loving, C.C. (2001). Defining "science" in a multicultural world: Implications for science education. *Science Education, 85*(1), 50–67. https://doi.org/10.1002/1098-237x(200101)85:1%3C50::aid-sce5%3E3.0.co;2-g

Cohen, G.L. (2003). Party over policy: The dominating impact of group influence on political beliefs. *Journal of Personality and Social Psychology, 85*(5), 808. https://doi.org/10.1037/0022-3514.85.5.808. Medline:14599246

Cohen, S.D. (2011). The art of public narrative: Teaching students how to construct memorable anecdotes. *Communication Teacher, 25*(4), 197–204. https://doi.org/10.1080/17404622.2011.601726

Collett, P. (2003). *The book of tells: How to read people's minds from their actions.* HarperCollins.

Collins, H., & Evans, R. (2007). *Rethinking expertise.* University of Chicago Press.

Comer, L.B., & Drollinger, T. (1999). Active empathetic listening and selling success: A conceptual framework. *Journal of Personal Selling & Sales Management, 19*(1), 15–29.

Cook, E., Kennedy, E., & McGuire, S.Y. (2013). Effect of teaching metacognitive learning strategies on performance in general chemistry courses. *Journal of Chemical Education, 90*(8), 961–967. https://doi.org/10.1021/ed300686h

Cook, M.P. (2006). Visual representations in science education: The influence of prior knowledge and cognitive load theory on instructional design principles. *Science Education, 90*(6), 1073–1091. https://doi.org/10.1002/sce.20164

Crameri, F., Shephard, G.E., & Heron, P.J. (2020). The misuse of colour in science communication. *Nature Communications, 11*(1), 1–10. https://doi .org/10.1038/s41467-020-19160-7. Medline:33116149

Crouch, C., Fagen, A.P., Callan, J.P., & Mazur, E. (2004). Classroom demonstrations: Learning tools or entertainment?. *American Journal of Physics, 72*(6), 835–838. https://doi.org/10.1119/1.1707018

Crow, D., & Jones, M. (2018). Narratives as tools for influencing policy change. *Policy & Politics, 46*(2), 217–234. https://doi.org/10.1332/030557318x15230061022899

Dahlstrom, M.F. (2014). Using narratives and storytelling to communicate science with nonexpert audiences. *Proceedings of the National Academy of*

Sciences, 111(Supplement 4), 13614–13620. https://doi.org/10.1073
/pnas.1320645111. Medline:25225368

Damasio, A.R. (1994). *Descartes' error: Emotion, rationality and the human brain.*
Putnam.

Damasio, A.R. (2003). *Looking for Spinoza: Joy, sorrow, and the feeling brain.*
Houghton Mifflin Harcourt.

Danielsen, S. (2013). Fracturing over creation care? Shifting environmental
beliefs among evangelicals, 1984–2010. *Journal for the Scientific Study of
Religion, 52*(1), 198–215. https://doi.org/10.1111/jssr.12017

Daston, L., & Galison, P. (2007). *Objectivity.* Princeton University Press.

Davies, S., McCallie, E., Simonsson, E., Lehr, J.L., & Duensing, S. (2009).
Discussing dialogue: Perspectives on the value of science dialogue events
that do not inform policy. *Public Understanding of Science, 18*(3), 338–353.
https://doi.org/10.1177/0963662507079760

Davis, K.C., Duke, J., Shafer, P., Patel, D., Rodes, R., & Beistle, D. (2017).
Perceived effectiveness of antismoking ads and association with quit
attempts among smokers: Evidence from the tips from former smokers
campaign. *Health Communication, 32*(8), 931–938. https://doi.org/10
.1080/10410236.2016.1196413. Medline:27435919

Dearing, J.W. (1995). Newspaper coverage of maverick science: Creating
controversy through balancing. *Public Understanding of Science, 4*(4),
341–361. https://doi.org/10.1088/0963-6625/4/4/002

Degner, L.F., Hack, T., O'Neil, J., & Kristjanson, L.J. (2003). A new approach
to eliciting meaning in the context of breast cancer. *Cancer Nursing,
26*(3), 169–178. https://doi.org/10.1097/00002820-200306000-00001.
Medline:12832949

De Laet, M., & Mol, A. (2000). The Zimbabwe bush pump: Mechanics of a
fluid technology. *Social Studies of Science, 30*(2), 225–263. https://doi.org
/10.1177/030631200030002002

Del Negro, C.A., Funk, G.D., & Feldman, J.L. (2018). Breathing matters.
Nature Reviews Neuroscience, 19(6), 351–367. https://doi.org/10.1038
/s41583-018-0003-6. Medline:29740175

Desai, R.H., Conant, L.L., Binder, J.R., Park, H., & Seidenberg, M.S. (2013).
A piece of the action: Modulation of sensory-motor regions by action
idioms and metaphors. *NeuroImage, 83*, 862–869. https://doi.org/10.1016
/j.neuroimage.2013.07.044. Medline:23891645

Devos, C., Boudrenghien, G., Van der Linden, N., Azzi, A., Frenay, M.,
Galand, B., & Klein, O. (2017). Doctoral students' experiences leading to
completion or attrition: A matter of sense, progress and distress. *European
Journal of Psychology of Education, 32*(1), 61–77. https://doi.org/10.1007
/s10212-016-0290-0

Dewey, J. (1910). Science as subject-matter and as method. *Science, 31*(787),
121–127. https://doi.org/10.1126/science.31.787.121. Medline:
17744061

Dickstein, L.S. (1980). Inference errors in deductive reasoning. *Bulletin of the Psychonomic Society, 16*(6), 414–416. https://doi.org/10.3758/bf03329585

Dieckmann, N.F., Gregory, R., Peters, E., & Hartman, R. (2017). Seeing what you want to see: How imprecise uncertainty ranges enhance motivated reasoning. *Risk Analysis, 37*(3), 471–486. https://doi.org/10.1111/risa.12639. Medline:27667776

Dillard, J.P., & Shen, L. (2005). On the nature of reactance and its role in persuasive health communication. *Communication Monographs, 72*(2), 144–168. https://doi.org/10.1080/03637750500111815

DiSessa, A.A. (1993). Toward an epistemology of physics. *Cognition and Instruction, 10*(2–3), 105–225. https://doi.org/10.1080/07370008.1985.9649008

DiSessa, A.A. (2014). A history of conceptual change research: Threads and fault lines. In R.K. Sawyer (Ed.), *The Cambridge handbook of the learning sciences* (pp. 88–108). Cambridge University Press.

Dixon, G.N., & Clarke, C.E. (2013). Heightening uncertainty around certain science: Media coverage, false balance, and the autism-vaccine controversy. *Science Communication, 35*(3), 358–382. https://doi.org/10.1177/1075547012458290

D'Olimpio, L. (2016, June 2). The trolley dilemma: Would you kill one person to save five? *The Conversation.* Retrieved from https://theconversation.com/the-trolley-dilemma-would-you-kill-one-person-to-save-five-57111

Druckman, J.N., & Bolsen, T. (2011). Framing, motivated reasoning, and opinions about emergent technologies. *Journal of Communication, 61*(4), 659–688. https://doi.org/10.1111/j.1460-2466.2011.01562.x

Dudo, A., & Besley, J.C. (2016). Scientists' prioritization of communication objectives for public engagement. *PLOS One, 11*(2), e0148867 https://doi.org/10.1371/journal.pone.0148867. Medline:26913869

Dudo, A., Brossard, D., Shanahan, J., Scheufele, D.A., Morgan, M., & Signorielli, N. (2011). Science on television in the 21st century: Recent trends in portrayals and their contributions to public attitudes toward science. *Communication Research, 38*(6), 754–777. https://doi.org/10.1177/0093650210384988

Dudo, A., Cicchirillo, V., Atkinson, L., & Marx, S. (2014). Portrayals of technoscience in video games: A potential avenue for informal science learning. *Science Communication, 36*(2), 219–247. https://doi.org/10.1177/1075547013520240

Duncan, S. (1972). Some signals and rules for taking speaking turns in conversations. *Journal of Personality and Social Psychology, 23*(2), 283. https://doi.org/10.1037/h0033031

Duncan, S., & Barrett, L.F. (2007). Affect is a form of cognition: A neurobiological analysis. *Cognition and Emotion, 21*(6), 1184–1211. https://doi.org/10.1080/02699930701437931. Medline:18509504

Dunning, D. (2011). The Dunning–Kruger Effect: On being ignorant of one's own ignorance. In M.P. Zanna & J.M. Olson (Eds.), *Advances in experimental social psychology* (Vol. 44, pp. 247–296). Academic Press.

Dunwoody, S., & Peters, H.P. (1992). Mass media coverage of technological and environmental risks: A survey of research in the United States and Germany. *Public Understanding of Science, 1*(2), 199–230. https://doi .org/10.1088/0963-6625/1/2/004

Durlak, J.A., & DuPre, E.P. (2008). Implementation matters: A review of research on the influence of implementation on program outcomes and the factors affecting implementation. *American Journal of Community Psychology, 41*(3), 327–350. https://doi.org/10.1007/s10464-008-9165-0. Medline:18322790

Dutton, D.G., & Aron, A.P. (1974). Some evidence for heightened sexual attraction under conditions of high anxiety. *Journal of Personality and Social Psychology, 30*(4), 510. https://doi.org/10.1037/h0037031. Medline: 4455773

Dweck, C. (2015). Carol Dweck revisits the growth mindset. *Education Week, 35*(5), 20–24.

Eddington, A.S. (1931). Presidential address, 1930: The end of the world (from the standpoint of mathematical physics). *The Mathematical Gazette, 15*(212), 316–324. https://doi.org/10.2307/3606671

Edelstein, B. (2018). *Thinking Shakespeare (revised edition): A working guide for actors, directors, students … and anyone else interested in the bard.* Theatre Communications Group.

Ehret, P.J., Van Boven, L., & Sherman, D.K. (2018). Partisan barriers to bipartisanship: Understanding climate policy polarization. *Social Psychological and Personality Science, 9*(3), 308–318. https://doi.org/10.1177 /1948550618758709

Eick, C.J., & King Jr., D.T. (2012). Nonscience majors' perceptions on the use of YouTube video to support learning in an integrated science lecture. *Journal of College Science Teaching, 42*(1), 26–30.

Ekman, P., & Friesen, W.V. (1969). The repertoire of nonverbal behavior: Categories, origins, usage, and coding. *Semiotica, 1*(1), 49–98. https://doi .org/10.1515/semi.1969.1.1.49

Ekman, P., & Friesen, W.V. (1974). Detecting deception from the body or face. *Journal of Personality and Social Psychology, 29*(3), 288. https://doi.org /10.1037/h0036006

Elliott, K.C., & Resnik, D.B. (2014). Science, policy, and the transparency of values. *Environmental Health Perspectives, 122*(7), 647–650. https://doi.org /10.1289/ehp.1408107. Medline:24667564

Engdahl, E., & Lidskog, R. (2014). Risk, communication and trust: Towards an emotional understanding of trust. *Public Understanding of Science, 23*(6), 703–717. https://doi.org/10.1177/0963662512460953. Medline:25414929

Ericsson, K.A. (2018). The differential influence of experience, practice, and deliberate practice on the development of superior individual performance of experts. In K.A. Ericsson, R.R. Hoffman, A. Kozbelt, & A.M. Williams (Eds.), *The Cambridge handbook of expertise and expert performance* (pp. 696–713). Cambridge University Press.

Estrada, M., Schultz, P.W., Silva-Send, N., & Boudrias, M.A. (2017). The role of social influences on pro-environment behaviors in the San Diego region. *Journal of Urban Health*, 2(94), 170–179. https://doi.org/10.1007/s11524-017-0139-0. Medline:28265806

Evans, J. (2018). *Morals not knowledge: Recasting the contemporary US conflict between religion and science.* University of California Press.

Evans, J.H., & Hargittai, E. (2020). Who doesn't trust Fauci? The public's belief in the expertise and shared values of scientists in the COVID-19 pandemic. *Socius*, 6, 2378023120947337. https://doi.org/10.1177/2378023120947337

Feasey, R. (2021). Meghan Markle and the royal pregnancy announcement: Media mis/reporting of advanced maternal age. *Journal of Gender Studies*, 1–13. https://doi.org/10.1080/09589236.2021.1934658

Ferrari, P.F., & Coudé, G. (2018). Mirror neurons, embodied emotions, and empathy. In K.Z. Meyza and E. Knapska (Eds.), *Neuronal correlates of empathy from rodent to human* (pp. 67–77). Academic Press.

Fine, P.E.M., & Clarkson, J.A. (1986). Individual versus public priorities in the determination of optimal vaccination policies. *American Journal of Epidemiology*, 124(6), 1012–1020. https://doi.org/10.1093/oxfordjournals.aje.a114471. Medline:3096132

Finson, K.D. (2002). Drawing a scientist: What we do and do not know after fifty years of drawings. *School Science and Mathematics*, 102(7), 335–345. https://doi.org/10.1111/j.1949-8594.2002.tb18217.x

Fischhoff, B. (1995). Risk perception and communication unplugged: twenty years of process. *Risk Analysis*, 15(2), 137–145. https://doi.org/10.1111/j.1539-6924.1995.tb00308.x. Medline:7597253

Fischhoff, B. (2015). The realities of risk-cost-benefit analysis. *Science*, 350(6260). https://doi.org/10.1126/science.aaa6516. Medline:26516286

Fischhoff, B., & Davis, A.L. (2014). Communicating scientific uncertainty. *Proceedings of the National Academy of Sciences*, 111(Supplement 4), 13664–13671. https://doi.org/10.1073/pnas.1317504111. Medline:25225390

Fischhoff, B., Slovic, P., Lichtenstein, S., Read, S., & Combs, B. (1978). How safe is safe enough? A psychometric study of attitudes towards technological risks and benefits. *Policy Sciences*, 9(2), 127–152. https://doi.org/10.1007/bf00143739

Fiske, S.T., & Dupree, C. (2014). Gaining trust as well as respect in communicating to motivated audiences about science topics. *Proceedings of the National Academy of Sciences*, 111(Supplement 4), 13593–13597. https://doi.org/10.1073/pnas.1317505111. Medline:25225372

Flusberg, S.J., Matlock, T., & Thibodeau, P.H. (2017). Metaphors for the war (or race) against climate change. *Environmental Communication, 11*(6), 769–783. https://doi.org/10.1080/17524032.2017.1289111

Flusberg, S.J., Matlock, T., & Thibodeau, P.H. (2018). War metaphors in public discourse. *Metaphor and Symbol, 33*(1), 1–18. https://doi.org/10.1080/10926488.2018.1407992

Foster, C.A., Witcher, B.S., Campbell, W.K., & Green, J.D. (1998). Arousal and attraction: Evidence for automatic and controlled processes. *Journal of Personality and Social Psychology, 74*(1), 86. https://doi.org/10.1037/0022-3514.74.1.86

Fowler, J.H., & Kam, C.D. (2007). Beyond the self: Social identity, altruism, and political participation. *Journal of Politics, 69*(3), 813–827. https://doi.org/10.1111/j.1468-2508.2007.00577.x

Fox-Glassman, K.T., & Weber, E.U. (2016). What makes risk acceptable? Revisiting the 1978 psychological dimensions of perceptions of technological risks. *Journal of Mathematical Psychology, 75*, 157–169. https://doi.org/10.1016/j.jmp.2016.05.003

Fragale, A.R., & Heath, C. (2004). Evolving informational credentials: The (mis) attribution of believable facts to credible sources. *Personality and Social Psychology Bulletin, 30*(2), 225–236. https://doi.org/10.1177/0146167203259933. Medline:15030635

Francek, M. (2013). A compilation and review of over 500 geoscience misconceptions. *International Journal of Science Education, 35*(1), 31–64. https://doi.org/10.1080/09500693.2012.736644

Frankel, F., & DePace, A.H. (2012). *Visual strategies: A practical guide to graphics for scientists & engineers.* Yale University Press.

Franklin, J. (2007). The end of science journalism. In M.W. Bauer & M. Bucchi (Eds.), *Journalism, science and society* (pp. 143–156). Routledge.

Fresnel, A.J., & Arago, F. (1900). *The wave theory of light: Memoirs of Huygens, Young and Fresnel.* American Book Company.

Furedi, A. (1999). Social consequences. The public health implications of the 1995 "pill scare." *Human Reproduction Update, 5*(6), 621–626. https://doi.org/10.1093/humupd/5.6.621. Medline:10652971

Gere, C. (2017). *Pain, pleasure, and the greater good: From the panopticon to the Skinner box and beyond.* University of Chicago Press.

Gericke, N.M., & Smith, M.U. (2014). Twenty-first-century genetics and genomics: Contributions of HPS-informed research and pedagogy. In M.R. Matthews (Ed.), *International handbook of research in history, philosophy and science teaching* (pp. 423–467). Springer.

Gick, M.L., & Holyoak, K.J. (1983). Schema induction and analogical transfer. *Cognitive Psychology, 15*(1), 1–38. https://doi.org/10.1016/0010-0285(83)90002-6

Gigerenzer, G. (2007). *Gut feelings: The intelligence of the unconscious.* Penguin.

Gigerenzer, G. (2015a). On the supposed evidence for libertarian paternalism. *Review of Philosophy and Psychology, 6*(3), 361–383. https://doi.org/10.1007/s13164-015-0248-1. Medline:26213590

Gigerenzer, G. (2015b). *Simply rational: Decision making in the real world.* Oxford University Press.

Gigerenzer, G., Gaissmaier, W., Kurz-Milcke, E., Schwartz, L.M., & Woloshin, S. (2007). Helping doctors and patients make sense of health statistics. *Psychological Science in the Public Interest, 8*(2), 53–96. https://doi.org/10.1111/j.1539-6053.2008.00033.x. Medline:26161749

Gigerenzer, G., & Galesic, M. (2012). Why do single event probabilities confuse patients?. *BMJ (Clinical Research ed.), 344*, e245. https://doi.org/10.1136/bmj.e245. Medline:22236599

Gigerenzer, G., Hoffrage, U., & Ebert, A. (1998). AIDS counselling for low-risk clients. *AIDS Care, 10*(2), 197–211. https://doi.org/10.1080/09540129850124451. Medline:9625903

Gilovich, T., Griffin, D., & Kahneman, D. (Eds.). (2002). *Heuristics and biases: The psychology of intuitive judgment.* Cambridge University Press.

Goldfarb, J.L., & Kriner, D.L. (2017). Building public support for science spending: Misinformation, motivated reasoning, and the power of corrections. *Science Communication, 39*(1), 77–100. https://doi.org/10.1177/1075547016688325

Goldsteen, R.L., Goldsteen, K., & Schorr, J.K. (1992). Trust and its relationship to psychological distress: The case of Three Mile Island. *Political Psychology*, 693–707.

Goleman, D. (1995). *Emotional intelligence: Why it can matter more than IQ.* Bantam.

Gowaty, P.A. (1982). Sexual terms in sociobiology: Emotionally evocative and, paradoxically, jargon. *Animal Behaviour, 30*(2), 630–631. https://doi.org/10.1016/s0003-3472(82)80079-1

Grecucci, A., Pappaianni, E., Siugzdaite, R., Theuninck, A., & Job, R. (2015). Mindful emotion regulation: Exploring the neurocognitive mechanisms behind mindfulness. *Biomed Research International, 2015*, 670724–670724. https://doi.org/10.1155/2015/670724. Medline:26137490

Greene, J.E. (2012). Goldilocks black holes. *Scientific American, 306*(1), 40–47. https://doi.org/10.1038/scientificamerican0112-40. Medline:22279833

Greeno, J.G. (1994). Gibson's affordances. *Psychological Review, 101*(2), 336–342. https://doi.org/10.1037/0033-295x.101.2.336. Medline:8022965

Groves, F.H. (1995). Science vocabulary load of selected secondary science textbooks. *School Science and Mathematics, 95*(5), 231–235. https://doi.org/10.1111/j.1949-8594.1995.tb15772.x

Gruber, H.E., & Vonèche, J.J. (Eds.). (1977). *The essential Piaget.* Routledge & Kegan Paul.

Guo, P.J., Kim, J., & Rubin, R. (2014, March). How video production affects student engagement: An empirical study of MOOC videos. In *Proceedings of the First ACM Conference on Learning@scale* (pp. 41–50). Association for Computing Machinery.

Gustafson, A., & Rice, R.E. (2019). The effects of uncertainty frames in three science communication topics. *Science Communication, 41*(6), 679–706. https://doi.org/10.1177/1075547019870811

Guyer, J.J., Fabrigar, L.R., & Vaughan-Johnston, T.I. (2019). Speech rate, intonation, and pitch: Investigating the bias and cue effects of vocal confidence on persuasion. *Personality and Social Psychology Bulletin, 45*(3), 389–405. https://doi.org/10.1177/0146167218787805. Medline:30084307

Hammer, D. (2000). Student resources for learning introductory physics. *American Journal of Physics, 68*(S1), S52–S59. https://doi.org/10.1119/1.19520

Han, P.K. (2016). The need for uncertainty: A case for prognostic silence. *Perspectives in Biology and Medicine, 59*(4), 567. https://doi.org/10.1353/pbm.2016.0049. Medline:28690246

Han, P.K., Klein, W.M., & Arora, N.K. (2011). Varieties of uncertainty in health care: A conceptual taxonomy. *Medical Decision Making, 31*(6), 828–838. https://doi.org/10.1177/0272989x10393976

Hansson, S.O. (2017). Five caveats for risk–risk analysis. *Journal of Risk Research, 20*(8), 984–987. https://doi.org/10.1080/13669877.2016.1147493

Hardin, G. (1968). The tragedy of the commons: The population problem has no technical solution; it requires a fundamental extension in morality. *Science, 162*(3859), 1243–1248. https://doi.org/10.1126/science.162.3859.1243. Medline:17756331

Harrigan, J.A., & Steffen, J.J. (1983). Gaze as a turn-exchange signal in group conversations. *British Journal of Social Psychology, 22*(2), 167–168. https://doi.org/10.1111/j.2044-8309.1983.tb00578.x

Hart, P.S. (2011). One or many? The influence of episodic and thematic climate change frames on policy preferences and individual behavior change. *Science Communication, 33*(1), 28–51. https://doi.org/10.1177/1075547010366400

Hart, P.S., & Nisbet, E.C. (2012). Boomerang effects in science communication: How motivated reasoning and identity cues amplify opinion polarization about climate mitigation policies. *Communication Research, 39*(6), 701–723. https://doi.org/10.1177/0093650211416646

Hart, W., Albarracín, D., Eagly, A.H., Brechan, I., Lindberg, M.J., & Merrill, L. (2009). Feeling validated versus being correct: A meta-analysis of selective exposure to information. *Psychological Bulletin, 135*(4), 555–588. https://doi.org/10.1037/a0015701. Medline:19586162

Hauser, D.J., & Schwarz, N. (2015). The war on prevention: Bellicose cancer metaphors hurt (some) prevention intentions. *Personality and Social Psychology Bulletin, 41*(1), 66–77. https://doi.org/10.1177/0146167214557006. Medline:25352114

Haynes, R. (2003). From alchemy to artificial intelligence: Stereotypes of the scientist in Western literature. *Public Understanding of Science, 12*(3), 243–253. https://doi.org/10.1177/0963662503123003

Haynes, R.D. (2016). Whatever happened to the "mad, bad" scientist? Overturning the stereotype. *Public Understanding of Science, 25*(1), 31–44. https://doi.org/10.1177/0963662514535689. Medline:24916194

Haywood, B.K., & Besley, J.C. (2014). Education, outreach, and inclusive engagement: Towards integrated indicators of successful program outcomes in participatory science. *Public Understanding of Science, 23*(1), 92–106. https://doi.org/10.1177/0963662513494560. Medline:23887249

Hebert, P.D., Cywinska, A., Ball, S.L., & DeWaard, J.R. (2003). Biological identifications through DNA barcodes. *Proceedings of the Royal Society of London. Series B: Biological Sciences, 270*(1512), 313–321. https://doi.org/10.1098/rspb.2002.2218. Medline:12614582

Hegarty, M. (2005). Multimedia learning about physical systems. In R. Mayer & R.E. Mayer (Eds.), *The Cambridge handbook of multimedia learning* (pp. 447–465). Cambridge University Press.

Heidig, S., Müller, J., & Reichelt, M. (2015). Emotional design in multimedia learning: Differentiation on relevant design features and their effects on emotions and learning. *Computers in Human Behavior, 44,* 81–95. https://doi.org/10.1016/j.chb.2014.11.009

Hendriks, F., Kienhues, D., & Bromme, R. (2016). Trust in science and the science of trust. In B. Blöbaum (Ed.), *Trust and communication in a digitized world* (pp. 143–159). Springer.

Hernán, M.A., Clayton, D., & Keiding, N. (2011). The Simpson's paradox unraveled. *International Journal of Epidemiology, 40*(3), 780–785. https://doi.org/10.1093/ije/dyr041. Medline:21454324

Hershey, D. (2003). Misconceptions about Helmont's willow experiment. *Plant Science Bulletin, 49*(3), 78–84.

Hoffrage, U., & Gigerenzer, G. (1998). Using natural frequencies to improve diagnostic inferences. *Academic Medicine, 73*(5), 538–540. https://doi.org/10.1097/00001888-199805000-00024. Medline:9609869

Hoffrage, U., Lindsey, S., Hertwig, R., & Gigerenzer, G. (2000). Communicating statistical information. *Science, 290*(5500), 2261–2262. https://doi.org/10.1126/science.290.5500.2261. Medline:11188724

Hofstede, G. (2011). Dimensionalizing cultures: The Hofstede model in context. *Online Readings in Psychology and Culture, 2*(1), 2307–0919. https://doi.org/10.9707/2307-0919.1014

Hoge, E.A., Bui, E., Palitz, S.A., Schwarz, N.R., Owens, M.E., Johnston, J.M., … & Simon, N.M. (2018). The effect of mindfulness meditation training on biological acute stress responses in generalized anxiety disorder. *Psychiatry Research, 262,* 328–332. https://doi.org/10.1016/j.psychres.2017.01.006. Medline:28131433

Hoh, Y.K. (2017). An instant update on telomeres and telomerase. *American Biology Teacher, 79*(8), 615–620. https://doi.org/10.1525/abt.2017.79.8.615

Hutchings, J.A., & Stenseth, N.C. (2016). Communication of science advice to government. *Trends in Ecology & Evolution, 31*(1), 7–11. https://doi.org/10.1016/j.tree.2015.10.008. Medline:26724100

Inzunza, E.R. (2020). Reconsidering the use of the passive voice in scientific writing. *American Biology Teacher, 82*(8), 563–565.

Ioannidis, J.P. (2005). Why most published research findings are false. *PLOS Medicine, 2*(8), e124. https://doi.org/10.1371/journal.pmed.0020124

Ivlev, I., Hickman, E.N., McDonagh, M.S., & Eden, K.B. (2017). Use of patient decision aids increased younger women's reluctance to begin screening mammography: A systematic review and meta-analysis. *Journal of General Internal Medicine, 32*(7), 803–812.

Jarvis, L. (2017, October 9). Driving cancer beyond the brink. *Chemical and Engineering News, 95*(40). Retrieved from https://cen.acs.org/articles/95/i40/Driving-cancer-beyond-brink.html

Jasanoff, S. (2005). *Designs on nature: Science and democracy in Europe and the United States.* Princeton University Press.

Jasanoff, S. (2009). Technologies of humility: Citizen participation in governing science. In B. Nerlich, R. Elliott, & B. Larson (Eds.), *Communicating biological sciences: Ethical and metaphorical dimensions* (pp. 29–48). Ashgate Publishing.

Jensen, J.D., & Hurley, R.J. (2010). Conflicting stories about public scientific controversies: Effects of news convergence and divergence on scientists' credibility. *Public Understanding of Science, 21*(6), 689–704. https://doi.org/10.1177/0963662510387759. Medline:23832155

Jensen, J.D., Pokharel, M., Scherr, C.L., King, A.J., Brown, N., & Jones, C. (2017). Communicating uncertain science to the public: How amount and source of uncertainty impact fatalism, backlash, and overload. *Risk Analysis, 37*(1), 40–51. https://doi.org/10.1111/risa.12600. Medline:26973157

Jensen, K.K. (2004). BSE in the UK: Why the risk communication strategy failed. *Journal of Agricultural and Environmental Ethics, 17*(4), 405–423. https://doi.org/10.1007/s10806-004-5186-3

Johnson, A.N., Sievert, R., Durglo Sr, M., Finley, V., Adams, L., & Hofmann, M.H. (2014). Indigenous knowledge and geoscience on the Flathead Indian Reservation, northwest Montana: Implications for place-based and culturally congruent education. *Journal of Geoscience Education, 62*(2), 187–202. https://doi.org/10.5408/12-393.1

Johnson, E.J., & Goldstein, D. (2003). Do defaults save lives? *Science, 302*(5649), 1338–1339. https://doi.org/10.1126/science.1091721. Medline:14631022

Johnson, E.J., & Tversky, A. (1983). Affect, generalization, and the perception of risk. *Journal of Personality and Social Psychology, 45*(1), 20. https://doi.org/10.1037/0022-3514.45.1.20

Johnstone, A.H. (1991). Why is science difficult to learn? Things are seldom what they seem. *Journal of Computer Assisted Learning, 7*(2), 75–83. https://doi.org/10.1111/j.1365-2729.1991.tb00230.x

Johnstone, A.H. (1993). The development of chemistry teaching: A changing response to changing demand. *Journal of Chemical Education, 70*(9), 701–705. https://doi.org/10.1021/ed070p701

Jones, J.M. (2019, January). Americans continue to embrace political independence. Gallup. Retrieved from https://news.gallup.com/poll /245801/americans-continue-to-embrace-political-independence.aspx

Jones, M.D. (2014). Cultural characters and climate change: How heroes shape our perception of climate science. *Social Science Quarterly, 95*(1), 1–39. https://doi.org/10.1111/ssqu.12043

Jones, M.D., & Radaelli, C.M. (2015). The narrative policy framework: Child or monster? *Critical Policy Studies, 9*(3), 339–355. https://doi.org/10.1080 /19460171.2015.1053959

Jost, J.T., & Amodio, D.M. (2012). Political ideology as motivated social cognition: Behavioral and neuroscientific evidence. *Motivation and Emotion, 36*(1), 55–64. https://doi.org/10.1007/s11031-011-9260-7

Juanchich, M., & Sirota, M. (2019). Not as gloomy as we thought: Reassessing how the public understands probability of precipitation forecasts. *Journal of Cognitive Psychology, 31*(1), 116–129. https://doi.org/10.1080/20445911 .2018.1553884

Juslin, P.N., & Laukka, P. (2003). Communication of emotions in vocal expression and music performance: Different channels, same code? *Psychological Bulletin, 129*(5), 770. https://doi.org/10.1037/0033-2909 .129.5.770. Medline:12956543

Kabat-Zinn, J. (2003). Mindfulness-based interventions in context: Past, present, and future. *Clinical Psychology: Science and Practice, 10*, 144–156. https://doi.org/10.1093/clipsy.bpg016

Kahan, D. (2010). Fixing the communications failure. *Nature, 463*(7279), 296–297. https://doi.org/10.1038/463296a. Medline:20090734

Kahan, D.M. (2013). Ideology, motivated reasoning, and cognitive reflection. *Judgment and Decision Making, 8*(4), 407–424. https://doi.org/10.1017 /s1930297500005271

Kahan, D.M., Jenkins-Smith, H., Tarantola, T., Silva, C.L., & Braman, D. (2015). Geoengineering and climate change polarization: Testing a two-channel model of science communication. *Annals of the American Academy of Political and Social Science, 658*(1), 192–222. https://doi.org/10.1177 /0002716214559002

Kahan, D.M., Peters, E., Wittlin, M., Slovic, P., Ouellette, L.L., Braman, D., & Mandel, G. (2012). The polarizing impact of science literacy and numeracy on perceived climate change risks. *Nature Climate Change, 2*(10), 732–735. https://doi.org/10.1038/nclimate1547

Kahlor, L.A., Dudo, A., Liang, M.C., Lazard, A.J., & AbiGhannam, N. (2016). Ethics information seeking and sharing among scientists: The case of nanotechnology. Science Communication, *38*(1), 74–98. https://doi.org /10.1177/1075547015617942

Kahneman, D. (2011). *Thinking, fast and slow*. Macmillan.

Kalma, A. (1992). Gazing in triads: A powerful signal in floor apportionment. *British Journal of Social Psychology, 31*(1), 21–39. https://doi.org/10.1111/j.2044-8309.1992.tb00953.x

Kamizasa, N., Terashima, Y., & Awaki, H. (2012). A new sample of candidate intermediate-mass black holes selected by X-ray variability. *Astrophysical Journal, 751*(1), 39. https://doi.org/10.1088/0004-637x/751/1/39

Kandel, E.R., Schwartz, J.H., & Jessell, T.M. (1991). *Principles of neural science*. Appleton & Lange.

Karlsson, N., Loewenstein, G., & Seppi, D. (2009). The ostrich effect: Selective attention to information. *Journal of Risk and Uncertainty, 38*(2), 95–115. https://doi.org/10.1007/s11166-009-9060-6

Kasperson, R.E., Slovic, P., Pidgeon, N., & Renn, O. (2017). Whose views really matter in the end? In R.E. Kasperson (Ed.), *Risk conundrums* (pp. 24–32). Routledge.

Kata, A. (2012). Anti-vaccine activists, Web 2.0, and the postmodern paradigm – An overview of tactics and tropes used online by the anti-vaccination movement. *Vaccine, 30*(25), 3778–3789. https://doi.org/10.1016/j.vaccine.2011.11.112. Medline:22172504

Katsumoto, Y., Fukuchi-Mizutani, M., Fukui, Y., Brugliera, F., Holton, T.A., Karan, M., ... & Tanaka, Y. (2007). Engineering of the rose flavonoid biosynthetic pathway successfully generated blue-hued flowers accumulating delphinidin. *Plant and Cell Physiology, 48*(11), 1589–1600. https://doi.org/10.1093/pcp/pcm131. Medline:17925311

Kearns, F. (2021). *Getting to the heart of science communication*. Island Press.

Keefer, L.A., Landau, M.J., Sullivan, D., & Rothschild, Z.K. (2014). Embodied metaphor and abstract problem solving: Testing a metaphoric fit hypothesis in the health domain. *Journal of Experimental Social Psychology, 55*, 12–20. https://doi.org/10.1016/j.jesp.2014.05.012

Keller, E.F. (2000). *The century of the gene*. Harvard University Press.

Kelly, R.P., Cooley, S.R., & Klinger, T. (2013). Narratives can motivate environmental action: The Whiskey Creek ocean acidification story. *Ambio, 43*(5), 592–599. https://doi.org/10.1007/s13280-013-0442-2. Medline:24081705

Kemper, S. (1984). The development of narrative skills: Explanations and entertainments. In S.A. Kuczaj (Ed.), *Discourse development* (pp. 99–124). Springer.

Kendon, A. (1967). Some functions of gaze-direction in social interaction. *Acta Psychologica, 26*, 22–63. https://doi.org/10.1016/0001-6918(67)90005-4. Medline:6043092

Keohane, R.O., Lane, M., & Oppenheimer, M. (2014). The ethics of scientific communication under uncertainty. *Politics, Philosophy & Economics, 13*(4), 343–368. https://doi.org/10.1177/1470594x14538570

Key, J.S., & Hendry, M. (2016). Defining gravity. *Nature Physics, 12*(6), 524–525. https://doi.org/10.1038/nphys3786

Kimmerle, J., Flemming, D., Feinkohl, I., & Cress, U. (2015). How laypeople understand the tentativeness of medical research news in the media: An experimental study on the perception of information about deep brain stimulation. *Science Communication, 37*(2), 173–189. https://doi.org/10.1177/1075547014556541

Kirby, D.A. (2017). The changing popular images of science. In K.H. Jamieson, D. Kahan, & D.A. Scheufele (Eds.), *The Oxford handbook of the science of science communication* (pp. 291–300). Oxford University Press.

Klar, S. (2013). The influence of competing identity primes on political preferences. *Journal of Politics, 75*(4), 1108–1124. https://doi.org/10.1017/s0022381613000698

Klar, S. (2014). Identity and engagement among political independents in America. *Political Psychology, 35*(4), 577–591. https://doi.org/10.1111/pops.12036

Knobloch-Westerwick, S., Johnson, B.K., Silver, N.A., & Westerwick, A. (2015). Science exemplars in the eye of the beholder: How exposure to online science information affects attitudes. *Science Communication, 37*(5), 575–601. https://doi.org/10.1177/1075547015596367

Knorr-Cetina, K. (1981). *The manufacture of knowledge: An essay on the constructivist and contextual nature of science.* Pergamon Press.

Koenigsberger, L. (1906). *Hermann von Helmholtz.* F.A. Welby (Trans.). Clarendon Press.

Kogut, T., & Beyth-Marom, R. (2008). Who helps more? How self-other discrepancies influence decisions in helping situations. *Judgment and Decision Making, 3*(8), 595. https://doi.org/10.1017/s1930297500001558

Kohl, P.A., Kim, S.Y., Peng, Y., Akin, H., Koh, E.J., Howell, A., & Dunwoody, S. (2016). The influence of weight-of-evidence strategies on audience perceptions of (un)certainty when media cover contested science. *Public Understanding of Science, 25*(8), 976–991. https://doi.org/10.1177/0963662515615087. Medline:26657318

Kotcher, J.E., Myers, T.A., Vraga, E.K., Stenhouse, N., & Maibach, E.W. (2017). Does engagement in advocacy hurt the credibility of scientists? Results from a randomized national survey experiment. *Environmental Communication, 11*(3), 415–429. https://doi.org/10.1080/17524032.2016.1275736

Krathwohl, D.R. (2002). A revision of Bloom's Taxonomy: An overview. *Theory into Practice, 41*(4), 212–218. https://doi.org/10.1207/s15430421tip4104_2

Krawczyk, A., Knäuper, B., Gilca, V., Dubé, E., Perez, S., Joyal-Desmarais, K., & Rosberger, Z. (2015). Parents' decision-making about the human papillomavirus vaccine for their daughters: I. Quantitative results. *Human Vaccines & Immunotherapeutics, 11*(2), 322–329. https://doi.org/10.1080/21645515.2014.1004030. Medline:25692455

Krawczyk, A., Perez, S., King, L., Vivion, M., Dubé, E., & Rosberger, Z. (2015). Parents' decision-making about the human papillomavirus

vaccine for their daughters: II. Qualitative results. *Human Vaccines &*
Immunotherapeutics, 11(2), 330–336. https://doi.org/10.4161/21645515
.2014.980708. Medline:25692507

Kuhn, T.S. (1993). Metaphor in science. In A. Ortony (Ed.), *Metaphor and*
thought (pp. 533–542). Cambridge University Press.

Kuhn, T.S. (1996). *The structure of scientific revolutions.* University of Chicago Press.

Kunda, Z. (1990). The case for motivated reasoning. *Psychological Bulletin,*
108(3), 480–498. https://doi.org/10.1037/0033-2909.108.3.480.
Medline:2270237

Laird, J.D. (1974). Self-attribution of emotion: The effects of expressive
behavior on the quality of emotional experience. *Journal of Personality*
and Social Psychology, 29(4), 475 https://doi.org/10.1037/h0036125.
Medline:4818323

Lakoff, G., & Johnson, M. (1980). *Metaphors we live by.* University of Chicago
Press.

Landau, M., Arndt, J., & Cameron, L. (2017). Do metaphors in health
messages work? Exploring emotional and cognitive factors. *Journal of*
Experimental Social Psychology, 74, 135–149. https://doi.org/10.1016/j
.jesp.2017.09.006. Medline:33833472

Larson, B. (2005). The war of the roses: Demilitarizing invasion biology.
Frontiers in Ecology and the Environment, 3(9), 495–500. https://doi.org/10
.1890/1540-9295(2005)003[0495:twotrd]2.0.co;2

Larson, B. (2009). Should scientists advocate? The case of promotional
metaphors in environmental science. In B. Nerlich, R. Elliott, & B. Larson
(Eds.), *Communicating biological sciences: Ethical and metaphorical dimensions*
(pp. 145–152). Ashgate Publishing.

Latour, B. (1987). *Science in action.* Harvard University Press.

Latour, B., & Woolgar, S. (1979). *Laboratory life: The social construction of*
scientific facts. Sage.

Laudan, L. (1983). The demise of the demarcation problem. In R.S. Cohen
(Ed.), *Physics, philosophy and psychoanalysis* (pp. 111–127). Springer.

Laukka, P., Linnman, C., Åhs, F., Pissiota, A., Frans, Ö., Faria, V., ... &
Furmark, T. (2008). In a nervous voice: Acoustic analysis and perception
of anxiety in social phobics' speech. *Journal of Nonverbal Behavior, 32*(4),
195–214. https://doi.org/10.1007/s10919-008-0055-9

Lave, J., & Wenger, E. (1991). *Situated learning: Legitimate peripheral*
participation. Cambridge University Press.

Leach, J., Driver, R., Scott, P., & Wood-Robinson, C. (1996). Children's ideas
about ecology 2: Ideas found in children aged 5-16 about the cycling of
matter. *International Journal of Science Education, 18*(1), 19–34. https://doi
.org/10.1080/0950069960180102

Leask, J., Chapman, S., & Robbins, S.C.C. (2010). "All manner of ills": The
features of serious diseases attributed to vaccination. *Vaccine, 28*(17), 3066–
3070. https://doi.org/10.1016/j.vaccine.2009.10.042. Medline:19879997

Lederman, N.G. (1992). Students' and teachers' conceptions of the nature of science: A review of the research. *Journal of Research in Science Teaching, 29,* 331–359. https://doi.org/10.1002/tea.3660290404

Lee, B.Y. (2021, August). Some may be getting COVID-19 vaccines in disguise to hide vaccination status. *Forbes.* Retrieved from www.forbes.com/sites /brucelee/2021/08/09/some-may-be-getting-covid-19-vaccines-in-disguise -to-hide-vaccination-status/?sh=3a22ce3c2ff3

Leeper, T.J., & Slothuus, R. (2014). Political parties, motivated reasoning, and public opinion formation. *Political Psychology, 35,* 129–156. https://doi.org /10.1111/pops.12164

Levenson, R.W., Ekman, P., & Friesen, W.V. (1990). Voluntary facial action generates emotion-specific autonomic nervous system activity. *Psychophysiology, 27*(4), 363–384. https://doi.org/10.1111/j.1469-8986.1990.tb02330.x . Medline:2236440

Levenson, R.W., & Ruef, A.M. (1992). Empathy: A physiological substrate. *Journal of Personality and Social Psychology, 63*(2), 234. https://doi.org /10.1037/0022-3514.63.2.234

Lewandowsky, S., Ecker, U.K., Seifert, C.M., Schwarz, N., & Cook, J. (2012). Misinformation and its correction: Continued influence and successful debiasing. *Psychological Science in the Public Interest, 13*(3), 106–131. https://doi.org/10.1177/1529100612451018. Medline:26173286

Lewandowsky, S., & Van Der Linden, S. (2021). Countering misinformation and fake news through inoculation and prebunking. *European Review of Social Psychology, 32*(2), 348–384. https://doi.org/10.1080/10463283.2021 .1876983

Lieberman, A., Schroeder, J., & Amir, O. (2022). A voice inside my head: The psychological and behavioral consequences of auditory technologies. Organizational Behavior and Human Decision Processes, *170,* 104133. https://static1.squarespace.com/static/5c171ac1710699e060ed3d94/t /61f9fdfb778cfe78c0480075/1643773435507/VoiceInsideMyHead.pdf

Lightman, A.P. (1989). Science: Magic on the mind physicists' use of metaphor. *American Scholar, 58*(1), 97–101.

Linklater, K. (2006). *Freeing the natural voice: Imagery and art in the practice of voice and language.* Nick Hern Books.

Linn, M.C., Eylon, B.S., & Davis, E.A. (2013). The knowledge integration perspective on learning. In M.C. Linn, E.A. Davis, & P. Bell (Eds.), *Internet environments for science education* (pp. 57–74). Routledge.

Linquist, S., & Bartol, J. (2013). Two myths about somatic markers. *British Journal for the Philosophy of Science, 64*(3), 455–484. https://doi.org/10 .1093/bjps/axs020

Lin-Siegler, X., Ahn, J.N., Chen, J., Fang, F.F.A., & Luna-Lucero, M. (2016). Even Einstein struggled: Effects of learning about great scientists' struggles on high school students' motivation to learn science. *Journal of Educational Psychology, 108*(3), 314–328.

Lipkus, I.M. (2007). Numeric, verbal, and visual formats of conveying health risks: Suggested best practices and future recommendations. *Medical Decision Making, 27*(5), 696–713. https://doi.org/10.1177/0272989x07307271. Medline:17873259

Lippman, W. (1922). *Public opinion.* Retrieved from https://hdl.handle.net /2027/uc1.b5232744

Litalien, D., & Guay, F. (2015). Dropout intentions in PhD studies: A comprehensive model based on interpersonal relationships and motivational resources. *Contemporary Educational Psychology, 41,* 218–231.

Llopart, M., & Esteban-Guitart, M. (2018). Funds of knowledge in 21st century societies: Inclusive educational practices for under-represented students. A literature review. *Journal of Curriculum Studies, 50*(2), 145–161. https://doi.org/10.1080/00220272.2016.1247913

Lockard, J.S., Allen, D.J., Schiele, B.J., & Wiemer, M.J. (1978). Human postural signals: Stance, weight-shifts and social distance as intention movements to depart. *Animal Behaviour, 26,* 219–224. https://doi.org/10 .1016/0003-3472(78)90021-0

Longino, H.E. (1990). *Science as social knowledge: Values and objectivity in scientific inquiry.* Princeton University Press.

Longino, H.E. (2013). *Studying human behavior.* University of Chicago Press.

Lönngren, J., & Van Poeck, K. (2021). Wicked problems: A mapping review of the literature. *International Journal of Sustainable Development & World Ecology, 28*(6), 481–502. https://doi.org/10.1080/13504509.2020 .1859415

Lord, C.G., Ross, L., & Lepper, M.R. (1979). Biased assimilation and attitude polarization: The effects of prior theories on subsequently considered evidence. *Journal of Personality and Social Psychology, 37*(11), 2098–2109. https://doi.org/10.1037/0022-3514.37.11.2098

Luokkanen, M., Huttunen, S., & Hildén, M. (2014). Geoengineering, news media and metaphors: Framing the controversial. *Public Understanding of Science, 23*(8), 966–981. https://doi.org/10.1177/0963662513475966. Medline:23825283

Mandelbrot, B. (1983). *The fractal geometry of nature.* W.H. Freeman and Company.

Manning, P. (2013). "No reefer madness please – we're British": Accounting for the remarkable absence of mediated drugs education in post-war Britain 1945–1985. *Media History, 19*(4), 479–495. https://doi.org/10.1080 /13688804.2013.844893

Manski, C.F. (2020). The lure of incredible certitude. *Economics & Philosophy, 36*(2), 216–245. https://doi.org/10.1017/ s0266267119000105

Martínez, A., & Mammola, S. (2021). Specialized terminology reduces the number of citations of scientific papers. *Proceedings of the Royal Society B, 288*(1948), 20202581. https://doi.org/10.1098/rspb.2020.2581. Medline: 33823673

Masaoka, Y., Izumizaki, M., & Homma, I. (2014). Where is the rhythm generator for emotional breathing? *Progress in Brain Research, 209*, 367–377. https://doi.org/10.1016/b978-0-444-63274-6.00019-9. Medline:24746058

Matlock, T., Coe, C., & Westerling, A.L. (2017). Monster wildfires and metaphor in risk communication. *Metaphor and Symbol, 32*(4), 250–261. https://doi.org/10.1080/10926488.2017.1384273

Mattys, S.L., & Melhorn, J.F. (2007). Sentential, lexical, and acoustic effects on the perception of word boundaries. *Journal of the Acoustical Society of America, 122*(1), 554–567. https://doi.org/10.1121/1.2735105. Medline: 17614511

Mayer, R.E. (2014). Incorporating motivation into multimedia learning. *Learning and Instruction, 29*, 171–173. https://doi.org/10.1016/j.learninstruc.2013.04.003

Mayer, R.E., Bove, W., Bryman, A., Mars, R., & Tapangco, L. (1996). When less is more: Meaningful learning from visual and verbal summaries of science textbook lessons. *Journal of Educational Psychology, 88*(1), 64–73. https://doi.org/10.1037/0022-0663.88.1.64

Mayer, R.E., & Estrella, G. (2014). Benefits of emotional design in multimedia instruction. *Learning and Instruction, 33*, 12–18. https://doi.org/10.1016/j.learninstruc.2014.02.004

Mayer, R.E., & Moreno, R. (2003). Nine ways to reduce cognitive load in multimedia learning. *Educational Psychologist, 38*(1), 43–52. https://doi.org/10.1207/s15326985ep3801_6

McDonnell, L., Barker, M.K., & Wieman, C. (2016). Concepts first, jargon second improves student articulation of understanding. *Biochemistry and Molecular Biology Education, 44*(1), 12–19. https://doi.org/10.1002/bmb.20922. Medline:26537537

McGuire, W.J., & Papageorgis, D. (1961). The relative efficacy of various types of prior belief-defense in producing immunity against persuasion. *Journal of Abnormal and Social Psychology, 62*(2), 327. https://doi.org/10.1037/h0042026. Medline:13773992

McKenzie, C.R., & Nelson, J.D. (2003). What a speaker's choice of frame reveals: Reference points, frame selection, and framing effects. *Psychonomic Bulletin & Review, 10*(3), 596–602. https://doi.org/10.3758/bf03196520. Medline:14620352

Mead, M. and Métraux, R. (1957). Image of the scientist among high-school students. *Science, 126*, 384–390. https://doi.org/10.1126/science.126.3270.384. Medline:17774477

Meadows, D., Sweeney, L.B., & Mehers, G.M. (2016). *The climate change playbook: 22 systems thinking games for more effective communication about climate change.* Chelsea Green Publishing.

Meadows, G., & Wiesenmayer, R.L. (1999). Identifying and addressing students' alternative conceptions of the causes of global warming: The need for cognitive conflict. *Journal of Science Education and Technology, 8*(3), 235–239.

Medawar, P. (1999). Is the scientific paper a fraud? In E. Scanlon, R. Hill, & K. Junker (Eds.), *Communicating science: Professional contexts* (pp. 27–31). Routledge. (Original work published in 1963.)

Mehrabian, A. (1972). *Nonverbal communication*. Aldine Atherton.

Méndez, D.I., & Alcaraz, M.Á. (2015). Astrophysics titles in *Scientific American* magazine (1990–2014): Linguistic and discourse practices. *International Journal of Applied Linguistics and English Literature, 4*(6), 39–51. https://doi .org/10.7575/aiac.ijalel.v.4n.6p.39

Menon, A. (2019). Brexit and public opinion 2019. Retrieved from https:// ukandeu.ac.uk/new-report-reveals-brexit-identities-stronger-than-party -identities/

Mercer, S.W., Higgins, M., Bikker, A.M., Fitzpatrick, B., McConnachie, A., Lloyd, S.M., … & Watt, G.C. (2016). General practitioners' empathy and health outcomes: A prospective observational study of consultations in areas of high and low deprivation. *Annals of Family Medicine, 14*(2), 117–124. https://doi.org/10.1370/afm.1910. Medline:26951586

Merton, R.K. (1973). *The sociology of science: Theoretical and empirical investigations*. University of Chicago Press.

Miles, S., & Frewer, L.J. (2003). Public perception of scientific uncertainty in relation to food hazards. *Journal of Risk Research, 6*(3), 267–283. https:// doi.org/10.1080/1366987032000088883

Miller, C.H., Lane, L.T., Deatrick, L.M., Young, A.M., & Potts, K.A. (2007). Psychological reactance and promotional health messages: The effects of controlling language, lexical concreteness, and the restoration of freedom. *Human Communication research, 33*(2), 219–240. https://doi.org/10.1111 /j.1468-2958.2007.00297.x

Miller, G.A. (1956). The magical number seven, plus or minus two: Some limits on our capacity for processing information. *Psychological Review, 63*(2), 81. https://doi.org/10.1037/h0043158

Minstrell, J. (1982). Explaining the "at rest" condition of an object. *The Physics Teacher, 20*(1), 10–14. https://doi.org/10.1119/1.2340924

Minstrell, J. (1992). Facets of students' knowledge and relevant instruction. In R. Duit, F. Goldberg, & H. Niedderer (Eds.), *Research in Physics Learning: Theoretical Issues and Empirical Studies* (pp. 110–128). IPN.

Molek-Kozakowska, K. (2017). Communicating environmental science beyond academia: Stylistic patterns of newsworthiness in popular science journalism. *Discourse & Communication, 11*(1), 69–88. https://doi.org/10 .1177/1750481316683294

Montero-Marin, J., Garcia-Campayo, J., Pérez-Yus, M.C., Zabaleta-del-Olmo, E., & Cuijpers, P. (2019). Meditation techniques v. relaxation therapies when treating anxiety: A meta-analytic review. *Psychological Medicine, 49*(13), 2118–2133. https://doi.org/10.1017/s0033291719001600. Medline:31322102

Montibeller, G., & Von Winterfeldt, D. (2015). Cognitive and motivational biases in decision and risk analysis. *Risk Analysis, 35*(7), 1230–1251. https://doi.org/10.1111/risa.12360. Medline:25873355

Moreno, R. (2006). Learning in high-tech and multimedia environments. *Current Directions in Psychological Science, 15*(2), 63–67. https://doi.org/10 .1111/j.0963-7214.2006.00408.x

Moreno, R., & Mayer, R.E. (1999). Cognitive principles of multimedia learning: The role of modality and contiguity. *Journal of Educational Psychology, 91*(2), 358–368. https://doi.org/10.1037/0022-0663.91.2.358

Moreno, R., & Mayer, R.E. (2000). A coherence effect in multimedia learning: The case for minimizing irrelevant sounds in the design of multimedia instructional messages. *Journal of Educational Psychology, 92*(1), 117–125. https://doi.org/10.1037/0022-0663.92.1.117

Mossler, M.V., Bostrom, A., Kelly, R.P., Crosman, K.M., & Moy, P. (2017). How does framing affect policy support for emissions mitigation? Testing the effects of ocean acidification and other carbon emissions frames. *Global Environmental Change, 45*, 63–78. https://doi.org/10.1016/j.gloenvcha.2017.04.002

Moyer-Gusé, E., & Nabi, R.L. (2010). Explaining the effects of narrative in an entertainment television program: Overcoming resistance to persuasion. *Human Communication Research, 36*(1), 26–52. https://doi.org/10.1111/j .1468-2958.2009.01367.x

Moynihan, R., Bero, L., Ross-Degnan, D., Henry, D., Lee, K., Watkins, J., ... & Soumerai, S.B. (2000). Coverage by the news media of the benefits and risks of medications. *New England Journal of Medicine, 342*(22), 1645–1650. https://doi.org/10.1056/nejm200006013422206. Medline:10833211

Murphy, A.H., Lichtenstein, S., Fischhoff, B., & Winkler, R.L. (1980). Misinterpretations of precipitation probability forecasts. *Bulletin of the American Meteorological Society, 61*(7), 695–701. https://doi.org/10.1175 /1520-0477(1980)061%3C0695:moppf%3E2.0.co;2

Myers, T.A., Nisbet, M.C., Maibach, E.W., & Leiserowitz, A.A. (2012). A public health frame arouses hopeful emotions about climate change. *Climatic Change, 113*(3), 1105–1112. https://doi.org/10.1007/s10584-012-0513-6

Nakhleh, M.B. (1992). Why some students don't learn chemistry: Chemical misconceptions. *Journal of Chemical Education, 69*(3), 191. https://doi.org /10.1021/ed069p191

National Academies of Sciences, Engineering, and Medicine. (2017). *Communicating science effectively: A research agenda.* National Academies Press.

National Academy of Sciences and Institute of Medicine. (2008). *Science, evolution and creationism.* National Academies' Press. https://doi.org /10.17226/11876

National Commission for the Protection of Human Subjects of Biomedical and Behavioral Research. (1979, April 18). The Belmont report: Ethical principles and guidelines for the protection of human subjects research. Department of Health Education, and Welfare. Retrieved from

www.hhs.gov/ohrp/regulations-and-policy/belmont-report/read-the
-belmont-report/index.html

National Research Council. (1996). *Understanding risk: Informing decisions in a democratic society*. National Academies Press.

National Research Council. (2012). *A framework for K-12 science education: Practices, crosscutting concepts, and core ideas*. The National Academies Press.

National Science Board. (2016). Science and engineering indicators. Retrieved from www.nsf.gov/statistics/2016/nsb20161/#/

Nazish, N. (2019, May). How to de-stress in 5 minutes or less, according to a Navy SEAL. *Forbes*. Retrieved from www.forbes.com/sites/nomanazish /2019/05/30/how-to-de-stress-in-5-minutes-or-less-according-to-a-navy -seal/?sh=4e3484f53046

Nelkin, D. (1995). *Selling science: How the press covers science and technology*. Freeman.

Nelkin, D. (2001). Molecular metaphors: the gene in popular discourse. *Nature Reviews Genetics, 2*(7), 555–559. https://doi.org/10.1038/35080583. Medline:11433362

Nerlich, B., & James, R. (2009). "The post-antibiotic apocalypse" and the "war on superbugs": Catastrophe discourse in microbiology, its rhetorical form and political function. *Public Understanding of Science, 18*(5), 574–590. https://doi.org/10.1177/0963662507087974. Medline:20027773

Nersessian, N.J. (2008). Model-based reasoning in scientific practice. In R.A. Duschl & R.E. Grandy (Eds.), *Teaching scientific inquiry: Recommendations for research and implementation* (pp. 57–79). Sense Publishers.

Newman, E.J., & Schwarz, N. (2018). Good sound, good research: How audio quality influences perceptions of the research and researcher. *Science Communication, 40*(2), 246–257. https://doi.org/10.1177 /1075547018759345

Nickerson, R.S. (1998). Confirmation bias: A ubiquitous phenomenon in many guises. *Review of General Psychology, 2*(2), 175–220. https://doi .org/10.1037/1089-2680.2.2.175

Niebert, K., & Gropengießer, H. (2015). Understanding starts in the mesocosm: Conceptual metaphor as a framework for external representations in science teaching. *International Journal of Science Education, 37*(5–6), 903–933. https://doi.org/10.1080/09500693.2015.1025310

Nisbet, E.C., Cooper, K.E., & Garrett, R.K. (2015). The partisan brain: How dissonant science messages lead conservatives and liberals to (dis)trust science. *Annals of the American Academy of Political and Social Science, 658*(1), 36–66. https://doi.org/10.1177/0002716214555474

Nisbet, M. (2009). Communicating climate change: Why frames matter for public engagement. *Environment: Science and Policy for Sustainable Development, 51*(2), 12–23. https://doi.org/10.3200/envt.51.2.12-23

Nisbet, M. (2018). *Scientists in civic life: Facilitating dialogue-based communication*. American Association for the Advancement of Science. Retrieved from www.aaas.org/programs/dialogue-science-ethics-and-religion/resources -engaging-scientists-project

Nisbet, M., & Markowitz, E.M. (2014). Understanding public opinion in debates over biomedical research: Looking beyond political partisanship to focus on beliefs about science and society. *PLOS One, 9*(2), e88473. https://doi.org/10.1371/journal.pone.0088473. Medline:24558393

Núñez, R. (2008). A fresh look at the foundations of mathematics: Gesture and the psychological reality of conceptual metaphor. In A.J. Cienki & Cornelia Mülller (Eds.), *Metaphor and gesture* (pp. 93–114). John Benjamins.

Nyhan, B., & Reifler, J. (2010). When corrections fail: The persistence of political misperceptions. *Political Behavior, 32*(2), 303–330. https://doi.org/10.1007/s11109-010-9112-2

Ojalehto, B.L., Medin, D.L., & García, S.G. (2017). Grounding principles for inferring agency: Two cultural perspectives. *Cognitive Psychology, 95*, 50–78. https://doi.org/10.1016/j.cogpsych.2017.04.001. Medline:28441519

Olson, R. (2015). *Houston, we have a narrative: Why science needs story.* Chicago: University of Chicago Press.

Ong, M., Wright, C., Espinosa, L., & Orfield, G. (2011). Inside the double bind: A synthesis of empirical research on undergraduate and graduate women of color in science, technology, engineering, and mathematics. *Harvard Educational Review, 81*(2), 172–209. https://doi.org/10.17763/haer.81.2.t022245n7x4752v2

Oreskes, N. (2003). The role of quantitative models in science. In C.D. Canham, J.J. Cole & W.K. Lauenroth (Eds.), *Models in ecosystem science* (pp. 13–31). Princeton University Press.

Oreskes, N. (2004). Science and public policy: What's proof got to do with it? *Environmental Science & Policy, 7*(5), 369–383. https://doi.org/10.1016/j.envsci.2004.06.002

Oreskes, N., & Conway, E.M. (2010). Defeating the merchants of doubt. *Nature, 465*(7299), 686–687. https://doi.org/10.1038/465686a. Medline:20535183

Osborne, J. (2014). Teaching scientific practices: Meeting the challenge of change. *Journal of Science Teacher Education, 25*(2), 177–196. https://doi.org/10.1007/s10972-014-9384-1

Osborne, J., Collins, S., Ratcliffe, M., Millar, R., & Duschl, R. (2003). What "ideas-about-science" should be taught in school science? A Delphi study of the expert community. *Journal of Research in Science Teaching, 40*(7), 692–720. https://doi.org/10.1002/tea.10105

Osborne, J., Simon, S., & Collins, S. (2003). Attitudes towards science: A review of the literature and its implications. *International Journal of Science Education, 25*(9), 1049–1079. https://doi.org/10.1080/0950069032000032199

Patterson, K., Grenny, J., McMillan, R., & Switzler, A. (2002). *Crucial conversations: Tools for talking when stakes are high.* McGraw-Hill.

Pearce, R.M. (1912). Chance and the prepared mind. *Science, 35*(912), 941–956. https://doi.org/10.1126/science.35.912.941. Medline:17792643

Pearce, W., Brown, B., Nerlich, B., & Koteyko, N. (2015). Communicating climate change: Conduits, content, and consensus. *Wiley Interdisciplinary Reviews: Climate Change, 6*(6), 613–626. https://doi.org/10.1002/wcc.366

Peter, C., & Koch, T. (2015). When debunking scientific myths fails (and when it does not): The backfire effect in the context of journalistic coverage and immediate judgments as prevention strategy. *Science Communication, 38*(1), 1–23. https://doi.org/10.1177/1075547015613523

Peterson, E.B., Chou, W.Y.S., Kelley, D.E., & Hesse, B. (2020). Trust in national health information sources in the United States: Comparing predictors and levels of trust across three health domains. *Translational Behavioral Medicine, 10*(4), 978–988. https://doi.org/10.1093/tbm/ibz066. Medline:31116400

Pew Research Center. (2014). The Pew religious landscape study. Retrieved from www.pewforum.org/about-the-religious-landscape-study/

Pew Research Center. (2015). Americans, politics and science issues. Retrieved from www.pewresearch.org/science/2015/07/01/americans -politics-and-science-issues/

Pew Research Center. (2017). The partisan divide on political values grows even wider. Retrieved from www.pewresearch.org/politics/2017/10/05 /the-partisan-divide-on-political-values-grows-even-wider/

Pew Research Center. (2018). The age gap in religion around the world. Retrieved from www.pewforum.org/2018/06/13/the-age-gap-in-religion -around-the-world/

Phillips, D.P., Kanter, E.J., Bednarczyk, B., & Tastad, P.L. (1991). Importance of the lay press in the transmission of medical knowledge to the scientific community. *New England Journal of Medicine, 325*(16), 1180–1183. https:// doi.org/10.1056/nejm199110173251620. Medline:1891034

Pielke Jr, R.A., & Conant, R.T. (2003). Best practices in prediction for decision-making: Lessons from the atmospheric and earth sciences. *Ecology, 84*(6), 1351–1358. https://doi.org/10.1890/0012-9658(2003)084[1351: bpipfd]2.0.co;2

Pigliucci, M., & Boudry, M. (2011). Why machine-information metaphors are bad for science and science education. *Science & Education, 20*(5), 453–471. https://doi.org/10.1007/s11191-010-9267-6

Pinker, S. (2021). *Rationality: What it is, why it seems scarce, why it matters.* Viking.

Pinto, M.F. (2015). Tensions in agnotology: Normativity in the studies of commercially driven ignorance. *Social Studies of Science, 45*(2), 294–315. https://doi.org/10.1177/0306312714565491. Medline:26477209

Pintrich, P.R., Marx, R.W., & Boyle, R.A. (1993). Beyond cold conceptual change: The role of motivational beliefs and classroom contextual factors in the process of conceptual change. *Review of Educational Research, 63*(2), 167–199. https://doi.org/10.3102/00346543063002167

Plass, J.L., Heidig, S., Hayward, E.O., Homer, B.D., & Um, E. (2014). Emotional design in multimedia learning: Effects of shape and color on

affect and learning. *Learning and Instruction, 29,* 128–140. https://doi.org
/10.1016/j.learninstruc.2013.02.006

Poland, C.M., Jacobson, R.M., Opel, D.J., Marcuse, E.K., & Poland, G.A.
(2015). Political, ethical, social, and psychological aspects of vaccinology.
In G.N. Milligan & A.D.T. Barrett (Eds.), *Vaccinology: An essential guide*
(pp. 335–357). Wiley.

Poland, G.A., & Jacobson, R.M. (1994). Failure to reach the goal of measles
elimination: Apparent paradox of measles infections in immunized
persons. *Archives of Internal Medicine, 154*(16), 1815–1820. https://doi.org
/10.1001/archinte.154.16.1815

Polya, G. (1957). *How to solve it: A new aspect of mathematical method.* Princeton
University Press.

Popper, K.R. (1959). *Logic of scientific discovery.* Basic Books.

Posner, G.J., Strike, K.A., Hewson, P.W., & Gertzog, W.A. (1982).
Accommodation of a scientific conception: Toward a theory of conceptual
change. *Science Education, 66*(2), 211–227. https://doi.org/10.1002/sce
.3730660207

Potter, S. (2011). Retrospect: January 15, 1919: Boston molasses flood.
Weatherwise, 64(1), 10–11. https://doi.org/10.1080/00431672.2011.536113

Priest, S., Goodwin, J., & Dahlstrom, M.F. (Eds.). (2018). *Ethics and practice in
science communication.* University of Chicago Press.

Priest, S.H., Bonfadelli, H., & Rusanen, M. (2003). The "trust gap" hypothesis:
Predicting support for biotechnology across national cultures as a function
of trust in actors. *Risk Analysis: An International Journal, 23*(4), 751–766.
https://doi.org/10.1111/1539-6924.00353. Medline:12926568

Pronin, E. (2009). The introspection illusion. *Advances in Experimental Social
Psychology, 41,* 1–67. https://doi.org/10.1016/s0065-2601(08)00401-2

Pronin, E., & Kugler, M.B. (2007). Valuing thoughts, ignoring behavior:
The introspection illusion as a source of the bias blind spot. *Journal of
Experimental Social Psychology, 43*(4), 565–578. https://doi.org/10.1016
/j.jesp.2006.05.011

Rabin, J.M., Burgasser, A., Bussey, T.J., Eggers, J., Lo, S.M., Seethaler, S., ... &
Weizman, H. (2021). Interdisciplinary conversations in STEM education:
can faculty understand each other better than their students do?
International Journal of STEM Education, 8(1), 1–10. https://doi.org
/10.1186/s40594-020-00266-9

Reber, R., & Schwarz, N. (1999). Effects of perceptual fluency on judgments
of truth. *Consciousness and Cognition, 8*(3), 338–342. https://doi.org/10
.1006/ccog.1999.0386. Medline:10487787

Reich, J.W., & Robertson, J.L. (1979). Reactance and norm appeal in anti-
littering messages. *Journal of Applied Social Psychology, 9*(1), 91–101. https://
doi.org/10.1111/j.1559-1816.1979.tb00796.x

Reichenbach, H. (1938). *Experience and prediction.* University of Chicago Press.

Resnik, D.B., & Elliott, K.C. (2016). The ethical challenges of socially responsible science. *Accountability in Research, 23*(1), 31–46. https://doi.org/10.1080/08989621.2014.1002608. Medline:26193168

Reynolds, A.S. (2018). *The third lens: Metaphor and the creation of modern cell biology.* University of Chicago Press.

Rickinson, M. (2001). Learners and learning in environmental education: A critical review of the evidence. *Environmental Education Research, 7*(3), 207–320. https://doi.org/10.1080/13504620120065230

Riskind, J.H., & Gotay, C.C. (1982). Physical posture: Could it have regulatory or feedback effects on motivation and emotion? *Motivation and Emotion, 6*(3), 273–298. https://doi.org/10.1007/bf00992249

Ritov, I., & Baron, J. (1990). Reluctance to vaccinate: Omission bias and ambiguity. *Journal of Behavioral Decision Making, 3*(4), 263–277. https://doi.org/10.1002/bdm.3960030404

Rocha Souza, R., Dorn, A., Piringer, B., & Wandl-Vogt, E. (2019, September). Towards a taxonomy of uncertainties: Analysing sources of spatio-temporal uncertainty on the example of non-standard German corpora. In *Informatics, 6*(3), 34. Multidisciplinary Digital Publishing Institute.

Rock, I., & Palmer, S. (1990). The legacy of Gestalt psychology. *Scientific American, 263*(6), 84–91. https://doi.org/10.1038/scientificamerican1290-84. Medline:2270461

Rogers, C.R. (1959). A theory of therapy, personality, and interpersonal relationships: As developed in the client-centered framework. In S. Koch (Ed.), *Psychology: A study of a science* (pp. 184–256). McGraw-Hill.

Roozenbeek, J., & Van der Linden, S. (2019). The fake news game: actively inoculating against the risk of misinformation. *Journal of Risk Research, 22*(5), 570–580. https://doi.org/10.1080/13669877.2018.1443491

Roser, M.E., & Gazzaniga, M.S. (2006). The interpreter in human psychology. In T.M. Preuss & J.H. Kaas (Eds.), *The evolution of primate nervous systems* (pp. 503–508). Academic Press.

Ross, S. (1962). Scientist: The story of a word. *Annals of Science, 18*(2), 65–85. https://doi.org/10.1080/00033796200202722

Rothman, J. (2020, October 5). How does science really work? *New Yorker.* Retrieved from www.newyorker.com/magazine/2020/10/05/how-does-science-really-work

Ruiz, J.B., & Bell, R.A. (2014). Understanding vaccination resistance: Vaccine search term selection bias and the valence of retrieved information. *Vaccine, 32*(44), 5776–5780. https://doi.org/10.1016/j.vaccine.2014.08.042. Medline:25176640

Ryan, J.N. (1985). The language gap: Common words with technical meanings. *Journal of Chemical Education, 62*(12), 1098. https://doi.org/10.1021/ed062p1098

Ryder, J., Leach, J., & Driver, R. (1999). Undergraduate science students' images of science. *Journal of Research in Science Teaching 36*(2), 201–219. https://doi.org/10.1002/(sici)1098-2736(199902)36:2%3C201::aid -tea6%3E3.0.co;2-h

Sacks, H., Schlegoff, I., & Jefferson, G. (1974). A simplest systematics for the organization of turn-taking in conversation. *Language, 50*, 696–735. https://doi.org/10.1353/lan.1974.0010

Salovey, P., & Mayer, J.D. (1990). Emotional intelligence. *Imagination, Cognition and Personality, 9*(3), 185–211. https://doi.org/10.2190/dugg -p24e-52wk-6cdg

Saltelli, A., & Funtowicz, S. (2014). When all models are wrong. *Issues in Science and Technology, 30*(2), 79–85.

Sanders, L.D., & Neville, H.J. (2000). Lexical, syntactic, and stress-pattern cues for speech segmentation. *Journal of Speech, Language, and Hearing Research, 43*(6), 1301–1321. https://doi.org/10.1044/jslhr.4306.1301. Medline:11193954

Sarewitz, D. (2011). Anticipatory governance of emerging technologies. In G.E. Marchant (Ed.), *The growing gap between emerging technologies and legal-ethical oversight* (pp. 95–105). Springer.

Schachter, S., & Singer, J. (1962). Cognitive, social, and physiological determinants of emotional state. *Psychological Review, 69*(5), 379. https:// doi.org/10.1037/h0046234. Medline:14497895

Scharrer, L., Rupieper, Y., Stadtler, M., & Bromme, R. (2017). When science becomes too easy: Science popularization inclines laypeople to underrate their dependence on experts. *Public Understanding of Science, 26*(8), 1003– 1018. https://doi.org/10.1177/0963662516680311. Medline:27899471

Schneps, M.H., & Sadler, P.M. (2010). A private universe online resources. *Science in School, 17*. Retrieved from www.scienceinschool.org/wp-content /uploads/2014/11/issue17_privateuniverse.pdf

Schoenfeld, A.H. (1988). Problem solving in context. In R. Charles & E.A. Silver (Eds.), *The teaching and assessing of mathematical problem solving* (pp. 82–92). Lawrence Erlbaum Associates

Schooler, J.W. (2014). Metascience could rescue the "replication crisis." *Nature, 515*(7525), 9–9.

Schultz, P.W., Nolan, J.M., Cialdini, R.B., Goldstein, N.J., & Griskevicius, V. (2007). The constructive, destructive, and reconstructive power of social norms. *Psychological Science, 18*(5), 429–434. https://doi.org/10.1111 /j.1467-9280.2007.01917.x. Medline:17576283

Schüz, N., Schüz, B., & Eid, M. (2013). When risk communication backfires: Randomized controlled trial on self-affirmation and reactance to personalized risk feedback in high-risk individuals. *Health Psychology, 32*(5), 561. https://doi.org/10.1037/a0029887. Medline:23646839

Schwartz, D., Fischhoff, B., Krishnamurti, T., & Sowell, F. (2013). The Hawthorne effect and energy awareness. *Proceedings of the National*

Academy of Sciences, 110(38), 15242–15246. https://doi.org/10.1073/pnas
.1301687110. Medline:24003110

Schwartz, R.S., Lederman, N.G., & Crawford, B.A. (2004). Developing views of
nature of science in an authentic context: An explicit approach to bridging
the gap between nature of science and scientific inquiry. *Science Education,
88*(4), 610–645. https://doi.org/10.1002/sce.10128

Schwarz, N. (2011). Feelings-as-information theory. In P.A.M. Van Lange,
A.W. Kruglanski & E.T. Higgins (Eds.), *Handbook of theories of social
psychology* (pp. 289–308). Sage Publications.

Schwarz, N., Sanna, L.J., Skurnik, I., & Yoon, C. (2007). Metacognitive
experiences and the intricacies of setting people straight: Implications
for debiasing and public information campaigns. *Advances in Experimental
Social Psychology, 39*, 127–161. https://doi.org/10.1016/s0065-2601(06)
39003-x

Seethaler, S. (2016a). Five things chemists (and other science faculty) should
know about the education research literature. *Journal of Chemical Education,
93*(1), 9–12. https://doi.org/10.1021/acs.jchemed.5b00109

Seethaler, S. (2016b). Shades of grey in vaccination decision making:
Tradeoffs, heuristics, and implications. *Science Communication, 38*(2),
261–271. https://doi.org/10.1177/1075547016637083

Seethaler, S., Czworkowski, J., & Wynn, L. (2018). Analyzing general chemistry
texts' treatment of rates of change concepts in reaction kinetics reveals
missing conceptual links. *Journal of Chemical Education, 95*(1), 28–36.
https://doi.org/10.1021/acs.jchemed.7b00238

Seethaler, S., & Linn, M. (2004). Genetically modified food in perspective:
an inquiry-based curriculum to help middle school students make sense
of tradeoffs. *International Journal of Science Education, 26*(14), 1765–1785.
https://doi.org/10.1080/09500690410001673784

Seymour, E., & Hewitt, N.M. (1997). *Talking about leaving: Why undergraduates
leave the sciences.* Westview.

Sfard, A. (1998). On two metaphors for learning and the dangers of choosing
just one. *Educational Researcher, 27*(2), 4–13. https://doi.org/10.3102/0013
189x027002004

Shah, A.K., & Oppenheimer, D.M. (2008). Heuristics made easy: An effort-
reduction framework. *Psychological Bulletin, 134*(2), 207. https://doi.org
/10.1037/0033-2909.134.2.207. Medline:18298269

Shepherd, S., & Kay, A.C. (2012). On the perpetuation of ignorance:
System dependence, system justification, and the motivated avoidance of
sociopolitical information. *Journal of Personality and Social Psychology, 102*(2),
264. https://doi.org/10.1037/a0026272. Medline:22059846

Sherman, S.J., Cialdini, R.B., Schwartzman, D.F., & Reynolds, K.D. (1985).
Imagining can heighten or lower the perceived likelihood of contracting a
disease: The mediating effect of ease of imagery. *Personality and Social Psychology
Bulletin, 11*(1), 118–127. https://doi.org/10.1177/0146167285111011

Shindell, D.T., Rind, D., & Lonergan, P. (1998). Increased polar stratospheric ozone losses and delayed eventual recovery owing to increasing greenhouse-gas concentrations. *Nature, 392*(6676), 589–592. https://doi .org/10.1038/33385

Shulman, L.S. (1986). Those who understand: Knowledge growth in teaching. *Educational Researcher, 15*(2), 4–14. https://doi.org/10.3102/0013189 x015002004

Signorini, P., Wiesemes, R., & Murphy, R. (2009). Developing alternative frameworks for exploring intercultural learning: A critique of Hofstede's cultural difference model. *Teaching in Higher Education, 14*(3), 253–264. https://doi.org/10.1080/13562510902898825

Simpson, D.Y., Beatty, A.E., & Ballen, C.J. (2021). Teaching between the lines: Representation in science textbooks. *Trends in Ecology & Evolution, 36*(1), 4–8. https://doi.org/10.1016/j.tree.2020.10.010. Medline:33187728

Simpson, E.H. (1951). The interpretation of interaction in contingency tables. *Journal of the Royal Statistical Society: Series B (Methodological), 13*(2), 238–241. https://doi.org/10.1111/j.2517-6161.1951.tb00088.x

Sjöberg, L. (2000). Perceived risk and tampering with nature. *Journal of Risk Research, 3*(4), 353–367. https://doi.org/10.1080/13669870050132568

Slovic, P. (1993). Perceived risk, trust, and democracy. *Risk Analysis, 13*(6), 675–682. https://doi.org/10.1111/j.1539-6924.1993.tb01329.x

Slovic, P. (1999). Trust, emotion, sex, politics, and science: Surveying the risk-assessment battlefield. *Risk Analysis, 19*(4), 689–701. https://doi.org/10 .1111/j.1539-6924.1999.tb00439.x

Slovic, P. (2000). *The perception of risk.* Earthscan Publications.

Smith, S.J., & Harvey, E.E. (2014). K-12 online lesson alignment to the principles of universal design for learning: The Khan Academy. *Open Learning: The Journal of Open, Distance and E-Learning, 29*(3), 222–242. https://doi.org/10.1080/02680513.2014.992402

Smithson, M. (1989). *Ignorance and uncertainty: Emerging paradigms.* Springer-Verlag Publishing.

Sniderman, P.M., & Bullock, J. (2004). A consistency theory of public opinion and political choice: The hypothesis of menu dependence. In W.E. Saris and P.M. Sniderman (Eds.), *Studies in public opinion: Attitudes, nonattitudes, measurement error, and change* (pp. 337–358). Princeton University Press.

Sniderman, P.M., & Theriault, S.M. (2004). The structure of political argument and the logic of issue framing. In W.E. Saris and P.M. Sniderman (Eds.) *Studies in public opinion: Attitudes, nonattitudes, measurement error, and change* (pp. 133–165). Princeton University Press.

Snow, C.P. (1959). Two cultures. *Science, 130*(3373), 419–419. https://doi.org /10.1126/science.130.3373.419. Medline:17817735

Sopory, P., & Dillard, J.P. (2002). The persuasive effects of metaphor: A meta-analysis. *Human Communication Research, 28*(3), 382–419. https://doi.org /10.1111/j.1468-2958.2002.tb00813.x

Southerland, S.A., Abrams, E., Cummins, C.L., & Anzelmo, J. (2001). Understanding students' explanations of biological phenomena: Conceptual frameworks or p-prims? *Science Education*, *85*(4), 328–348. https://doi.org/10.1002/sce.1013

Starr, C. (1969). Social benefit versus technological risk: What is our society willing to pay for safety? *Science*, *165*(3899), 1232–1238. https://doi.org /10.1126/science.165.3899.1232. Medline:5803536

Stefan, M. (2010). A CV of failures. *Nature*, *468*(7322), 467–467. https://doi .org/10.1038/nj7322-467a

Stern, F., & Kampourakis, K. (2017). Teaching for genetics literacy in the post-genomic era. *Studies in Science Education*, *53*(2), 193–225. https://doi.org /10.1080/03057267.2017.1392731

Stibe, A., & Cugelman, B. (2016, April). Persuasive backfiring: When behavior change interventions trigger unintended negative outcomes. In *Proceedings of the 11th International Conference on Persuasive Technology-Volume 9638* (pp. 65–77).

Story, M.F. (2001). Principles of universal design. In W.F.E. Preiser & E. Ostroff (Eds.), *Universal design handbook* (pp. 4.1–4.12). McGraw-Hill.

Strauss, S. (2009). Metaphor contests and contested metaphors: From webs spinning spiders to barcodes to DNA. In B. Nerlich, R. Elliott, & B. Larson (Eds.), *Communicating biological sciences: Ethical and metaphorical dimensions* (pp. 153–166). Ashgate Publishing.

Stuckey, M., Hofstein, A., Mamlok-Naaman, R., & Eilks, I. (2013). The meaning of "relevance" in science education and its implications for the science curriculum. *Studies in Science Education*, *49*(1), 1–34. https://doi .org/10.1080/03057267.2013.802463

Stucki, I., & Sager, F. (2018). Aristotelian framing: logos, ethos, pathos and the use of evidence in policy frames. *Policy Sciences*, *51*(3), 373–385. https:// doi.org/10.1007/s11077-018-9322-8

Sucharov, M. (2019). *Public influence: A guide to op-ed writing and social media engagement.* University of Toronto Press.

Sumner, P., Vivian-Griffiths, S., Boivin, J., Williams, A., Venetis, C.A., Davies, A., … & Chambers, C.D. (2014). The association between exaggeration in health related science news and academic press releases: Retrospective observational study. *BMJ (Clinical Research ed.)*, *349*, g7015–g7015. https:// doi.org/10.1136/bmj.g7015. Medline:25498121

Sverdlik, A., Hall, N.C., McAlpine, L., & Hubbard, K. (2018). The PhD experience: A review of the factors influencing doctoral students' completion, achievement, and well-being. *International Journal of Doctoral Studies*, *13*(1), 361–388.

Taber, C.S., & Lodge, M. (2006). Motivated skepticism in the evaluation of political beliefs. *American Journal of Political Science*, *50*(3), 755–769. https:// doi.org/10.1111/j.1540-5907.2006.00214.x

Taber, K.S. (2001). When the analogy breaks down: modelling the atom on the solar system. *Physics Education*, *36*(3), 222–226. https://doi.org /10.1088/0031-9120/36/3/308

Taber, K.S., & García-Franco, A. (2010). Learning processes in chemistry: Drawing upon cognitive resources to learn about the particulate structure of matter. *Journal of the Learning Sciences, 19*(1), 99–142. https://doi.org/10.1080/10508400903452868

Tannen, D. (1981a). New York Jewish conversational style. *International Journal of the Sociology of Language, 30*, 133–149. https://doi.org/10.1515/ijsl.1981.30.133

Tannen, D. (1981b). Indirectness in discourse: Ethnicity as conversational style. *Discourse Processes, 4*(3), 221–238. https://doi.org/10.1080/01638538109544517

Tannen, D. (2005). *Conversational style: Analyzing talk among friends.* Oxford University Press.

Tasker, R. (2016). ConfChem conference on interactive visualizations for chemistry teaching and learning: Research into practice – Visualizing the molecular world for a deep understanding of chemistry. *Journal of Chemical Education, 93*(6), 1152–1153. https://doi.org/10.1021/acs.jchemed.5b00824

Thaler, R.H., & Sunstein, C.R. (2008). *Nudge: Improving decisions about health, wealth, and happiness.* Yale University Press.

Thibodeau, P.H., & Boroditsky, L. (2011). Metaphors we think with: The role of metaphor in reasoning. *PLOS One, 6*(2), e16782. https://doi.org/10.1371/journal.pone.0016782. Medline:21373643

Thibodeau, P.H., Hendricks, R.K., & Boroditsky, L. (2017). How linguistic metaphor scaffolds reasoning. *Trends in Cognitive Sciences, 21*(11), 852–863. https://doi.org/10.1016/j.tics.2017.07.001. Medline:28789831

Thompson, C. (2016, July). How data won the west: Early infographics saved soldiers' lives, debunked myths about slavery and helped Americans settle the frontier. *Smithsonian Magazine,* 23–27.

Timmons, B.H., & Ley, R. (Eds.). (1994). *Behavioral and psychological approaches to breathing disorders.* Plenum Press.

Tippett, C.D. (2010). Refutation text in science education: A review of two decades of research. *International Journal of Science and Mathematics Education, 8*(6), 951–970. https://doi.org/10.1007/s10763-010-9203-x

Toulmin, S. (1972). *Human understanding.* Princeton University Press.

Trevors, G.J., Muis, K.R., Pekrun, R., Sinatra, G.M., & Winne, P.H. (2016). Identity and epistemic emotions during knowledge revision: A potential account for the backfire effect. *Discourse Processes, 53*(5–6), 339–370. https://doi.org/10.1080/0163853x.2015.1136507

Tudor, A. (1989). Seeing the worst side of science. *Nature, 340*(6235), 589–592. https://doi.org/10.1038/340589a0

Tufte, E. (1983). *The visual display of quantitative information.* Graphics Press.

Tufte, E. (2006). *The cognitive style of PowerPoint: Pitching out corrupts within.* Graphics Press.

Turner, S., & Sullenger, K. (1999). Kuhn in the classroom, Lakatos in the lab: Science educators confront the nature-of-science debate.

Science, Technology, & Human Values, 24(1), 5–30. https://doi.org/10.1177/016224399902400102

Tversky, A., & Kahneman, D. (1971). Belief in the law of small numbers. *Psychological Bulletin, 76*(2), 105–110. https://doi.org/10.1037/h0031322

Tversky, A., & Kahneman, D. (1974). Judgment under uncertainty: Heuristics and biases: Biases in judgments reveal some heuristics of thinking under uncertainty. *Science, 185*(4157), 1124–1131. https://doi.org/10.1126/science.185.4157.1124. Medline:17835457

Tversky, A., & Kahneman, D. (1981). The framing of decisions and the psychology of choice. *Science, 211*(4481), 453–458. https://doi.org/10.1126/science.7455683. Medline:7455683

Tversky, B., Morrison, J.B., & Betrancourt, M. (2002). Animation: Can it facilitate? *International Journal of Human-Computer Studies, 57*(4), 247–262. https://doi.org/10.1006/ijhc.2002.1017

Umeda, N., & Coker, C.H. (1974). Allophonic variation in American English. *Journal of Phonetics, 2*(1), 1–5. https://doi.org/10.1016/s0095-4470(19)31174-x

United Nations (1948). Universal declaration of human rights. *UN General Assembly, 302*(2), 14–25. https://doi.org/10.1163/9789047412878_003

Van Asselt, M., & Rotmans, J. (2002). Uncertainty in integrated assessment modelling. *Climatic Change, 54*(1), 75–105. https://doi.org/10.1023/a:1015783803445

Van Bavel, J.J., & Pereira, A. (2018). The partisan brain: An identity-based model of political belief. *Trends in Cognitive Sciences, 22*(3), 213–224. https://doi.org/10.1016/j.tics.2018.01.004. Medline:29475636

Van Boven, L., Ehret, P.J., & Sherman, D.K. (2018). Psychological barriers to bipartisan public support for climate policy. *Perspectives on Psychological Science, 13*(4), 492–507. https://doi.org/10.1177/1745691617748966. Medline:29961412

Van der Bles, A.M., Van der Linden, S., Freeman, A.L., Mitchell, J., Galvao, A.B., Zaval, L., & Spiegelhalter, D.J. (2019). Communicating uncertainty about facts, numbers and science. *Royal Society Open Science, 6*(5), 181870. https://doi.org/10.1098/rsos.181870. Medline:31218028

Van der Linden, S., Leiserowitz, A., Rosenthal, S., & Maibach, E. (2017). Inoculating the public against misinformation about climate change. *Global Challenges, 1*(2), 1600008. https://doi.org/10.1002/gch2.201600008. Medline:31565263

Van Zant, A.B., & Berger, J. (2019). How the voice persuades. *Journal of Personality and Social Psychology, 118*(4), 661–682. https://doi.org/10.1037/pspi0000193. Medline:31192632

Vollmer, G. (1984). Mesocosm and objective knowledge. In F.M. Wuketits (Ed.), *Concepts and approaches in evolutionary epistemology* (pp. 69–121). Springer.

Vosniadou, S., & Brewer, W.F. (1992). Mental models of the earth: A study of conceptual change in childhood. *Cognitive Psychology, 24*(4), 535–585. https://doi.org/10.1016/0010-0285(92)90018-w

Vygotsky, L. (1978). Interaction between learning and development. In M. Gauvain & M. Cole (Eds.). *Readings on the development of children* (pp. 34–40). Scientific American Books.

Wagner, C.H. (1982). Simpson's paradox in real life. *American Statistician, 36*(1), 46–48. https://doi.org/10.1080/00031305.1982.10482778

Wagner, W., Fisher, E., & Pascual, P. (2018). Whose science? A new era in regulatory "science wars." *Science, 362*(6415), 636–639. https://doi.org/10.1126/science.aau3205. Medline:30409870

Wailoo, K. (2021). *Pushing cool: Big tobacco, racial marketing, and the untold story of the menthol cigarette.* University of Chicago Press.

Wakefield, M., Terry-McElrath, Y., Emery, S., Saffer, H., Chaloupka, F.J., Szczypka, G., ... & Johnston, L.D. (2006). Effect of televised, tobacco company–funded smoking prevention advertising on youth smoking-related beliefs, intentions, and behavior. *American Journal of Public Health, 96*(12), 2154–2160. https://doi.org/10.2105/ajph.2005.083352. Medline:17077405

Walker, M.B. (1982). Smooth transitions in conversational turn-taking: Implications for theory. *Journal of Psychology, 110*(1), 31–37. https://doi.org/10.1080/00223980.1982.9915322

Walker, M.B., & Trimboli, C. (1983). The expressive function of the eye flash. *Journal of Nonverbal Behavior, 8*(1), 3–13. https://doi.org/10.1007/bf00986326

Walker, W.E., Harremoës, P., Rotmans, J., Van Der Sluijs, J.P., Van Asselt, M.B., Janssen, P., & Krayer von Krauss, M.P. (2003). Defining uncertainty: A conceptual basis for uncertainty management in model-based decision support. *Integrated Assessment, 4*(1), 5–17. https://doi.org/10.1076/iaij.4.1.5.16466

Wall, M. (2016, February 11). Epic gravitational wave detection: How scientists did it. Space.Com. Retrieved from www.space.com/31913-how-scientists-detected-gravitational-waves-ligo.html

Walters, J. (2016, February 12). Explain it to me like I'm a kid: Scientists try to make sense of gravitational waves. *The Guardian.* Retrieved from www.theguardian.com/science/2016/feb/12/gravitational-waves-explained

Watson, J. (1968). *The double helix: A personal account of the structure of DNA.* Harvard University Press.

Watson, J.D., & Crick, F.H. (1953). Molecular structure of nucleic acids: A structure for deoxyribose nucleic acid. *Nature, 171*(4356), 737–738. https://doi.org/10.1038/171737a0. Medline:13054692

Weber, J.R., & Schell Word, C. (2001). The communication process as evaluative context: What do nonscientists hear when scientists speak? *BioScience, 51*(6), 487–495. https://doi.org/10.1641/0006-3568(2001)051[0487:tcpaec]2.0.co;2

Weingart, P., Muhl, C., & Pansegrau, P. (2003). Of power maniacs and unethical geniuses: Science and scientists in fiction film. *Public Understanding of Science, 12*(3), 279–287. https://doi.org/10.1177/0963662503123006

Weinstein, N.D. (1989). Optimistic biases about personal risks. *Science, 246*(4935), 1232–1233. https://doi.org/10.1126/science.2686031. Medline:2686031

Weisberg, D.S., Landrum, A.R., Hamilton, J., & Weisberg, M. (2021). Knowledge about the nature of science increases public acceptance of science regardless of identity factors. *Public Understanding of Science, 30*(2), 120–138. https://doi.org/10.1177/0963662520977700. Medline:33336623

Weisberg, S.M., & Newcombe, N.S. (2017). Embodied cognition and STEM learning: Overview of a topical collection in CR: PI. *Cognitive Research: Principles and Implications, 2*(1), 1–6. https://doi.org/10.1186/s41235-017-0071-6. Medline:28959709

Welch, H.G., Schwartz, L.M., & Woloshin, S. (2000). Are increasing 5-year survival rates evidence of success against cancer? *JAMA, 283*(22), 2975–2978. https://doi.org/10.1001/jama.283.22.2975. Medline:10865276

Wheeler, L.B., Mulvey, B.K., Maeng, J.L., Librea-Carden, M.R., & Bell, R.L. (2019). Teaching the teacher: Exploring STEM graduate students' nature of science conceptions in a teaching methods course. *International Journal of Science Education, 41*(14), 1905–1925.

White, B.Y., & Frederiksen, J.R. (1998). Inquiry, modeling, and metacognition: Making science accessible to all students. *Cognition and instruction, 16*(1), 3–118. https://doi.org/10.1207/s1532690xci1601_2

Wiens, J.D., Dugger, K.M., Higley, J.M., Lesmeister, D.B., Franklin, A.B., Hamm, K.A., ... & Sovern, S.G. (2021). Invader removal triggers competitive release in a threatened avian predator. *Proceedings of the National Academy of Sciences, 118*(31). https://doi.org/10.1073/pnas.2102859118. Medline:34282032

Wiggins, G., & McTighe, J. (2005). *Understanding by design* (2nd ed.). Association for Supervision and Curriculum Development.

Wilkinson, A.M. (1992). Jargon and the passive voice: Prescriptions and proscriptions for scientific writing. *Journal of Technical Writing and Communication, 22*(3), 319–325. https://doi.org/10.2190/4hur-13kr-k1df-b52d

Winter, S., Krämer, N.C., Rösner, L., & Neubaum, G. (2015). Don't keep it (too) simple: How textual representations of scientific uncertainty affect laypersons' attitudes. *Journal of Language and Social Psychology, 34*(3), 251–272. https://doi.org/10.1177/0261927x14555872

Witte, K., & Allen, M. (2000). A meta-analysis of fear appeals: Implications for effective public health campaigns. *Health Education & Behavior, 27*(5), 591–615. https://doi.org/10.1177/109019810002700506. Medline:11009129

Wolske, K.S., Gillingham, K.T., & Schultz, P.W. (2020). Peer influence on household energy behaviours. *Nature Energy, 5*(3), 202–212. https://doi .org/10.1038/s41560-019-0541-9

Wong-Parodi, G., Krishnamurti, T., Davis, A., Schwartz, D., & Fischhoff, B. (2016). A decision science approach for integrating social science in climate and energy solutions. *Nature Climate Change, 6*(6), 563–569. https://doi.org/10.1038/nclimate2917

Wood, T., & Porter, E. (2019). The elusive backfire effect: Mass attitudes' steadfast factual adherence. *Political Behavior, 41*(1), 135–163. https:// doi.org/10.1007/s11109-018-9443-y

Wood, W., & Rünger, D. (2016). Psychology of habit. *Annual Review of Psychology, 67*, 289–314. https://doi.org/10.1146/annurev-psych-122414 -033417. Medline:26361052

Wright, L.K., Cardenas, J.J., Liang, P., & Newman, D.L. (2017). Arrows in biology: Lack of clarity and consistency points to confusion for learners. *CBE – Life Sciences Education, 17*(1), ar6. https://doi.org/10.1187/cbe.17 -04-0069. Medline:29351909

Wynne, B. (1989). Sheep farming after Chernobyl: A case study in communicating scientific information. *Environment, Science and Policy for Sustainable Development, 31*(2), 10–39. https://doi.org/10.1080/00139157 .1989.9928930

Yaqub, O. (2018). Serendipity: Towards a taxonomy and a theory. *Research Policy, 47*(1), 169–179. https://doi.org/10.1016/j.respol.2017.10.007

Yaseen, Z.S., & Foster, A.E. (2019). What is empathy? In A.E. Foster and Z.S. Yaseen (Eds.), *Teaching empathy in healthcare: Building a new core competency* (pp. 3–16). Springer.

Yong, E. (2018). *I spent two years trying to fix the gender imbalance in my stories. The Atlantic.* Retrieved from http://bit.ly/2LjE9DZ.

Zee, E.H.V., & Minstrell, J. (1997). Reflective discourse: Developing shared understandings in a physics classroom. *International Journal of Science Education, 19*(2), 209–228. https://doi.org/10.1080/0950069970190206

Zehr, S. (2000). Public representations of scientific uncertainty about global climate change. *Public Understanding of Science, 9*(2), 85–103. https://doi .org/10.1088/0963-6625/9/2/301

Zehr, S. (2017). Scientific uncertainty in health and risk messaging. In *Oxford research encyclopedia of communication.* Oxford University Press. https://doi .org/10.1093/acrefore/9780190228613.013.215

Zeidan, F., Johnson, S.K., Diamond, B.J., David, Z., & Goolkasian, P. (2010). Mindfulness meditation improves cognition: Evidence of brief mental training. *Consciousness and Cognition, 19*(2), 597–605. https://doi.org/10 .1016/j.concog.2010.03.014. Medline:20363650

Zillmann, D. (1993). Mental control of angry aggression. In D.M. Wegner and J.W. Pennebaker (Eds.), *Handbook of mental control* (pp. 370–392). Prentice Hall.

Ziman, J. (2000). *Real science: What it is and what it means.* Cambridge University Press.

Zimmerman, M. (n.d.). The clergy letter project. www.theclergyletterproject .org

Zuwerink Jacks, J., & Cameron, K.A. (2003). Strategies for resisting persuasion. *Basic and Applied Social Psychology, 25*(2), 145–161. https://doi.org/10.1207 /s15324834basp2502_5

Index

Note: Page numbers in *italics* indicate a table or a figure.

Printed and bound by CPI Group (UK) Ltd, Croydon, CR0 4YY

31/08/2025

14727215-0002